SECOND SUNS

TWO TRAILBLAZING DOCTORS AND
THEIR QUEST TO CURE BLINDNESS,
ONE PAIR OF EYES AT A TIME

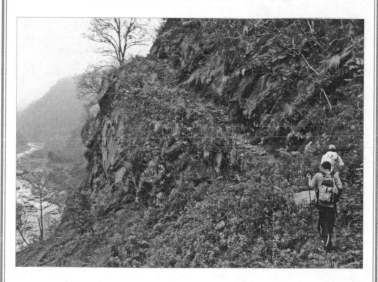

David Oliver Relin

Foreword by Paul Farmer
Afterword by Dr. Geoffrey Tabin

THE EXPERIMENT

NEW YORK

To Dawn, who brightens my days

The Experiment, LLC, 220 East 23rd Street, Suite 301, New York, NY 10010-4674
www.theexperimentpublishing.com

Many of the designations used by manufacturers and sellers to distinguish their products are claimed as trademarks. Where those designations appear in this book and The Experiment was aware of a trademark claim, the designations have been capitalized.

The Experiment's books are available at special discounts when purchased in bulk for premiums and sales promotions as well as for fundraising or educational use. For details, contact us at info@theexperimentpublishing.com.

Library of Congress Cataloging-in-Publication Data

Names: Relin, David Oliver, author.
Title: Second suns : two trailblazing doctors and their quest to cure blindness, one pair of eyes at a time / David Oliver Relin.
Description: New York : The Experiment, [2016] | Originally published: New York : Random House, c2013.
Identifiers: LCCN 2016018508 (print) | LCCN 2016025838 (ebook) | ISBN 9781615193622 (pbk.) | ISBN 9781615193639 (ebook)
Subjects: LCSH: Cataract--Surgery--Nepal. | Cataract--Surgery.
Classification: LCC RE31 .R45 2016 (print) | LCC RE31 (ebook) | DDC 617.7/42059--dc23
LC record available at https://lccn.loc.gov/2016018508

ISBN 978-1-61519-362-2
Ebook ISBN 978-1-61519-363-9

Cover design by Sarah Smith
Cover photograph by Ace Kvale
Spine image © Lonely | Shutterstock
Text design by Victoria Wong

Manufactured in the United States of America
Distributed by Workman Publishing Company, Inc.
Distributed simultaneously in Canada by Thomas Allen and Son Ltd.

First printing September 2016
10 9 8 7 6 5 4 3 2 1

Contents

When the Bandages Come Off

by Paul Farmer

Anyone who isn't deeply moved by this book must have a heart of stone. *Second Suns*, by the late David Oliver Relin, offers much more than its subtitle promises, which is to tell the tale of "two trail-blazing doctors and their quest to cure blindness." The story is richer than that. The two doctors in question—Sanduk Ruit of Nepal and the American Geoff Tabin, both ophthalmologists—don't even meet until halfway through the book. Relin's account unfurls like a good and true story should, and he lays out their encounter and subsequent collaboration, Ruit as mentor to Tabin, as both serendipitous and inevitable. The goal of this collaboration is to end blindness among the poor, first in Ruit's native Nepal and then, well, everywhere.

This goal would be unlikely if Sanduk Ruit had not developed new microsurgical methods of replacing cataracts with artificial lenses, which he and his protégés install in the blink of an eye and without the fuss and risk and sutures that until recently characterized the surgical treatment of cataracts. Even acknowledging this innovation, the goal might still be seen as immodest, since development of revolutionary new therapies is not the same thing as a revolution in delivering them to people living in poverty. Cataracts are, after all, the leading cause of blindness in much of the world. But Ruit and his ever-enlarging team have worked across Nepal, scrambling up to most Himalayan villages, like the one in which he was born, to do just that. Discovery, in this instance, was followed by development and refinement, then by delivery. That's how medicine should work.

Just that story alone—restoring vision to Sherpas and others living near the top of the world, but near the bottom as far as access to health care goes—would be an inspiring one. But that's just for starters. Since scrambling up the icy scree of the Himalayas is the sort of thing Geoff Tabin does before breakfast, the long-ago collision of the energetic young American and the reserved and courtly doctor from Nepal is a bit more plausible. Collision is, we learn, the right word: "If Tabin thought his credentials from Yale, Oxford, Harvard, Brown, and Melbourne would dazzle a surgeon from the medical backwater of Nepal— one who had hailed from a village without a school—he was mistaken." Relin's account offers plenty of detail about their clashing manners. "Truly, when I first met Geoff, I wasn't impressed," Ruit says unsparingly. "He was so hyperactive he made everyone nervous. And his surgical technique was still pretty lousy. Lots of foreign doctors came round in those days. Most wanted to do a little bit of work and have a nice mountain vacation in Nepal. I chalked him up as just another one of those jokers."

But Tabin, enamored as he was (and is) of climbing and rappelling and all manner of dangerous sport, was (and is) not at all a joker when it came to learning from a great man like Ruit. Nor was Tabin about to turn away from the great suffering caused by blindness in the high and precarious villages where the Nepal teams worked. Besides, the conviction that bound these doctors together was greater, as Ruit and his coworkers learned and as Tabin already knew, than the obvious stylistic differences between them. What inspires Ruit and Tabin, and the book's many protagonists, is the simple and still contrary belief that people should not be blinded or maimed or sickened by poverty. That's why they're still working together almost twenty years after their first collision.

Ruit and Tabin's belief can be nurtured in just about any place as long as there's the staff, stuff, and space to respond to sickness. Ruit and his teams had to make do with too few of these ingredients. As for staff, Ruit was a teacher for a reason, and he had a growing following throughout the world by the time Tabin had finished his training (occasionally put on hold by his obsession with the aptly termed extreme sports that were his second passion). As for space, the Nepalis had already shown they could operate safely in monasteries, police stations, schools, and even, in a pinch and with enough light, the occasional dirt-floored hut. The requisite stuff, however, was harder to come by. The new microsurgical procedures may not have required sutures, but they required operating scopes and intraocular lenses. Lots and lots of lenses. Buying these for poor patients required sustained financial support, always difficult to secure. As time went by, and as his trainees came into their own, Ruit and colleagues had allies that included Sherpas, armies of monks, an ambassador or two, a handful of well-to-do business folk, professors of ophthalmology in Australia and the United States, and even the Fourteenth Dalai Lama. Ruit and his team had also shown themselves able to make good with a heady mix of Marxists, monarchists, and Maoists in order to restore sight.

But innovation like this shouldn't be hidden away in villages at the top of the world or even in Kathmandu, nor could the doctors reach their goal working only from Nepal. Like the Lord Buddha, also from these parts, the team needed to take the show on the road if the Gospel According to Ruit was to reach millions shut out from medical modernity on three continents. That's what the book's protagonists set out to do, from Nepal to Rwanda, from Vietnam to Australia and Bhutan. It's impossible to put *Second Suns* down, in part because it shows them achieving such astounding success in their work, in all these places and in many others, but also in university hospitals on at least three continents and at the professional meetings, such as the World Ophthalmology Congress, where reputations are made and sometimes unmade. These are the settings in which this narrative unfolds, and the details will make you believe that Ruit and Tabin and their fellow travelers are in this fight to win.

Even after learning of their doggedness and astounding results, some may still find Ruit and Tabin's vision of a world without untreated cataracts to be naively utopian given that sixty million people suffer from them. And that's only one blinding affliction among many and far from the leading killer of young adults. The poorest Nepalis live in a medieval medical world, having to rely on their own devices and cunning and knowledge in order to respond to illness or injury. That's why so many of them live short lives; their "own devices" do not include intra-ocular lenses or antibiotics or surgical care. That's why, as Ruit notes, half of his parents' children died during childhood from what were, at the time of their deaths, readily treatable infections. The slow decline and death of a beloved sister, almost surely from drug-resistant tuber-culosis, marked his early life, stiffening his resolve to pursue a career in medicine.

But as formidable as the tasks before us are, I wouldn't bet against a team that included the quiet and determined prophet of a new religion and an irrepressible evangelist with boundless energy. There are a cou-ple of other developments likely to help make this vision of health equity a reality. Advances in medical technology would permit rapid advances in the health and well-being of the poor, were they distrib-uted justly, which was rarely true before the mid-twentieth century. In the course of two decades of working together, Ruit and Tabin—and Relin, too—noticed that their patients in Nepal were increasingly to be found among the elderly. This is because addressing the backlog of neglected patients with failing sight led to a rapid decline in unad-dressed need, a fairly shocking and welcome outcome in a country as poor as Nepal. After all, the period during which the protagonists in this book worked—along with many unnamed others who helped them or pursued similar projects—was not marked by massive improvements in infrastructure, such as roads or clinics, nor was it marked by some sudden and mysterious change in Nepali culture—to note only a cou-ple of the oft-asserted hypothetical prerequisites of rapid improvement in health status. What it was marked by was the removal of barriers to technological innovation—in this case, the microsurgical treatment of cataract disease, rather than the cumbersome and expensive and complication-prone method that preceded it—and modest efforts to promote the spread of the innovation in a manner that addressed the needs of the destitute sick. Lowering the high cost of artificial lenses will be critical to reducing the burden of blindness due to cataracts in Nepal and elsewhere in the poorer reaches of the world.

A second reason these two doctors are making headway is that they understand how best to harness advances in medical technology and promote training. They're cultivating an army of technicians—scrub nurses, ophthalmic assistants, eye doctors, even lens manufacturers—to take this work to scale. The places in which doctors train matters, too. With surgical skills like his, Sanduk Ruit could have worked and taught anywhere, and the path of least resistance would have been to take a job in Australia or the United States or India, and bring trainees from Nepal to him. But Ruit did not wish to proceed this way, in spite of powerful incentives to do so.

One of the heroes of this story is Ruit's father, who plied, along with his yaks and across narrow mountain trails, one of the region's caravan routes. Insisting that his son attend school when they lived in a village bereft of one, he first had to deposit him in Darjeeling, India—a fifteen-day trek away.

Another hero is, in my view, Geoff Tabin. I've known him for a long time, and I was proud to read of some of the lessons learned at the knee of his tough-minded and sometimes reproving senior colleague. On one occasion, in the far west of Nepal on a mission to (diplomatically) help a couple of old-school eye doctors improve their surgical technique, still-green Tabin shamed them instead. Ruit rang him on the phone and let him have it. I can't count the number of times I've seen young American physicians (and sometimes nurses) behave this way in settings from Haiti to Rwanda, believing that they care much more about their patients than their new and temporary colleagues. But Tabin took his scolding, and many others, because he knew in his heart it was true: No one from the States (or anywhere else) was going to make a difference in the lives of the sick-poor of Nepal without being part of a long game that included efforts to develop local capacity.

It was likely his ardent desire to avoid such errors—which I never saw, Tabin having learned those lessons long ago—that led him to seek out, in Rwanda, John Nkurikiye, a Rwandan ophthalmologist. I'd introduced him to Tabin, relates Relin, "as one of the most dedicated doctors I know of in Africa." My compliment was not because Nkurikiye, who grew up in a refugee camp in Burundi, was, upon finishing his training in South Africa, one of Rwanda's three ophthalmologists. Nor was it because he was one of the few refugees awarded a scholarship to medical school in Burundi, nor the fact that, fresh out of medical school, he volunteered to join the rebel force that would end the genocide. The violence was far from over when his battalion reached Kigali after a five-day march under fire and Nkurikiye helped set up a field hospital for the wounded in a city under attack by *genocidaires*. He doesn't much like to talk about those days, as voluble as he can be when talking about the corneal transplants he's been doing in Kigali, with Tabin's help. The Rwandan doctor had, observed Relin, "no time to talk about history. He was making it."

David Relin died in 2012, and I'm sorry I was never able to thank him for *Second Suns*. It must have been hard to track down these hyperheroes and to trek all over creation with them. But I'm pretty sure Relin felt plenty thanked. "Since I'd been writing about Ruit and Tabin," he notes near the elegiac end of his book, "the incomparable moment each morning when a patient's bandages were removed and they were again able to see had made whatever hardships we'd encountered while traveling seem worthwhile."

PAUL FARMER
July 2016

PAUL FARMER, medical anthropologist and physician, is a founding director and the chief strategist of Partners In Health, an international nonprofit organization that provides direct health care services to those living in poverty. He is the Kolokotrones University Professor and the chair of the Department of Global Health and Social Medicine at Harvard Medical School; he is also chief of the Division of Global Health Equity at Brigham and Women's Hospital, Boston. Additionally, Dr. Farmer serves as the United Nations Special Adviser to the Secretary-General on Community-Based Medicine and Lessons from Haiti.

SECOND SUNS

CHAPTER 1

See You

This world is blinded by darkness. Few can see. . . .
Become a lamp unto yourself.
—Siddhartha Gautama, the Buddha, from the last teaching

There is the Nepal of myth, the ice-and-rock realm of Mount Everest, the roof of the world. Then there is the country where most Nepalese actually live. I was still unfamiliar with that other, more earthly, Nepal when I first came to the Khumbu.

I had hiked up to the village of Thame, at twelve thousand feet, with Apa Sherpa. He stood a wiry five foot three and weighed perhaps 120 pounds. Apa's hair was cropped close, and his head was a thing of beauty—smooth and sun-browned like an exotic nut. Looking at him, you'd never guess he was one of the world's greatest athletes. But by the age of fifty, Apa had climbed to the top of Everest twenty times; no one had ever stood on the sharp peak of the earth's highest point more often.

Apa had invited me to Thame to meet his family and gather material about his career in the mountains, hoping that I would write a book about him. I was intrigued, not simply because of his high-altitude achievements but because, unlike many publicity-seeking Western mountaineers, Apa, like most Sherpas, climbed not for glory but to feed his family. He had also dedicated his most recent expeditions to raising money for the schools that surrounded the mountain his people know as Chomolungma, Goddess Mother of the World, and to raising awareness of the toll that global warming was taking on the Khumbu's receding glaciers.

By the time I arrived, the five-room school Sir Edmund Hillary had built in Apa's village was planning to lay off two of its teachers because of funding shortages, which would force the older students to walk six hours each day if they wanted to continue attending classes. And the lower portion of Thame had recently been washed away when a lake of glacial meltwater overran its rim and thundered through the valley where Apa had been raised. His family's home had been spared. So had the house next door, which belonged to the family of Tenzing Norgay, the first person to step onto the summit of Everest, alongside Hillary, in 1953.

Apa Sherpa had taken advantage of his prominence as a mountaineer to move his family from Nepal to suburban Salt Lake City, where his three children could count on a quality education. But his American dream hadn't panned out as he'd expected; Apa's attempt to create a line of outdoor clothing had crash-landed shortly after its launch. When he emailed me to introduce himself, he was working in a metal shop, stamping out road signs for Utah's highways. Apa wasn't bitter. He described his achievements on Everest with such matter-of-fact modesty that I agreed to accompany him to Nepal on his next expedition.

As the stone and ice immensities of the Himalaya thrust into view around every twist in the trail, Apa led me over swaying suspension bridges and up steep rock staircases with effortless grace. And as we traveled together, he proved to be one of the kindest people I'd ever met. Whenever my breathing became ragged, he'd put a hand on my shoulder. "Slowly, slowly," he'd say, guiding me to a seat on the nearest stone wall or to a bench at a tea house, where he'd pretend that he, too, was anxious to rest.

At altitude, the air was beautifully crisp, the peaks fairy-tale white. The sky draped over the low stone homes of Thame was the unblemished blue of tourist brochures. Each morning I'd wake to the gentle alarm of yak bells. Cocooned in my warm sleeping bag, I'd open my eyes, peer through puffs of my breath, and watch wood smoke from breakfast fires drift across low stone walls that divided pastures from potato fields. On one side, shaggy black pack animals foraged for grass shoots with delicate lips. On the other, slender plants angled toward the sun, pale green with new growth.

I interviewed Apa's elderly mother as she spun her prayer wheel and kept my tin mug of butter tea topped up. I also spoke with Apa's climbing partners, brothers, aunts, uncles, and cousins. I was so enchanted by Thame that I lingered there for several days, resisting the conclusion that was becoming as clear to me as the air above the village: that writing a book about a man climbing the same mountain twenty times, even the world's highest mountain, even for admirable reasons, was not something I could do well.

Apa was preparing for another attempt on Everest, and though I protested that I could find my way back down the trail to the airstrip at Lukla, where I planned to catch a small plane to Kathmandu, he insisted on accompanying me for the three-day trek. His middle-aged sister-in-law served as our porter, carrying, by a strap balanced across her broad forehead, the expedition bag I could barely lift. And with each step closer to the world of cities, with each foot of altitude lost, I felt more acutely how lucky I had been to get a glimpse into the life of this gentle man, and how much I regretted failing him.

Apa left me at Lukla. I promised that when he returned from Everest, we'd hold a fund-raiser together for the Thame School, which we managed to do a few months later. And I delayed telling him about my pessimistic view of the book's future. I didn't want him carrying that disappointment on his way back to the top of the world.

I spent a day sitting on a foggy airstrip, feeling like I'd been cast out of a kind of paradise, waiting for a window to open in the weather so a Yeti Airlines propeller plane could land. Dreadlocked European trekkers lounged against their backpacks, smoking hash or playing hacky sack on the empty runway, killing the hours. Sheets of fog blew by like possibilities, blanketing all of us in gloom, or opening narrow boreholes that revealed the snowfields of the high peaks, hinting at and then denying the splendor that surrounded us. The runway tilted steeply downhill, and everything felt out of balance. Though I was looking up, whenever I got a glimpse of clear sky I felt I was staring down into the ice-blue depths of a glacier.

The sight of those mountains made me think of a promise I'd made to another climber.

I'd met Dr. Geoffrey Tabin late one night the previous winter, in Utah. He approached me in the ballroom of the Cliff Lodge, at the Snowbird ski resort, after I'd given a lecture. Tabin waited until the crowd thinned out. Then he pounced. He told me about his considerable achievements as a climber, which included scaling the Seven Summits, the highest points on each continent. Before inviting me to dinner the following evening, he spoke of his current passion, working with a Nepalese surgeon named Sanduk Ruit to cure blindness in the developing world. Tabin was as tenacious and outgoing as Apa was modest and reserved. I agreed to join him for a meal only because he made it nearly impossible to say no.

We met for Mexican food the next night in Salt Lake City, where Tabin works, when he isn't overseas, as director of the International Ophthalmology Division at the University of Utah's Moran Eye Center. Or, rather, I watched as the bundle of nervous energy that is Geoff Tabin ticked in his seat like a time bomb and told implausible stories that turned out to be true—he really had been part of a group of adrenaline addicts at Oxford University who invented bungee jumping—while inhaling all his food and half of mine.

"A lot of climbers get all weird and competitive," Tabin said, his voice high-pitched, his cheeks bulging with *carne asada*. "I try to take the golden retriever approach to life. Try to be friendly to everyone. You get more done that way." I could see, even then, that he was more terrier than retriever. Tabin is compact, thickly muscled, and has a habit, once he gets something in his teeth, of not letting go. We spoke of my upcoming trip to Nepal with Apa, and he urged me to look in on his partner in Kathmandu if I had a few hours free. He said proudly that Tilganga, the eye hospital Dr. Ruit had built, was the finest medical facility in Nepal, an assembly line turning out minor miracles of healing. He assured me I'd find Ruit fascinating, if a little intimidating. Tabin's enthusiasm was infectious, but I couldn't escape the sensation that I was becoming lodged in the terrier's teeth.

On the airstrip, I waited seven hours with no sign of an arriving plane. Lukla is one of the world's most dangerous airports, and closures can last for days. Six months after I left, in similar weather, a Yeti Airlines Twin Otter crash-landed just short of the runway, killing two crew members and all sixteen passengers. Toward dusk, I was losing hope when a chartered helicopter touched down to pick up United Nations staff, and I was able to buy my way onboard.

We flew low, beneath the clouds, tracing the contours of the land. For me, Nepal was Kathmandu and a collection of snow peaks. But as we floated slowly down toward the capital, I saw that the barren, brick-colored hills in between were densely populated. Every slope, no matter its pitch, seemed to have been stripped of trees for cooking fires and sculpted into terraced fields. I observed small figures, bent to their labors, working to draw nourishment from depleted soil. Far below, rust-colored runoff from eroded hillsides pooled like blood where it met what had once been unspoiled mountain streams, staining them with evidence of overpopulation.

With my head leaning against the helicopter's scuffed window, I felt deflated, as the book I'd come halfway around the world hoping to write receded into the fog like the high peaks of the Himalaya. Dipping beneath storm clouds, we passed over the hill dwellers so closely that I could see our rotor blast ruffle their mud-spattered clothes. But they rarely looked up at us, and I had a peculiar sense of disconnection—that the six of us gliding over their heads in our aluminum capsule were living not only in a different world but in a different century.

Sullenly, I watched the poverty of the mid-hills slide past my window. The thatched huts fastened by pillars of felled trees to denuded hilltops, the men hacking terraces from the dirt with hoes, the women carrying water up from fouled streams that trickled an hour's hike beneath their homes, the underfed cattle and skinny dogs—all of it scrolled by like a documentary I didn't want to see. I couldn't know then how much of the next three years I'd be spending in that landscape, that the brick-red soil of the mid-hills would seep into my clothing and flesh and stain the way I saw not only Nepal but the world.

The air down at four thousand feet felt hot and wet. With each breath I was aware of dense vegetal decay. Despite its powerful engine, our Land Cruiser crept along, averaging only twenty miles an hour on the road from Kathmandu to Rasuwa. The drive had looked like a simple matter on the map I'd studied before setting out. But after hours of crawling first through maddening city traffic, then up a switchback road that climbed out of the smog-filled bowl of the Kathmandu Valley, we were still only beginning our journey, on a long, grinding descent to the Trishuli River.

Our driver, La La, and his young assistant took turns twisting every knob and dial on the dashboard. They had yet to master the operation of the air conditioner, so the windows were open to the scent of manure baking on the steep, terraced fields, and rotting plant matter where the jungle had not yet been slashed and burned. "This vehicle is brand-new," La La said cheerfully. "Only fifteen days, actually. A lot of the controls is unknown!"

I was sitting in the backseat, next to Sanduk Ruit. Up front, Ruit's wife, Nanda, leaned her forearms on the windowsill, her blue sari bright against the brown hillsides. Next to her sat one of their daughters. At seventeen, Serabla clearly asserted her status as a modern, emancipated woman. She wore Levi's, running shoes, and a track jacket.

"Not a bad way to travel, eh, Mommy," Ruit said to Nanda, who nodded dreamily. The white Land Cruiser had been a gift from a Chinese Australian donor, and Ruit was clearly delighted by it. "When we began these remote surgical camps, we used to ride on the tops of buses with all our cases of gear, isn't it?"

Each blind turn down the mountain road took me farther from the wood-fired pizza and glass of wine at an Italian restaurant I'd been anticipating in the capital, a small reward I'd been promising myself to dilute the taste of my failed trip to the Khumbu. But when I met Ruit, at Tilganga, he was preparing to leave immediately for a rural area, to perform free cataract surgeries, and, impulsively, he invited me along. I had no sense of Tilganga's merits as a hospital yet, and didn't have a handle on Ruit either, but Tabin had been right about at least one thing: Sanduk Ruit was intimidating. He held his large, craggy head high over his barrel chest, and a thatch of thick black hair sat on top of his scalp like a heavy woolen hat. And though he was affectionate with his wife and daughter, he spoke to me gruffly. In brief sentences. Without meeting my eyes.

Ruit was treating our conversation like an interview, so I took out my notepad and conducted one. "We'll be operating for three days," he explained. "With luck, we'll see two hundred cases."

"Why are we going to Rasuwa?"

"Because there are blind people there," Ruit said, without a trace of humor.

"But why Rasuwa particularly?" I asked, trying to keep the frustration from my voice.

Ruit exhaled, his eyelids lowered, indicating the effort it took to answer such an obvious question, and then he began to lecture. Rasuwa was one of the poorest regions of Nepal. The Tamang people who lived there were mostly subsistence farmers. Their lands were set unprofitably apart from the commercial center of Kathmandu, to the south, and the tourist magnet of the Khumbu, to the east. Ruit said he had conducted half a dozen free surgical camps in the area and still he was just draining an ocean of need, one teaspoon at a time. "The Tamang of Rasuwa are the most downtrodden people on earth," he said. "Also the most deserving."

I was weighing Ruit's words when La La jammed the Land Cruiser's brake pedal to the floor. A large Indian-made Tata bus, swinging wide around a hairpin turn, was bearing down on us. On its roof, dozens of wide-eyed passengers clutched goats, lambs, and children to their chests, bracing for impact as the bus's brakes shrieked. The psychedelic-colored snout of the Tata drew closer, filling our windscreen completely. I could see, in slow motion, the silver T-shaped hood ornament homing in on us like the nose cone of a missile . . . and then the squealing of the Tata's brakes went silent . . . and though only inches separated our bumpers, we were still intact. Flanking the Tata logo, someone had painted carefully, in flowing scarlet letters, "See . . . You." As in See you again? I wondered, or See you in the next life?

Both the Buddhists and the Hindus of Rasuwa believed, firmly, in reincarnation.

La La ground the gears, searching for reverse, then eased the Land Cruiser back, until we were pressed snug against a trash-strewn hillside, so the bus could pass. It inched forward, blowing hot diesel exhaust through our open windows. "Are you all right, my dear?" Ruit asked.

I presumed he was speaking to Nanda, until I realized he was examining me with the concern of a physician for a troubled patient.

"Sure," I said, shaken. "We're still here."

"We're always here," Ruit said, laughing. "But some conditions of existence are more painful than others."

Our brush with impermanence seemed to warm Ruit toward me, and to the task of telling the first few strands of his story. He was born in Olangchungola, a village built at ten thousand feet, near Kangchenjunga, a towering white wall in eastern Nepal, the world's third-tallest mountain. Ruit's father was a trader, leading horse and yak caravans to Tibet, bringing paint and rice and ready-made clothing up from the plains of India, and carrying yak-hair blankets, preserved meat, and salt down from the high plateau.

Olangchungola had no schools, so at age seven Ruit was sent away to study in India. "I knew that being a backward fellow from the mountains, you see, I had to work hundred times as hard to prove myself," he said as we rolled past fields of Tamang women in bright red headscarves, stooping to plant rice, shoot by shoot. Ruit worked hard enough to earn a college scholarship and gain admission to one of Asia's top medical schools.

We crossed the Trishuli, where another brightly colored Tata bus was parked in the shallows, the slow-moving current brushing its axles. The crew, stripped to their undershorts, flung buckets of tea-colored water against the dusty sides of the vehicle, washing it, while the passengers looked languidly out the windows or squatted on the hot metal roof, clutching their bundles, with a patience I found heartbreaking, a patience I could never quite muster, no matter how often I found myself in places where it was required.

Despite the trickling river, or perhaps because of its meagerness, the entire landscape looked scorched. Tamang women beating clothes against distant rocks blurred into points of color in the heat haze. And when we began to climb on the far side of the river, La La managed to raise the power windows only after we were all coated with a fine brick-colored dust. Up this dirt track on the other side of the river, into the parched hills of Rasuwa, the Land Cruiser bucked from side to side, crawling over boulders half the height of our tires. Every leaf, every twig along the roadside was filmed with red-brown dust. We rolled at walking pace, pressing our hands against the ceiling to stay in our seats.

The hours passed as we climbed, and I was lulled into daydreaming, staring at the houses of scavenged tin, the skimpy vegetable gardens hacked clear of bristling jungle, and bony cows tethered to posts by the more prosperous-looking homes. I thought about the endurance required to survive in a place like this. But where would you find the drive to do more than that? How much will and how many unlikely factors would have to line up, I wondered, to launch a boy from one of these homes to the frontier of medical innovation?

CHAPTER 2

Wound Construction

When facing two paths, if you are strong enough,
always choose the hardest one.
—Nepalese proverb, repeated to Sanduk Ruit by his father, Sonam

I woke, rubbed the dust out of my eyes, and studied the soldiers block-ing our way. Their Kalashnikovs were slung over their shoulders. They wore fatigue pants, blue windbreakers with red ironed-on ham-mers and sickles, and plastic shower sandals.

When Ruit rolled down the tinted window and showed his face, they stepped respectfully aside and opened an iron gate. After the soli-tude of the road, we pulled in to the courtyard of a concrete building where a crowd of expectant patients had gathered. Ruit said we had arrived in the village of Kalikasthan, at the heart of the Rasuwa Dis-trict. I saw no buildings other than the one in front of which we parked. Rutted dirt trails led away from it into sparse eucalyptus and pine for-est. The two-story cinder-block structure was a gift from Seventh-Day Adventists who had built it as a clinic, Ruit explained. The Maoists admired the solidity of the construction. They waited until the builders hung the fluorescent lights, bolted dentist's chairs to the concrete floor, and installed Western toilets. Then they liberated the building by force and turned it into a makeshift military post.

"The Maoists have a bad reputation, yet they're not so unreason-able," Ruit said, climbing out of the Land Cruiser. "They don't like religion. But they appreciate architecture."

A few months earlier, being an American in Rasuwa might have been awkward, because the Bush administration had branded the Maoists terrorists after 9/11 and had supplied weapons to the government they were trying to overthrow. But while I was with Apa, Maoist candidates had successfully appealed to the long-suffering majority of the Nepalese people and swept the national elections. They'd fanned out across the country, even appearing in the high villages of the Khumbu on foot, carrying microphones and speakers powered by car batteries, and had given fiery speeches promising the 81 percent of the country's citizens who labored as subsistence farmers a better life if they were in charge. Though they'd yet to hammer out the fine points of governance, the Maoists now ruled Nepal. What had started in the western district of Rolpa and had then spread to Rasuwa and other rural areas as an armed rebellion to free peasants from a powerful and wealthy Kathmandu elite now had to reinvent itself as a national party capable of improving the lives of the poor. Perhaps that's one reason why they'd allowed Ruit to turn their military post into a temporary eye hospital.

Ruit left to scrub for surgery, and I picked my way through the crowd of women in red and orange saris and men in *topi*s and turbans, gripping hand-carved canes. On the unlit second floor I found Ruit's advance team hard at work processing a long line of patients, who shuffled forward with varying degrees of vision. I saw not only elderly people but children as young as five, their arms extended for balance, slowly groping their way along.

In wealthy countries, cataracts, the clouding of the clear lens of the eye, typically affect older people. But in the developing world, poor nutrition, exposure to unfiltered ultraviolet rays, and the numbing range of physical traumas afflicting those who live at the subsistence level, compounded by a lack of basic medical care, all combine to make cataracts the leading cause of preventable blindness among the world's poor. That was who filled the second floor of this temporary hospital: the world's poor. The line of patients inched politely onward, oblivious to any Western notion of personal space, the chest of one person pressing into the bony shoulder blades of the next. The cloying smell of body odor and infection clung to many of the patients like the patched and sun-faded clothing most of them wore. Their battered hands and feet were maps of hardship. Though most had walked hours on rocky trails for the right to wait in this dank cement room, many were barefoot.

As they cleared the line, Ruit's staff prepped each patient for surgery. A female medical technician gently trimmed eyelashes with a pair of tapered scissors. Others simply scrubbed Rasuwa's red dust from patients' faces.

Beside a door leading to the operating room, a small video monitor sat on the floor. On the screen, with a clarity I hoped the visually impaired patients couldn't discern, a crescent-shaped blade pierced a large, unblinking eyeball.

The Nepalese waiting their turn beneath that blade stared calmly at the screen for a moment or two at a time, or chatted with their neighbors. Ruit told me that when he began working in rural Nepal, more than two decades earlier, rumors that he practiced enucleation—that is, removing the entire eyeball—had frightened prospective patients away. "I put the monitor there so my trainees can watch, but also because it relaxes the patients," Ruit explained. "They see that cataract surgery is in fact a very simple procedure, and they know what to expect."

I squatted next to two boys, nine and thirteen, who couldn't be anything but brothers. They were both squinting at the monitor and leaning their heads together while the younger boy, whose cataracts were less mature, described the surgery. With Ruit's daughter Serabla translating, I asked them their names and ages. Birbahadur, the thirteen-year-old, interrupted to ask why we weren't speaking Nepali.

"You see, his cataracts are so advanced he can't tell you're a foreigner," Serabla said.

Voices raised in alarm drew my eyes to a thin, stooped woman wearing a ginger-colored silk blouse and a long, pink floral *guneo*, clothes noticeably finer than most of her peers', who stumbled as she was called to the eyelash station. She clutched at the air in front of her wildly and would have fallen if her husband hadn't rushed to steady her and lead her carefully across the room. The woman walked with the painful, jackknifed posture of someone with osteoporosis and clutched his arm like a life preserver.

Her name was Patali Nepali, she said, inclining her head in the direction of my voice. Her hair was long and dark, silvered with age, and tied back neatly with a ribbon. I looked into her eyes. She would have been beautiful if not for the pale, milky orbs the size of marbles where her irises would have been. I could see myself reflected on the blank surfaces, squatting in front of her. She wore an orange *tikka* at the center of her forehead, which Hindus believe stimulates the growth of the third eye. Certainly, her other two weren't doing her much good.

Wheezing asthmatically as she spoke, Patali said that she came from a village well over an hour's walk away, in a range of hills visible to our west. I'd assumed she was elderly, but she told me she was fifty-six and had spent most of her life as a seamstress. She'd worked until a year earlier, she said, her skills steadily deteriorating, until she was forced to admit she could no longer see well enough to sew. With the family reduced to one income, they tried to live on her husband's earnings as a woodcutter and hired laborer; they were Damai, members of one of the lowest, the untouchable castes, and owned no land themselves. They'd been forced to sell off many of their possessions, including their only cow, to feed their five children.

"This last year," Patali said, "I can do nothing useful. My own children have to wash me like a child. So we have been hungry. I eat only in the morning, but still there is never enough for my family."

A few weeks before our conversation, their eldest son, a seventeen-year-old on his way to Kathmandu to look for work, was injured in a bus accident. He'd been riding in the cheapest seat, on the roof, when the bus collided with a cement truck. Her son was more fortunate than some. He was thrown clear of the wreck but broke both his legs. "I was obliged to sell the last fine thing in my home to pay his medical bills," Patali told me. "My sewing machine."

I asked her husband how he had brought Patali to Rasuwa. "We took a taxi," he said. I realized how few vehicles I'd seen on the climb to Rasuwa and wondered if a village tucked even farther into these hills was reachable by road. "Basket taxi," he said, laughing, pointing to his strong woodcutter's back. "I'm the taxi!"

Ruit's team had done their best to turn a filthy military post into a sterile operating theater. They'd slit open black plastic trash bags and taped them over broken windows. Next to extinct fluorescent fixtures, bare lightbulbs hung over the two operating tables from extension cords cleverly taped to the ceiling. Cables snaked past medical equipment crowded into the room, toward a generator outdoors. The generator also powered the most critical equipment, two Zeiss surgical microscopes that had been delicately transported from Kathmandu.

Behind a mask, in a green gown and white latex gloves, Ruit seemed even more intimidating. But when he saw me, he waved me over warmly. "Come here, stand beside me, David," he said. "This is a rather challenging case." I stepped over a tangle of cables and balanced behind Ruit's left shoulder, my feet pressed together on a small patch of clear concrete, between a rusty fan plugged in to a power strip with bare wires and a bucket full of blood-soaked things I didn't want to look at too carefully.

I tried to meet the one functioning eye of the elderly-looking man on the table, but he couldn't see me. He was thin and grizzled and wore a necklace of heavy amber beads smoothed by time. In one socket, only a scarred blue-white mass remained from a youthful farming accident. The other eye was blinded by a large cataract. When I read his chart, I learned that Thulo Bahadur was fifty-two, another lesson in the way hardship can sculpt human features. Ruit asked me to remove the man's orange-and-pink cotton *topi*. When I did I saw how rarely, except to sleep, he must have taken the cap off. The skin on Thulo's forehead was several shades lighter than his browned and deeply lined face.

I've always loved watching any physical task performed flawlessly. I'm mesmerized by a gas station attendant who can clean a windshield with precise, confident strokes, or a woodsman capable of splitting firewood with a single clean blow. But Ruit was in another class altogether. He painted bright orange sterilizing solution briskly around the man's right eye, propped the lids open with a wire speculum, and whipped a surgical drape over his head, leaving the large cataract exposed through a perfectly aligned hole. As he delicately lowered the lens of the Zeiss and picked up his crescent blade, I felt a shiver of appreciation for the grace and economy of his movements, the flawless choreography of his instruments in motion.

Ruit beckoned me forward and encouraged me to watch the surgery on a monitor connected to the microscope. I leaned forward to look. Through the high-powered Zeiss, the moon-bright cataract, orbited by a faint ring of translucent cornea, looked more like a planetary body than part of a human. "This is a very, very, very large cataract," Ruit said. "This fellow would only perceive light and no light, but no forms. So we'll just get it out of the way."

Ruit urged the point of his blade gently upward into my field of view, piercing the outer surface of the eye, which flexed before tearing, and then carved slowly, from side to side, expanding his point of entry. "This is the wound construction," Ruit murmured. "I'm actually making a tunnel. You must make the passageway large enough to deliver the nucleus. The nucleus is like the yellow of the boiled egg, you know?" When he was satisfied, he inserted a Simcoe cannula, a combination probe, suction, and irrigating device. With the tip of the probe, he separated the spherical, cloudy lens of the eye from the filmy capsule that enclosed it. And using the cannula to direct a jet of sterile fluid at the orb, he succeeded in loosening the cataract until it spun in place, like a marble ball on a decorative water fountain. "This," Ruit said, with the reverence of a Buddhist monk chanting morning *pujas*, "is the 'hydro-dissection.'

"But now comes the little bit tricky part. Normally I would make a slightly smaller wound, but this fellow's cataract is so . . . " he trailed off in mid-sentence, concentrating. I would come to know these silences, and the difficult tasks they enveloped, intimately. Ruit fed the cannula back through the wound. It was scored with fine textural lines, like a file, allowing it to grip the cataract's smooth surfaces. He worked it under the cataract in tiny increments that seemed too precise for human hands to direct. He was humming, something catchy and minor key, unmistakably a tune from the subcontinent, perhaps from a recent Bollywood film.

When he had caught the cataract with the probe, he drew it slowly into the wide end of the funnel-shaped wound. I saw the clear tissue along the pathway bulge as he urged the cataract through the narrowing tunnel he'd designed. Ruit stopped humming, and I could feel him holding his breath as he coaxed the cataract completely out of the wound, which puckered shut after delivering the hardened tissue into the humid air of the operating room. "Perfect," Ruit said happily, gathering the cataract in a fold of gauze and flicking it toward the bucket at my feet. "But he won't be able to see until we insert an artificial lens."

While prepping patients for surgery, Ruit's technicians had measured the shape of each person's eyes with a device called a keratometer, so he could insert a lens of the correct power, a lens that would ensure that the patient's vision was as precise as possible after the cataracts were removed. A nurse held out a small plastic tray, and Ruit plucked an intraocular lens about the size of a child's fingernail from it with a miniature set of forceps. He slid it briskly through the wound until the lens was centered under his patient's dilated pupil. When I leaned forward to look at Thulo Bahadur's eye, it appeared clear and clean as a freshly washed window.

"So this is what we're calling sutureless surgery," Ruit said, the pride in his voice unmistakable. "The wound will seal itself and heal without stitches. And tomorrow the patient should see very, very well."

As Ruit folded and discarded the surgical drape, and the nurse taped a plastic eyecup over Thulo Bahadur's repaired eye, I glanced at my watch. The entire operation had taken seven minutes. For an unusually challenging cataract surgery. Seven minutes to restore a man's sight. My spine tingled like *it* was connected to the generator.

I watched a dozen cases more, some lasting only four or five minutes, until the patients were led away to a recovery room by Maoist soldiers who'd been assigned to help. Ruit handled his instruments with such ease and precision that the surgery began to seem simple, something that anyone, even I, could attempt. Then I stood behind the room's second operating table, observing Dr. Kim and Dr. Kim, two North Korean surgeons Ruit was training to bring his method to their banished country. Their instruments jerked and sawed with such relative violence that I could barely stand to watch. When they finally completed their single case, more than forty-five minutes after they'd started, I leapt at the chance to find a few breaths of fresh air.

By mistake I walked through a door that led not outside but into a room as hot and wet as a sauna. On a table cobbled together with two sheets of carpet-topped plywood and supported by cinder blocks, four patients were lying on their backs, receiving injections of local anesthesia, waiting for surgery. Along the opposite wall, two autoclaves, which I mistook at first for huge cooking pots, hissed and rattled over propane rings of flame, sterilizing surgical equipment.

Into this steam room, an unsteady Patali was led by her husband. Patali's thin legs were shaking, and I had Serabla ask him if he wanted me to find some food for his wife. "They already gave us dal and such," he said cheerfully. "Today, she is not suffering hunger, only fear."

Fortunately, Patali couldn't see the anesthetist's long needle as it approached her eye. After she felt the sting, her hands fluttered and twitched at her sides, like sparrows trapped inside the building. "I have to go!" she cried toward the spot where her husband had been standing, but nurses had already shooed him back to the waiting room.

"I think you should stay," I said, taking one of her hands. It felt tiny and cold despite the heat from the autoclaves. "Tell her Dr. Ruit is a good surgeon," I said to Serabla. "Tell her that when the bandages come off, she'll be able to see her children again."

On the operating table, Patali clutched my hand throughout the surgery on her left eye. Five minutes later, when I helped her sit up and repositioned her so her right eye faced Dr. Ruit, she was calm enough to release my hand. I stepped behind him, skirting the bucket now brimming with medical waste. Ruit had removed his hiking shoes, and his wide, bare foot lay on the pedal of the microscope, controlling fine focus. As he set to work on Patali's second eye, I leaned forward to watch, my fingers resting lightly on his shoulder.

"Don't touch me!" he barked.

I jumped back, accidentally kicking the microscope's power cord out of the socket. "Daayviid," Ruit said, his voice now low and sing-songy, the voice of someone calming a startled animal. "This lady would like to see out of both eyes, eventually. Do you think you might be good enough to plug my microscope back in?"

On the roof of the temporary hospital, Ruit's team had set up camp. Six tents were duct-taped to the concrete, lines of drying surgical scrubs hanging between them. Exhausted nurses and technicians sprawled on sleeping bags or darted inside to change into jeans and T-shirts. The esprit de corps of Ruit's team was obvious, and I was struck by the confidence of the professional women, compared with the meekness of most of the female patients I'd met. At dinner, one particularly sassy scrub nurse wore a tight T-shirt that declared, in bold letters: SHUT YOUR MOUTH WHEN YOU TALK TO ME.

I sat inside a low, open-ended mess tent across a camp table from Ruit, beside three Chinese Australian donors who'd come to determine what sort of investment they were getting for their money. I mopped the last of my dal and *aloo gobi* from a metal plate with my second freshly baked chapatti. Ruit swallowed his last bite and sighed contentedly. "It's important," he said, "to feed your army really, really well."

The crowns of eucalyptus trees rose just above the roofline of the building, stirring in the slight breeze. They flavored the dusk with herbal currents. Once it became fully dark, the cook's assistant removed our plates and replaced them with candles, which lent the glowing interior of the tent substance, separated it from the dim evening air.

The two North Korean surgeons were both named Kim, but they couldn't have been more different. One was small, shy, and bespectacled. The other was strapping, outgoing, and as handsome as a soldier on a Soviet-realist propaganda poster. When I was introduced as an American journalist, they found an excuse to slip out, and returned a few minutes later properly equipped. They had each fastened a pin depicting Kim Jong Il, the "Dear Leader," to their shirts.

Ruit reviewed the day's surgeries with them, drawing diagrams of the interior chamber of the eye on a page ripped from my notebook. He had performed forty-four perfect surgeries over the course of the afternoon. Between them, the Kims had struggled to complete seven. "The secret," Ruit said, sketching the ideal wound construction, "is to go slowly, slowly, slowly until you've mastered the technique, you see. You'll need to do about two hundred cases each before you really get the hang of it."

"How many cases have you done?" I asked. "More than two hundred, I imagine?"

"Oh, a few more," Ruit said, reaching for the bottle of rum he'd brought from Kathmandu.

"By his own hand, more than eighty thousand," said Nanda, the keeper of her husband's flame. The scale of what Ruit had achieved and what he was attempting struck me then, for the first time. One man had already restored sight to the equivalent of a football stadium's worth of people. Yet more than one hundred million people around the world who needed an ophthalmologist's services were still waiting. Beneath us, sleeping on mats in a recovery room, were fifty-one people who, if all went well, could no longer be counted among that number tomorrow. And when the Kims returned to North Korea, they would bring Ruit's technique with them and pass it on to their colleagues in one of the world's most isolated places. He was seeding not only Nepal and North Korea but much of the poorest ground in Asia with enthusiastic young surgeons like Kim and Kim. It was visionary.

Ruit poured a healthy splash of rum into each of our mugs, neatly quartered a bowl of limes with a sharp knife, and squeezed fresh juice into each of our drinks. Then he raised his mug. "What we do is hard," he said, with something like glee. "If it was easy, someone else could do it." Everyone sipped the citrusy rum, and we traded toasts in the half dozen languages of those assembled around the table. The Kims looked elated. The breeze picked up. Guttering candles threw sparks of light off our tin mugs, onto the canvas walls of the tent, and I felt something rare, something important, being kindled.

Early the next morning Ruit looked fresh in a crisply ironed white polo shirt and black trekking pants. Though we'd had only a few hours of sleep, he practically skipped, clear-eyed, toward another long day of surgery.

The fifty-one postoperative patients were gathered in a courtyard bordered by low stone walls, waiting with bandaged eyes, squatting on packed dirt with the same heartrending patience as the bus passengers stranded in the slow-moving Trishuli. Ruit conferred with his camp logistics manager, Khem Gurung, making sure the day's new cases were properly organized. Khem was one of the dozens of younger, clean-cut medical technicians who cheerfully endured the hardships of traveling and working with Ruit.

"I have to eat something and scrub in," Ruit told me. "Stay and see these bandages come off. You might find it interesting."

The day had a peculiar yellow cast. Shafts of storm light broke through scudding clouds to pick out individual potato and turnip fields on the laboriously terraced hillsides, and made certain stands of scrub pine smolder like they were about to ignite.

Patali had dressed for the occasion in a style befitting a master seamstress. She wore a crimson-colored silk blouse of her own design, and she had brushed her long black hair so thoroughly before tying it back with a matching silk ribbon that her silvered strands looked like reflections rather than evidence of age. Her husband waited outside the courtyard with the other family members, leaning anxiously over the stone wall. He murmured something reassuring, and her head tilted toward his voice like a plant tracking the sun's passage.

Ruit's team didn't wear uniforms. Most of the male staff favored polo shirts, like their leader. But what set them apart was their brisk efficiency, movements that must have been modeled on Ruit's. Khem Gurung's shirt was lime green, and his manner with patients mirrored Ruit's almost exactly. Khem knelt to peel off the first patient's bandages, then examined his eyes in the bright beam of a handheld slit lamp until he was satisfied the surgery had been a success. Thulo Bahadur blinked in the sunlight. Then he began to laugh.

"How many fingers am I holding?" Khem asked.

"Two," Thulo said, waggling his head dismissively, as if insulted to be asked such a simple question. "Two fingers. I can see that perfectly well." He looked across the courtyard, past the fifty other bandaged patients, toward the stand of eucalyptus; then his eyes focused on the battered cane he held clutched in both hands. He pulled himself up by it until he was standing and dropped the stick in the dirt by his bare feet like something unclean.

Nurses followed Khem down the line of patients, handing out eyedrops and instructions for keeping the wounds clean until they healed. The two young brothers squatted, stunned and motionless, after their bandages came off. Then Birbahadur saw his mother, a worn-looking woman in a red head scarf and heavy brass earrings, waving outside the wall. He waved back at her shyly. She covered her mouth with both hands and burst into tears.

I squatted in front of Patali with Khem. Ruit's initials had been neatly printed on her bandages with a felt marker. Khem peeled both bandages down until the blue plastic cups that had covered her eyes were dangling from her cheekbones. Patali blinked and blinked and didn't react at all. Her eyes were deeply bloodshot, and I feared the surgery had been a failure. Then her mouth widened into a grin at the vision kneeling before her; a sweaty, unshaven foreign journalist pointing a camera at you can't be the most inspiring thing to see at the moment you regain your sight. But she didn't seem to mind.

"If you can see clearly, why don't you touch his nose," Khem said.

Patali reached out with her forefinger and placed it squarely on the tip of my nose. All three of us laughed when she found her mark. "Wait," I said, scrambling over to her husband. I put out a hand and helped him over the wall. He squatted beside his wife and straightened his plain brown *topi* on his head. Patali studied his lined face.

"So, how does he look?" I asked.

"The same," Patali said. "Still handsome." Then she threw her thin arm over his solid shoulder. I watched Patali take in the world surgery had returned to her. I saw her gaze alight on a distant ridgeline, where a shaft of morning sun brushed the tips of terraced hills with a warm caramel color. They were only the dusty mid-hill ranges of Nepal, one of the poorest vistas the country could conjure, but she looked toward home as tenderly as Apa Sherpa had during our trek when we'd crested a ridge and he'd first sighted the distant summit of Everest. "Oh," she said, leaning against her husband, smiling fully for the first time since the bandages came off, "Look at the hills! Do you see how they shine?"

I watched Ruit's staff perform a few dozen small miracles more. The oldest patients seemed the most overwhelmed by the gift of second sight. Their joy was sudden and unfiltered. One elderly man, wearing a white turban and a shabby suit coat that hung to his knees, danced circles around his walking staff, singing to himself, drawing protests from patients whose feet he was too entranced to avoid.

All fifty-one of the previous afternoon's surgeries had been successful, Khem explained when he finished his examinations. Kim and Kim's patients had a bit more swelling and postoperative trauma, but for beginners their results were excellent, he said.

I watched 114 new patients being led into the hospital for the second day of surgery, many hunched over and staggering as unsteadily as Patali had the previous afternoon. Patients streamed past them out of the compound, dozens of the formerly blind hiking away toward their homes, navigating the uneven dirt trails that radiated out from the temporary hospital without the aid of the relatives who accompanied them.

Walking toward a rusted gate, I saw someone who looked like Patali. But this woman was standing straight up and striding confidently beside her husband. Her back hadn't been bent by osteoporosis at all, I realized, but by her sense of helplessness, by the weight of blindness. The transformation was startling, almost more than I could reasonably believe one day after seeing her squatting timidly on the concrete floor of the hospital, waiting for surgery.

I fumbled in my pockets for rupees, doing the math. Not enough. I scrounged through my camera bag, finding a thick wad of bills I'd saved for an emergency. I ran to the gate before she could begin the long walk home and pressed the money into her hands. "For a sewing machine," I said, unable to meet Patali's eyes.

On the roof of the building, leaning against a railing, Sanduk Ruit was watching his patients. He stood with one arm over the shoulder of Serabla, who looked on proudly at her father's handiwork. I pointed Ruit out to Patali, told her that the man on the roof was the one who had restored her sight. She bent low toward him, her hands clasped together in gratitude. "Thank you, Doctor *dai*," she said, even though we were much too far away for Ruit to hear. "Thank you." Then she took her husband's arm and they walked together up a dirt trail that led toward a pine grove, his basket immeasurably lighter. I watched until they entered the shade and were swallowed by shadows.

I looked up at the figure on top of the building, silhouetted against a borderless sky. Though his pitch had been full of self-promotion and bluster the night we'd had dinner, Tabin hadn't overstated the importance of his work with Ruit. The man on the roof was still a mystery to me, but I wondered if there was a single person on earth doing more measurable good for others.

The line had been cast in Salt Lake City and the hook set in the mid-hills. I had come to Nepal, lost one book on the trails of the Khumbu, and swerved, finding another. I felt the weight of the mostly empty notebook in my shirt pocket. "Well," I thought, flipping it open to a clean, blank page, "well."

CHAPTER 3

Here You Are

The greatest country, the richest country, is not that which has the most capitalists, monopolists, immense grabbings, vast fortunes . . . but the land in which . . . wealth does not show such contrasts high and low, where all men have enough . . . and no man is made possessor beyond the sane and beautiful necessities.
—Walt Whitman

I sat beside Geoff Tabin as we hurtled down Interstate 80, toward Salt Lake City, in his cramped, sticky-surfaced Ford Escape hybrid. The floor was piled high with cans of used tennis balls, medical journals, crushed paper coffee cups, and nearly empty sports drink containers. Tabin was on the phone to Ghana, confirming the dates for an upcoming trip he'd arranged to train local surgeons and operate on five hundred cataract patients. We were traveling at nearly eighty miles an hour around sweeping curves down a rocky canyon, and he seemed oblivious to the double- and triple-length tractor-trailers passing inches from our side mirrors as he drifted in and out of our lane.

He hung up and dialed Nepal. It was evening in Kathmandu, and he had to shout over the wind blast and the bad connection, trying to make himself understood to Ruit as they planned Tabin's next trip. "What's that? Ten! I can bring about ten fresh corneas!" Tabin said. "Today? The usual, trying not to blind anybody. Listen, we've got John Nkurikiye here from Rwanda. You remember I sent him to you last spring. Yes, I'll certainly say hello. He's very solid. I think John could be the person to really anchor eye care in Africa. Also, I'm talking with two ophthalmic technicians from Nigeria. I want to send them to you at Tilganga for a month or so." Tabin looked crestfallen as he listened, for a moment, to an objection Ruit had apparently voiced. "Okay, you know I always trust your judgment. We'll discuss it when I see you." Tabin signed off with "Love to Nanda and the kids."

By the time he hung up we had descended several thousand feet and were approaching the hilly eastern suburbs of Salt Lake, where the sparkling, glass-and-steel John A. Moran Eye Center was located on the University of Utah campus. Traffic ahead of us had slowed, but Tabin seemed not to notice the river of brake lights as he typed a text message to a mountaineer buddy he hoped would join us that evening for dinner. He looked up from his phone just in time and jammed on the brakes, slapping his forearm protectively against my chest as we stopped a foot from the rear mud flaps of a cattle transport.

"Hey, have you met Andrew McLean?" he asked. I would come to know this conversational lane change well, the lack of spaces in Tabin's speech before he veered at freeway speed toward an apparently unrelated subject. "Technically, he may not be the best skier in the world, but he'll ski lines no one else would think of touching. He's really fun," Tabin said. "Fun," I soon learned, was the doctor's highest compliment. "He should be there tonight. I'm thinking incredible, incredible steaks and my famous dirty martinis. Wait till you taste one. They'll knock you out!"

It was just after six in the morning.

In the surgeons' dressing room of the Moran, Tabin sniffed the armpits of the scrubs he'd worn earlier that morning while he'd attacked his home climbing gym, which peaked in difficulty on an overhanging pitch of 135 degrees. He'd started his workout long before I was awake, but I knew the angle of the slope because he'd given me a forced-march tour of the sprawling house where he and his family lived, on rangeland outside Park City, late the evening before. The only room where we'd lingered was his attic, where he'd pointed out the routes he'd set, the colorful resin holds that spread across the walls and ceiling like a peculiar formation of coral. Tabin told me that he tried to "get a quick burn" every morning and declared that his central philosophy in life was to keep that flame lit all day, to live every hour fully—or, as he put it precisely, to "keep the fun-o-meter in the red."

He peeled off his scrubs and pulled a clean, folded pair from the stack of fresh hospital laundry. His gold wedding ring hung from a scarlet cord around his neck, a talisman he'd had blessed by the Dalai Lama. At five foot eight, Tabin didn't have the long, wiry build common to many elite climbers. But you don't reach the highest point on each continent, or make the first ascent of Everest's Kangshung Face, without physical gifts. He had worked hard to sculpt and refine the modest material he'd been handed genetically. Even at fifty-two, Tabin had legs with the chiseled musculature of a bicycle racer's, and his forearms were comically large. Popeye large. They ended at hard, callused hands, hands that seemed blunt instruments for the manipulation of delicate surgical tools.

Dressed for surgery in scrubs and a sterile gown, Tabin walked so fast, trailed by his two ophthalmic residents and half a dozen medical students, that I had to jog to keep up. Shadowing Tabin and trying to answer questions he or any member of the hospital staff lobbed at them was a critical element of his trainees' education.

I fell into stride next to an African ophthalmologist on his way to watch Tabin perform cataract surgery. John Nkurikiye was a tall and handsome forty-four-year-old surgeon. He would have been imposing but for a cheerful spray of freckles across the bridge of his nose and eyes so wide open and optimistic they seemed to belong to a much younger man, not someone who had witnessed the worst of the Rwandan genocide.

I introduced myself and, to make conversation while we tried to keep pace with Tabin, made the mistake of inquiring whether his family was Tutsi or Hutu. Nkurikiye stiffened. "You know, those are artificial categories the Europeans created for us," he said. "We've had enough trouble because of those words. I prefer not to use them."

Tabin paused outside the swinging doors to the operating room, and Nkurikiye and I caught up to his entourage as he consulted with one of his trainees, Chris Kurz, who was completing his cornea fellowship with Tabin at the Moran. He and Tabin reviewed a recent corneal transplant Kurz had performed, a far more complex procedure than a cataract surgery, which Kurz said had gone well, except he'd had to sponge away more blood during the operation than he'd expected.

Tabin turned to face the rest of us, aiming his question toward the knot of students with pens and notebooks at hand. "Do you know how to tell, with one hundred percent certainty, if a plant is poison ivy?" Tabin asked.

No one ventured an opinion.

"Okay, you take a handful of the reddest leaves you can find and rub them on the thin strip of skin between your testicles and your anus. Then you wait two to three hours. If you experience extreme itching and discomfort, the plant is definitely poison ivy!"

There were a few embarrassed chuckles, and the pens hovered motionless over open notebooks.

"Likewise," Tabin continued, "if Dr. Kurz is operating on an eye, how does he know if he's cutting corneal tissue? The cornea, the clear surface at the front of the eye, is unique. It's the only tissue in the body that draws all the oxygen it needs from the air, not a network of capillaries. If Dr. Kurz cuts and it bleeds, he's cut not corneal tissue but the sclera, the tough white outer wall that covers the rest of the eye," Tabin said, driving his point home neatly, setting the students' pens in motion.

I imagined that during all the cramming they'd have to do one day for their medical boards, few of them would struggle to remember this particular lesson.

Tabin backed through a set of swinging doors and bent to a set of double sinks to scrub in. Four support staff lounged in front of crisp, flat-screen displays, calibrating equipment or browsing the Internet. From the ceiling, an octopus-like PrismAlix lighting array, with dazzling halogen discs held at the end of each tentacle, lit the adjustable chrome operating table brighter than a tropical beach at noon. Tabin, swaddled in a crisp green paper smock that had been tied behind his back by a nurse, took his place on a Stryker Surgistool, calibrated by a technician to the precise millimeter of height and forward lean the doctor preferred. The chromium stool, a mobile wonder of shock-absorbing arachnid legs, looked fully capable of jettisoning boosters, landing on Mars, and collecting soil samples.

I thought of the single 60-watt bulb taped to the ceiling over Ruit's plywood operating table in Rasuwa.

Travel frequently enough, dislocate yourself often enough at jet speed, and your culture shock mutates into something else: not the shock of the new or the unknown but the unsettling juxtaposition of the present and the very recent past. Here you are. But there you were. And all too often that contrast points, in my experience, to a gulf between meager resources and material excess too wide to comfortably accept.

Evidently John Nkurikiye was thinking along the same lines. "All of this for one patient, for one rather simple procedure," he said, shaking his head as a woman was wheeled through the double doors by orderlies and positioned before Tabin's gloved hands.

That made six medical staff in the room, and seven observers. Tabin's scrub nurse took no notice of me as she began to lay out surgical tools. But as soon as the operating theater manager confirmed Tabin's choice of jazz over soft rock for the sound system, she glanced in my direction. I looked away and turned toward Tabin's elderly patient. The day before, while I'd been watching Tabin remove a cataract at the VA hospital near the Moran, a nurse whose name tag read M. BIGWOOD had called me over for questioning. He was a large man, unsmiling. It might have been my inexpertly tied surgical mask; knotting a mask behind your head is like tying a bow tie behind your back, and I'd yet to fasten one convincingly. Or perhaps he'd simply chosen that moment to conduct a random pop quiz.

"Tell me," the man had asked, "how long has cataract surgery been practiced?"

I tried to recall fragments from the background reading I'd recently begun.

"Since about 2000 B.C.?" I said, fairly confident I had the right date.

"Excellent," he said. "They called it 'couching,' poking at the cataract with a needle. Not very helpful, and you can only imagine the infection rates, but they might have seen a bit of light after that, a little improvement."

I tried to peer over his large shoulders to watch Tabin work, but M. Bigwood wasn't done with me. "Where does the material for a modern IOL come from?"

My ability to recall precise details was degrading as I strained to see. I floundered for a moment, then said, "An airplane windshield?"

"What airplane?"

He had me there. I shrugged.

"A World War II Spitfire," he said. "Military surgeons noticed that shards of Spitfire windshield shattered by gunfire didn't react with tissue when they were embedded in pilot's eyes. So they knew the eye wouldn't reject lenses manufactured from the stuff. Intraocular lenses have been made of a similar material ever since."

Now I watched Tabin perform surgery on the elderly woman, taking care not to make eye contact with the female nurse in charge of the Moran's operating room and prompt questions from her. I looked everywhere but in her direction.

My eyes strayed to a flat-screen monitor at one of the technicians' desks. I noticed an article he was browsing through, titled "The 10 Most Stressful Jobs." Surgeon and anesthesiologist led the list, followed by smoke jumper and industrial deep-water diver. Tabin had told me a story the previous evening about a Boston surgeon who'd jumped to his death from the roof of a hospital after accidentally removing the uncancerous eye, the one healthy eye, from his preteen patient.

On the largest of the variously angled monitors mounted on the walls behind his head, I watched the sharp end of the modern tool Tabin was wielding to break up his patient's cataract. It was called a phacoemulsification device, or phaco for short. Tabin inserted the phaco tip into the capsule of the eye. Rather than coaxing out the cloudy lens of the eye whole, as Ruit had in Rasuwa, Tabin used phacoemulsification to pulverize the cataract with precisely directed ultrasound waves, then draw out the fragments with suction so that he could insert a foldable IOL through the tiny wound he'd created.

"Hey, you've got to see this," Tabin called to me. I joined Nkuri-kiye and the scribbling students ringing the operating table. A nurse handed Tabin an injector that tapered to a needle-thin point. Magnified on the monitor, it looked as thick as the neck of a beer bottle. Tabin fed the tip back up the tunnel he'd carved, depressed a plunger, and a translucent lens unfolded like a sea creature across the width of the eye, spreading thin arms, called "haptics," that held it in place.

Even I could tell how clear the patient's eye now appeared, projected many times the size of life across a bank of monitors, staring placidly at all the cardinal points, like the Buddha eyes I'd seen painted on nearly every smooth surface atop the temples of Kathmandu.

"That went just textbook!" Tabin said after nearly half an hour, which included a delay of fifteen minutes when his patient interrupted him from beneath her draping to ask for another injection of anesthesia. I noticed the light sheen of sweat on his forehead, and condensation on his rimless glasses. I pictured Tabin a few hours earlier, hanging from the ceiling of his attic by his fingertips. Those same fingers had just restored a woman's sight. What sort of adrenaline jolt, I wondered, did that provide to his system?

Assistants peeled off Tabin's paper surgical gown, cap, and mask, throwing them into a trash container along with his latex gloves. He dialed a series of contacts on his iPhone, trying to line up a partner for a late-afternoon rock climb, hoping to inject a few more hours of fun between the end of his workday and the beginning of the evening's festivities.

Nurses tossed the surgical tools and the mostly full bottles of IV fluids into the garbage, then stuffed in the disposable drapes that had covered the patient. Nkurikiye and I stood next to a trash can piled as high as my waist with the detritus of a single operation.

In Ruit's operating theater, all the surgical tools were sterilized and reused. IV fluids were consumed until the containers hang empty from their racks. Drapes and surgical gowns were laundered and boiled in autoclaves again and again until they disintegrated.

Nkurikiye stared at the trash, shaking his head.

"I know this is America, but this seems too wasteful even for a country as rich as yours. Do you know what those instruments cost? Do you know how hard they are for me to get in Rwanda? I'd jump into that can and steal them if it wouldn't land Dr. Geoff in warm water. Do you know I could treat one hundred patients—more!—with the contents of that trash?"

I knew. Or, rather, I was beginning to know, which, I realized, is not at all the same. Here you are. There you were.

CHAPTER 4

Burn the Day

More and more I want to write about people who cannot
modify themselves to reality, whose life looks like no one else's,
people who stain your life.
—James Salter

"Here we are," Tabin said, inching through a knot of admirers at the auditorium door, shaking hands, exchanging email addresses, and promising to look at résumés of those who hoped to work with him, before jogging down a sloping aisle toward the lectern.

I had spent a few days watching Tabin work by then, and had attended a specialized lecture he'd given to ophthalmology students, which had reinforced how little I still understood about the technical challenges required to cure blindness. It had also demonstrated just how often Tabin tended to dance along the border of socially unacceptable behavior. He'd begun by accidently projecting the wrong slide. Everyone in the classroom had gasped at a photo of an enormous naked man, lying facedown, presumably dead, on an urban sidewalk. "Whoops," Tabin had said as he'd fiddled with the cursor on his laptop, "wrong PowerPoint! That's from a slide show I mostly do for climbers. I used to call it 'Why fat people shouldn't bungee jump,' but people kept telling me that was in bad taste."

Tabin's noontime talk the next day was open to all the students at the University of Utah School of Medicine. His work with Ruit had been attracting increased media attention, and that had made Tabin a prominent figure on campus. The packed lecture hall was evidence of the Utah students' curiosity about how he'd managed to forge a career of world-changing work beyond the mainstream of medicine.

As a technician fiddled with his laptop, until a facsimile of his overcrowded desktop loomed on the screen behind his head, Tabin crackled with energy, rocking from foot to foot in a pair of trail-running shoes still speckled with red dirt from a single-track mountain bike ride the previous afternoon. He'd changed into khakis and a well-worn, pale blue short-sleeved button-down that appeared to have been cut from material the precise shade and texture of the scrubs he'd worn into surgery. From where I sat, next to Nkurikiye in the third row, I could see threads protruding where his shoulder seams were separating.

"We've got a lot to cover, so let's get going," Tabin said. A file folder bloomed open, and an image of a stark, black-banded mountain filled the screen, spindrift blowing from the summit. "I was in the middle of my first year at Harvard Medical School when I was invited along by a team attempting the last unclimbed face of this. I sent my academic adviser a postcard, telling him I was off to Mount Everest, and to hold my spot," Tabin said, and the crowd laughed. "I don't recommend you try anything like that if you want to have a career in medicine. I came back from an unsuccessful expedition to find myself out of Harvard."

Tabin clicked through a few dozen more slides of mountains and the scruffy groups of climbers, whose tribe, it was clear from his enthusiasm, he had joined just as proudly as he had the medical community. The photos of bare-chested young men posing on glaciers or dangling from overhanging ledges on slender ropes were full of bravado. And unlike so many public figures who are required to repeat canned speeches, Tabin evinced a pleasure at sharing snapshots from his former life that seemed anything but forced, especially when he paused on a two-decade-old slide of himself, bearded, obviously exhausted, his oxygen mask pulled aside to reveal his triumphant grin on top of the world.

"I shouldn't do this," he said, caught up in the moment, and in the palpable buzz of appreciation he'd extracted from his audience. He flipped to a photo of Everest taken from a distance, towering above the neighboring peaks, and explained that his team, which had succeeded in putting America's first female mountaineer on the summit, had trekked toward it, through deep mud, during the monsoon. "We wore these nylon tights, not so much to get in touch with our feminine side and bond with our female teammates, but to keep off the leeches. There's a poem I wrote. It's rather good, actually. It's called 'Leech on My Dingus.' Would you like to hear it?"

A few of the students hooted, urging him on.

"On second thought, I probably shouldn't perform it in front of a full audience," Tabin said, and as he hit the brakes, I was relieved to see that there were some borders of bad taste he had the sense not to cross. "But if anyone wants to stay after the lecture, and promises not to be offended, I'll give a private recitation."

Then, with no change in tone or intake of breath, Tabin executed another one of those conversational swerves at freeway speed. With Everest's granite pyramid still hovering over his head, he detailed the extent of blindness worldwide: The latest survey from the International Agency for the Prevention of Blindness had concluded that 40 million people in the world were blind, unable, even, to count fingers at a distance of ten feet. If you included people who were severely visually disabled, the number leapt to 161 million. Three out of four of them, Tabin said, could easily have their sight restored if only they received the kind of medical care people in countries like America take for granted. He switched to a pie chart depicting leading causes of preventable blindness worldwide. "As you can see," he said, "more than half of the preventable blindness in the world is caused by cataract disease, which is simple to treat. But there's a problem with my profession," he explained. Most ophthalmologists are more interested in the latest high technology than in curing that massive backlog of blind people. "Why?" he asked, before answering his own question. "Because most of those blind people live in poor countries. And even if millions of them are so disabled by their blindness that they can't work, they can't walk on uneven ground, all they can do is sit in the corner of their homes, hoping to be fed, it's a lot more profitable to charge people in wealthy countries thousands of dollars for minor procedures like cataract surgery or Lasik, so they can drive a bit better at night, or follow the path of their golf ball a little better, than to provide life-changing care to those who need it most."

Tabin's passion was infectious, or would have been, had dozens of pizzas not just then been placed on a table ten feet in front of his lectern. But he was oblivious to their arrival. He was staring at the crags and contours of the mountain of information he was trying to convey, and losing his hungry audience. I stood up and drew his attention to the steaming towers of cardboard boxes. When everyone except Tabin had inhaled a few slices of cheese or pepperoni, he resumed his talk.

He spoke of returning from the top of the world, of meeting a surgeon named Sanduk Ruit, who'd been born among Nepal's high peaks but now lived in Kathmandu. He spoke of Ruit's determination to focus on conquering the backlog, case by case, of the world's needlessly blind. "What if I told you that Dr. Ruit pioneered a simple way to do cataract surgery," Tabin said. "That he's able, in about four minutes, to do a high-quality procedure, with results just as good as the outcome I can achieve here, for about twenty dollars a patient?" There was a murmur throughout the lecture hall. "Well, it's a fact. And I believe, dollar for dollar, it's the single most effective medical intervention on earth. After Dr. Ruit taught me this amazing thing was possible, I knew I had to dedicate my life to working with him." Tabin presented a slide of Ruit at an eye camp in rural Nepal, grinning Buddha-like as he untaped the bandaged eyes of a woman who squinted up at him, hopefully. "So this man here's become my partner in everything I do."

Tabin talked about the organization he founded with Ruit, the Himalayan Cataract Project. He spoke of the 500,000 low-cost, high-quality surgeries the HCP and the organizations it partnered with had already performed in some of the world's poorest, most isolated communities since 1995. He detailed the HCP's emphasis on training, saying they had taught Ruit's technique to hundreds of surgeons in the developing world. He presented flow charts and maps, but almost everyone's eyes remained on the small man with the outsized forearms, his chin nodding vigorously as he made each fresh point from the podium, as if underscoring the foolishness of disagreeing with such obvious truths.

He said that the few ophthalmologists in developing countries tended to live in cities, but that most blind people were subsistence farmers and laborers in remote rural areas. He said that other ophthalmic organizations were doing excellent work for the poor of the developing world, and he declared that the HCP's greatest innovation, and challenge, was streamlining and simplifying surgical procedures, so they could effectively organize mobile outreach efforts to remote areas in two dozen countries, from Tibet to North Korea to Ethiopia and Rwanda. Finally, Tabin laid out the lofty goal he and Ruit had set for themselves, a goal that involved more sustained effort and logistical intricacy than any expedition to the world's high places. They were attempting to cure preventable blindness. Everywhere on earth.

After the applause had faded, and most students had shuffled off to labs or classes or insomniacal hospital shifts, I wondered how many who had listened to Tabin's speech might be swayed to choose less lucrative fields of medicine. How many would forgo late-model German sedans and second homes in the world's beauty spots to assume challenges that would take them to the world's dustier posts and away from the guaranteed payday of practicing in affluent cities. At least a few, it seemed, judging from the number who'd remained to hear Tabin's poem.

"Okay, I promise you'll be glad you waited for this," he said, clearing his throat theatrically, then reciting in a Monty Pythonesque English accent:

> Leech on my dingus. Leech on my dingus.
> You gave me quite a scare
> This morning before breakfast when I found you *there*.
> I even wore nylons to keep you away,
> But they ran at the crotch hiking yesterday.

Leech on my dingus. Leech on my dingus.
You crawled in through that hole
And made a beeline, straight for my pole.
Why is it I who must suffer the hex
Of an engorged leech feeding at my sex?

Leech on my dingus. Leech on my dingus.
I don't wish to be intimate anymore.
To me you are nothing but a @#$%-sucking whore.
And no matter how much you suck my dingus
I will never reciprocate with leechalingus.

His climactic line brought scattered applause. I noticed a few strained looks of good cheer on the faces of the female students, and I was glad, for his sake, that he'd resisted the urge to present "Leech on My Dingus" to the entire audience.

"Well, John," Tabin said to the dignified Dr. Nkurikiye, who'd listened with an attentive, unreadable expression on his face. "What did you think of my poem?"

"You know, Geoff," Nkurikiye replied in his elegant East African English, "I don't really speak American."

Four examination rooms at the Moran's clinic contained patients, most of them elderly, waiting to see Tabin. Lights flashed from small monitors outside each door, alerting him to their presence. Tabin tapped these lights off each time he entered a room; then he examined the patient's eyes through a slit lamp and recommended antibiotic eyedrops for infection or, in several cases, corrective surgery.

For the next two hours, Tabin jogged from room to room, snatching handfuls of lunch from a bowl of M&M's on the reception desk. Nkurikiye and I hustled to keep pace with him. He punched dim one last flashing light and entered the darkened room where an elderly woman named Betty squinted up at us from a wheelchair.

Betty shifted uncomfortably in her chair. She had recently begun treatment for breast cancer. Her left foot was in a cast, broken when she'd stumbled on the stairs in her home. Tabin had already operated on her eyes, transplanting corneas from a cadaver, with limited success, and he suspected that underlying damage to her retinal tissue had caused the transplants to fail. He was preparing to try the surgery again.

Betty looked so frail it was hard to imagine her walking even with a healed foot. "You have to wait until you get so old and everything goes at once," she said quietly. "The broken leg, the cancer, I can stand. But going blind . . ." She trailed off. "That's the worst. Any more you feel dead even though you're still breathing."

Tabin had his hand on her shoulder and was kneading it gently as she spoke. I'd noticed how often he put his hands on all of his patients, as if the healing process started with simple contact.

"Am I going to be able to see again, Doctor?" Betty asked. "Are you going to make this better?"

"I hope so," Tabin said, "but there are no guarantees. The eye is like a camera. The clear front of the eye is like a lens, and the retina at the back of the eye is like film that processes the image. We don't know if the film at the back of your eye is still capable of making images. But the good news," he added, now rubbing her knee, "is you don't have much to lose by trying surgery again. And you may have a lot to gain."

"Thank you, Doctor," Betty said, pressing her mouth into a thin, resolute line.

In the Moran's soaring glass atrium, a tall, strikingly handsome young medical student named Andrew Dorais was waiting for Tabin with a bag of climbing gear slung over his shoulder. Given Tabin's growing international reputation, there was intense competition among medical students, residents, and fellows to apprentice with him. Already, I'd noticed that a suspicious number of these candidates were fit, young rock climbers.

Tabin had completed his medical duties for the day, and, displaying the same disarming speed with which he shifted conversational topics, he turned his attention from work to play, chatting enthusiastically with Dorais about a multipitch climb they were planning in the canyons above the University of Utah campus. "The view from the top is just outstanding," Tabin said. "Ten out of ten. You're not going to believe what you'll see!"

Tabin retrieved his climbing gear from his Ford, crammed it into Dorais's car, and tossed me the keys. "Why don't you and John have a cup of coffee—I should be done by five forty-five." He asked if I'd wait for him in the parking lot of a Phillips 66 gas station a few miles up-canyon, so he wouldn't have to waste ten minutes driving back down after his climb and we'd have time to shop for the dinner party he had planned.

Nkurikiye and I drank coffee at a café on the Moran's top floor. He frowned at his white foam cup. "You must visit Rwanda," he said. "Our coffee . . ." He paused, tactfully, to edit his criticism. "Our coffee compares rather favorably with this."

Nkurikiye was Rwandan, but like so many of his fellow citizens, he had been forced into exile by the periodic waves of violence that had washed over his country for much of the twentieth century. He'd been educated in Burundi and South Africa and, after becoming a doctor, had volunteered as a medical officer in the Rwandan Patriotic Front, the rebel army that had watched the gathering genocidal storm brewing from its camps in Uganda, on Rwanda's northern border. In 1994, when word of mass executions by machete had reached his encampment, he'd joined a group of soldiers, led by future president Paul Kagame, who'd fought their way to the capital, Kigali, and tried to put an end to the killing. Nkurikiye told his story in the barest possible outline, only hinting at his personal trauma and loss, politely redirecting the conversation to the puzzling blandness of much of the American food he'd sampled so far.

On one subject he was extremely talkative: the bounty of American material life. He considered Salt Lake supermarkets overwhelming, because they contained more choices—from entire aisles of cereal or potato chips—than anyone could reasonably expect. But he found them enchanting, too. "Anything you can dream of is there," he said, "if you know where to look."

Nkurikiye felt that America's abundance threaded through every aspect of our national life, including his encounters with patients. "In Rwanda," he said, "you would never hear patients speaking to doctors the way they do here. Dr. Tabin is a renowned surgeon. Yet his patients question everything, second-guess much of the medical advice he gives them. In my country there are so few doctors, patients are simply grateful to see you. Here, they can always wheel their cart to another aisle of medical experts if they don't like what you have to say."

I asked him if he found that frustrating. "It is an adjustment," he said. "The threshold here for problems is very low. But I'm not complaining. Perfection is not bad, if it's possible. In fact, it's wonderful, if you can afford it. As a doctor, nothing would make me happier than to have these choices, these resources, for Rwanda's people."

We hit a lull in the conversation, and both of us looked out through the café's floor-to-ceiling windows, over Salt Lake City's eastern suburbs, to the lines of jumbo-sized SUVs idling at lights, to the curving rows of five-thousand-square-foot homes terraced into neatly landscaped hillsides, watered lawns sparkling gem green among the baked brown hills.

"If you had these resources, what would you do in Rwanda?" I asked.

"We're a small country, a country just beginning to recover from catastrophe," he said. "We'll never be anything like this. But Nepal is a good model for us. I'd like, one day, to become something like the Ruit of Rwanda. My dream is to build an eye hospital on the Tilganga model, not run by a bureaucratic government—private, but not for profit. I'd like to create a training center that can change eye care, that can reverse blindness across East Africa. With Dr. Geoff and Dr. Ruit's help, I think we could make that happen."

Nkurikiye left with a medical student who'd offered to drive him home to the spartan rental house that the Moran had provided for him. I stood in the parking lot, jingling Tabin's overloaded key chain, and looked up at the concave glass façade of the Moran, curved like the functional retina of an enormous eye, reflecting the light of the lowering sun. Betty might not have her sight returned to her here, but thousands of other patients certainly would. And from this building containing the latest medical technology, where the ceaseless energy of

Dr. Tabin combined with the boundless optimism of international visitors like Dr. Nkurikiye, who came to glimpse the possibility of perfection, what other visions might be achieved?

At the Phillips 66 station, I slumped in the driver's seat of Tabin's Ford. There was no sign of him at 5:45, or 6:00, or 6:15. Finally, just before 6:30, Dorais's car arrived and Tabin slung his gear in the back and switched places with me, taking the wheel. "That was fun, fun, fun," he said, easing into traffic. "Andrew's not quite world-class, but he's a *darn* good climber." Tabin's nose was sunburned and one elbow bloodied, bits of gravel clinging to a fresh abrasion. He seemed as oblivious to the wound as he was to his late arrival.

We roared up the sweeping curves of I-80 toward Park City while Tabin fiddled with his phone, scanning emails and text messages. "Shit!" he said. "Shit! I forgot I've got a tennis match." He asked if I could drop him at the Park City Racquet Club and shop for dinner while he played. He peeled off his sweat-stained climbing clothes in the club parking lot. Standing in his boxer shorts among the rows of Swedish and German cars, he fished around for a tennis outfit, pulling on a reeking pair of gray gym shorts and a wrinkled, once-white T-shirt advertising antibiotic eyedrops.

"There should be ten of us, maybe twelve," he said after directing me to his grocer of choice. "So why don't you get twelve great steaks— whatever looks best, maybe rib eye. Also some salad stuff, some veggies for the grill, some wine, actually lots of wine with this group. We'll stop by my house for martini fixings on the way." He didn't mention money. I agreed to pick him up an hour later.

I stashed the groceries among the sports gear in Tabin's truck and watched the end of his match through the long glass window of the racquet club's waiting room. He was playing doubles, and the other three men on his court wore clean, color-coordinated outfits. One of his opponents had recently played on the pro tour. Tabin's partner had once been an All-American at Arizona State. But despite his wrinkled gray clothes, the doctor held his own, hitting crisp baseline drives to the far corners of the court, chasing down drop shots with the same tenacity with which he pursued all the other passions of his life.

Three decades earlier, Tabin had been captain of the Yale tennis team. The summer before he began studying at Oxford as a Marshall Scholar, he'd played in several professional European tournaments, leaving the world of pro tennis only after calculating that his odds of success in it were slight. Still: medicine, mountaineering, tennis. It seemed unfair for a person to excel in so many fields, to have the ability and energy to jam so much bristling life into every hour of the day. But I wondered, as Tabin dove for and missed a hard, angled passing shot, if the doctor's life might not involve some form of sacrifice, at the very least for the members of his family who hoped to share meaningful amounts of his time.

Tabin jogged into his chaotic house, past a pack of barking rescue dogs—dogs his wife, Jean, had taken in during his last trip—to fetch supplies. Without showering, he changed into long pants and a bright orange bicycle jersey. He threw vodka, vermouth, olives, oil, vinegar, and half a head of lettuce into a cardboard box, leaned over his daughter Sara, eleven, and son, Daniel, nine, at the kitchen table to give a cursory glance at their homework, and kissed his wife on his way out. "You sure you don't want to come?" he asked.

"You misbehave with your climbing buddies," Jean said, sticking out her knee while closing the door to prevent the dogs from escaping.

As Tabin drove, I could see the lifts of the Canyons ski area, stilled by summer, and, beyond them, the towers of Olympic ski jumps, silhouetted against a darkening sky. Fifteen minutes later, we approached the modern glass-and-timber house belonging to Tabin's friend Bill Crouse. With our arms full of meat and liquor, we squeezed through the front hall, threading our way past a fleet of mountain bikes, road bikes, and racks of climbing gear.

The party had started without us, and half a dozen open wine bottles stood on the kitchen counter. Tabin greeted everyone, from his closest friends to casual acquaintances, with precisely the same short, sharp yelp of pleasure. He commandeered the stereo, turned up the electric blues he'd selected, and mixed a giant batch of dirty martinis.

I thought I'd seen Tabin in his element that morning, leaning forward on his Surgistool, surrounded by a team of technicians. But this was clearly his element, too. I stood awkwardly, holding both the glass of red wine someone had passed me and the martini Tabin had jammed into my other hand, meeting people with nods rather than handshakes. Everyone seemed to be a skier, cyclist, or climber. Crouse was a former mountain guide who had summited Everest six times. The conversation revolved not around regular work but first ascents of obscure peaks, the condition of single-track trails near Park City, and planned trips to ski or climb new routes in Greenland and Antarctica.

Tabin introduced me to Andrew McLean, who had pioneered a form of backcountry skiing so technical he'd had to invent the tools to make many of his first descents practical. As a product designer at the outdoor company Black Diamond, he'd dreamed up and manufactured the Whippet, a ski pole with an ice ax built into the grip for "fall and you die" terrain, slopes so steep you could perish unless you had a sharp tool at hand to arrest your slide. McLean, like Tabin, appeared physically unimpressive at first glance. He was skinny and wore unflattering glasses over a toothy grin too large to fit his narrow face. Then I noticed the prominent veins in his limbs, so corded and twined that it seemed he was capable of pumping twice the volume of blood that ordinary humans could circulate. "Geoff makes a fantastic martini, but as a skier, he's just passable," McLean said, sipping his drink. "I'll admit he's got a good motor, though. Maybe that's what got him up all those mountains."

"Can you keep up with Andrew?" I asked Tabin.

"No one can keep up with Andrew," Tabin said, his chin once again nodding emphatically after he'd finished speaking, as he often did when hammering home a fact he considered indisputable. "Hey, is the grill ready?" he shouted to someone over his shoulder. "I'm starving!" I spoke with McLean awhile longer, as Tabin ran onto the deck and threw a dozen rib eyes over the coals, sending up flames that lit his beaming face the same fiery shade as his shirt. McLean seemed to know Tabin as a mountaineer first and a doctor only distantly second. Nearly everyone I spoke to at the party seemed to view Tabin primarily as the fourth person to climb the Seven Summits. Of his higher goals in medicine, they had only the haziest perspective.

Someone turned the music up even louder, and Muddy Waters's throaty baritone made the windows rattle like a second set of drums. I felt, at that moment, very far from the quiet evening on the roof of the makeshift hospital in Rasuwa with Ruit. How had these two fundamentally different men managed to work as partners for more than a decade? How could someone as calm, deliberate, and disciplined as Ruit possibly mesh with an impulsive extrovert like Tabin, who burned every waking hour of his days?

Tabin had run back inside, leaving the grill unattended, and was telling a lengthy, uninterruptible joke from the supply he always had on tap, shouting over the music, the needle of his fun-o-meter surging into the red. Could the secret of Ruit and Tabin's success be found in the way their personalities, and their radically different upbringings, complemented each other? I suspected so, but I realized I needed to stop simply grazing the present and start excavating. I sipped from my left hand, then my right. Like Ruit and Tabin, the combination was odd but effective. I was definitely becoming drunk.

Was the doctors' shared vision really a force capable of curing much of the preventable blindness on earth? I stood unsteadily, listening to Tabin labor up a long ridge toward his punch line, and watching the fire I could clearly see flaring up over his shoulder turn several hundred dollars of prime, aged steak into cinders.

CHAPTER 5

Down from the Moon

*This country is said to present a very elevated, rugged tract of lofty
mountains, sparingly snowed, uninhabitable by man or domestic animals.*
—Notation written across a blank spot on an 1858 British colonial map of
northeastern Nepal, the region where Sanduk Ruit was born

Cold. The kind of cold you can't escape. That is Sanduk Ruit's first
memory. Not the faces of his five brothers and sisters. Not the
silver bird-shaped buckle that fastened the striped *pangi* his mother
wore around her waist, or his father's ruddy complexion, perpetually
windburned from his days on the trail to Tibet. Those memories come
later. But the cold, so relentless you could almost see waterfalls of ice-
blue air crashing down canyon walls from the snow peaks, pooling in
the shadowed Tamor River gorge, and steeping his village in glacial
chill.

Perhaps that's why the pot of boiling water proved so irresistible. In
Ruit's small wood-plank house, as in similar homes across the eastern
Himalaya, where humans lived at the limit of what altitude allows, a
fire was always burning, hot water always at hand to cook *tsampa*, boil
a potato, or brew tea. Sanduk Ruit, aged four, climbed up on a bundle
of split cooking wood and stared down into the steam. The warmth was
delicious, and he wanted more of it. Pushing up the sleeve of his homespun sweater of heavy brown yak hair, he lowered his left arm, up to his
elbow, into the fire-blackened pot.

Ruit doesn't remember the pain, only voices raised in alarm, the
skin of his left forearm forming a movable crust like boiled milk, and
frantic consultations between his parents and neighbors. Finally, he

recalls his mother strapping him to his father's back, and being carried up, up, toward the palace at the top of the world. "All-seeing Buddha," his father chanted, repeating the *puja* as he climbed the steep path past the black-and-white *mani* stones, through a forest of flapping prayer flags affixed to poles, mindful of the son he'd already lost, chanting until his voice grew hoarse: "All-knowing Buddha, let all the winds and suns and soil help the boy be well."

Diki Chhyoling monastery sat five hundred feet above Olangchungola, chiseled into the canyon wall, an aerie for peculiar crimson-robed creatures who chose to live exposed to the wind and weather. To the right of the path were rhododendron bushes whose small, bloodred blooms thrived, improbably, at altitude. To the left was the windswept river gorge. Ruit looked down when he dared, seeing how close his father placed his feet to the edge of the narrow path, aware that one stumble could send them both on a dizzying plunge. But his father's footing was sure, a product of his treks into Tibet, carrying paint and fabric and sugar from the plains of India, and returning with yak-wool blankets and heavy sacks of salt, cargo far more unwieldy than a four-year-old son. Ruit felt the wind probing at his thin clothes with sharp fingernails, and buried his face in his father's long hair, taking shelter within his warmth and strength.

From the narrow veranda on the second floor of his home, Ruit had often watched the setting sun brush the monastery's gleaming rust-colored walls, throw golden sparks from the stores of treasure he pictured stacked there. From the village, Diki Chhyoling, one of Nepal's oldest Buddhist monasteries, looked like a vision from the stories his father told, stories of men who became so wise they no longer struggled to eat, or to stay warm, or bothered to live tethered to the ground but floated, at first, inches from the earth, then up between these palaces hanging from the clouds.

When Ruit left the shelter of his father's hair and was lowered onto a rocky ledge outside the monastery courtyard, his legs were unsteady. From this height, he was confused to see that Olangchungola, the center of the world, where more than seventy families chopped wood and carried water and tended their ponies, yaks, and *dzos*, had vanished in the canyon's shadowed depth. Weathered brass urns standing astride the entrance seemed too grand and intimidating to simply walk between. Ruit was disappointed to see that the feet of the elderly monk who invited them inside didn't float but stepped firmly on packed dirt as he led them through the entrance, held a scarlet curtain aside, and beckoned them in out of the wind.

In the prayer hall of the monastery, Ruit squeezed his eyes shut in terror. *Thangkas* dense with scenes of earthly suffering hung in the gloom, their details picked out with terrible clarity by sunlight lancing through chinks in the stone walls. Above the dusty Tibetan carpet where his father laid him down, Ruit found one of these paintings too awful to look at for long. A grinning blue-skinned devil, wearing a necklace of human heads, stood tending a pot of boiling water. In it were dozens of people, their open mouths forming howls Ruit could almost hear.

Perhaps that's why he'd been brought here. His father was always talking about fate, about how past actions predicted your future as reliably as the sun rising over the rhododendrons each morning. "Our fate is written on our foreheads," Sonam often said. Maybe putting his arm in the pot had stirred the machinery of that fate into motion. Maybe it meant a blue-skinned demon lurking somewhere nearby would now have to finish the job, and boil the rest of him like a potato.

But no demon appeared from the shafts of darkness behind painted columns carved with skulls and snakes. Only a younger monk with close-cropped hair and a kind face. Ruit stared at the framed centerpiece of Diki Chhyoling's shrine, a mushroom, nearly two feet wide, reputed to have been found in the forest with the words *om mani padme om* clearly visible on its cap. The monk spread a white silk *kata* under Ruit's damaged arm, scooped a ladle into a wooden jug, and smoothed cool yellow yak butter from Ruit's hand to his elbow. Then he wound the *kata* carefully around Ruit's arm, while the older monk dipped a horsehair brush into a stone cistern and, by the light of butter lamps, chanted healing *pujas* while he shook drops of water believed to have been blessed by Guru Rinpoche himself, showering them down onto Ruit's uplifted head. Ruit's arm healed without infection, but the skin remained puckered and discolored, as if a wrinkled rose-hued silk sheath had been permanently fastened to his flesh.

The following year, when he was five, Ruit broke his other arm.

He was attempting to ride the village's most fearsome *dzo*. Egged on by a pack of friends, he climbed onto the animal and grabbed the rough hair on either side of its neck. Another boy yanked the *dzo's* tail, and the yak-cow hybrid shot forward like it had been shocked, bucking and twisting, galloping down the path of paving stones that divided the village of Olangchungola.

Ruit landed on his right arm and felt it crack against a stone, snapping his forearm cleanly. This time his father wasn't as worried, or as sympathetic, finishing his butter tea before carrying Ruit back up to the monastery, lecturing him all the way, and during the painful process of having the monks straighten, then set, his arm in bamboo splints, about taming his mischievous impulses.

"I *was* very, very naughty," Ruit says, laughing with a hint of pride. "But there's so little for children to do in a place like Olangchungola. We had no school. And I was too young to work. So we ran around like little devils."

As Ruit grew older, he realized how fragile life could be in his village. There was a traditional healer who did what he could with medicinal herbs, but the nearest doctor was a six-day walk south, toward India. His parents spoke in short, clipped sentences about his older brother, who'd died before Ruit had formed any memory of him, at age four, from severe diarrhea. Ruit came of age intensely aware that at any moment forces beyond human control could snuff a life out. Ruit's mother, Kasang, told him about the time his own life was endangered as an infant, when a high fever threatened to kill her second son just months after the loss of his elder brother. She told and retold the story, while stirring *tsampa* or making his favorite pounded-corn cakes, of how she'd bundled him up in her warmest yak-hair blanket and carried him a day's walk over the Tiptala into Tibet, to visit the sacred hot springs.

"There, my jewel," she'd say, breaking the corner off a still-cooling cake for him, her words as smooth and practiced as prayer, describing how she had undressed, lowered herself through the freezing air into the center of the most powerful pool, held him on her lap, and ladled hot water over his pink skin, chanting *pujas* to Buddha and Guru Rinpoche, and the spirits of the rocks and the sky and the earth, just to be safe, until she felt sure her son would survive. In Olangchungola, as in much of the eastern Himalaya, Buddhist practice is blended with the traditions of Bon, the older, animist faith that had dominated the mountains until the teachings of Siddhartha Gautama were carried north by Guru Rinpoche.

Each spring, when the winter snows that silted the high passes to Tibet shut began to melt and the trading caravans prepared to set out once again, the village would gather in the courtyard of the monastery for the Phutuk festival. The monks would dance, and Ruit's father, Sonam, would watch them appraisingly, joining in when invited. Like most second sons, Sonam had been sent to study for the monkhood. But the death of his elder brother had brought his career down from Diki Chhyoling to the dusty business of the world. And even though his hair grew out and he wore the black robes of a trader rather than crimson, he knew all the prayers, and Sanduk was proud to see how expertly he danced alongside the monks, how lightly he moved for such a thick and powerful man.

Sanduk watched, enthralled, as the monks, accompanied by drums, bellowing bass horns curved up like elephants' trunks, and clashing cymbals, chanted the history of his father's favorite deity, Padmasambhava. Known to the Walung as Guru Rinpoche, he was the founder of Tantric Buddhism who flew from his home in Pakistan's Karakoram Mountains to Tibet on a tiger, defeating demons with the power of his awakened mind and wielding his *vajra*, a five-pointed thunderbolt that eradicates ignorance. Guru Rinpoche had seeded remote villages of the range with monasteries like Diki Chhyoling, the monks chanted, so humans like the Walunga could learn it was possible to free oneself from the cycle of birth and death, rebirth and suffering, and that compassion was the highest human quality.

Other learning, in a village so remote, was hard to come by. Sonam taught his son to write the Tibetan alphabet. The Nepalese customs officer, stationed in the village to levy import duties on caravans coming down from Tibet, taught Sanduk simple math and the rudiments of written Nepali. By seven, Sanduk was watching, fascinated, over his grandfather's shoulder as he read from sacred scrolls in Pali, picking up a smattering of that ancient tongue. But a child as bright as Sanduk quickly grew unsatisfied with these basic lessons, so a family meeting was convened to decide what to do with this uncontainable boy who caromed from one end of Olangchungola to the other, breaking and burning his arms, like a fledgling Guru Rinpoche attempting to take flight.

Sanduk's maternal grandfather was Dori Namgyal Ukyab, the village *gova*, or chief, a bear of a man with a dense black mustache who had hereditary authority to arbitrate all disputes short of murder in the five Walung villages along the Tamor River. There were no roads to the distant capital, Kathmandu, where schools were plentiful, and there was no simple solution. The *gova* retired to his *lha-kang*, or "god's room," drew a scroll from a shelf, smoothed it flat, and studied it, hoping for inspiration. When he returned to join his family by the fire, the *gova* leaned down to squeeze his grandson's plump cheeks, his solid brass earrings dangling like manifestations of his certainty. "Darjeeling," he said.

Hard trekking over high passes meant courting disaster, Sonam knew from long experience, so he took every possible precaution. With the *gova*, he consulted the scrolls for an auspicious day to depart. He climbed to a ledge high above the monastery, where he could see the snow peak standing at the north end of the valley, the blade-shaped mountain the Walunga called Throne of the Gods, marking the border where Nepal met Tibet. He stacked stones to form a cairn at the edge of a sheer drop. Seeking guidance, Sonam placed rice cakes on the uppermost stone, then retreated to sit and wait.

He and the boy would face fifteen days of difficult travel to the southeastern border of Nepal, then across into India, and he didn't know if Sanduk was strong enough to make the trip. He worried that leaving his seven-year-old son in another country to study among strangers, far from his place at the heart of the Walunga, might be too much for either of them to bear.

A raven swooped down from the heights, landed on the uppermost stone, and pecked, authoritatively, at the rice. Sonam stood up, brushed his hands on his heavy black *chuba*, and started home. The definitive way the raven ate answered the question he'd asked. It was settled.

Sanduk Ruit waited on the balcony of his home. His mother stood behind him, sniffling, clutching his shoulders as his father and his helper, Dharkay, fussed with the straps securing the loads to their yaks. Ruit inspected the small felt shoulder bag his mother had made for him. She'd dyed it red, decorated it with coins and tiny bells, and filled it with cubes of a dried yak cheese called *churpa* and a freshly baked batch of his favorite corn cakes.

Every possible precaution had been taken. Sonam had seen to it that the lamas chanted *pujas* for their safe travel and draped white silk *katas* around their necks to protect them. No one in the Ruits' home had used a broom in the days before their departure, lest they stir up sluggish demons that might stalk them on lonely trails. Kasang had filled a silver cup with water and set it by the hearth, assuring her son that she'd keep it full for him until he returned, an extravagance in a place where all water had to be carried up from the Tamor. Finally, the yaks coughed and stamped with impatience, and it was time to leave.

"Let the boy go," Sonam said.

Sanduk looked up at his mother, trying not to cry. Then he looked down at the first store-bought objects he'd ever owned in his life: a pair of drab green canvas sneakers, manufactured by the Chinese military. He put one in front of the other.

They tried to follow the Tamor. But the river twisted down and away from them, a coil of cold smoke, diving out of sight over boulders, hiding where it was blown by the spirits' breath in the depths of canyons, while they had to follow the trail and climb over gaspingly steep rock headlands before descending into each new valley.

Several times Sonam offered to let his son ride a yak. "It was really hard going," Ruit says. "Sometimes even for my father. Hour after hour we would sweat, climbing to the top of a stairs of stone only to see yet a steeper one waiting round the bend. Then the cold and wind as we crossed passes was almost more than I could bear." Sanduk accepted a few rides on the broad, swaying backs of the animals, fragrant with the sacks of roasted barley they carried for the *tsampa* they stirred over cooking fires. But he saw the pleasure in his father's eyes when he pushed uphill on his own, and so he refused to ride whenever he was able, laboring up each ridge powered by his Chinese sneakers alone.

"I was worried whether Sanduk was old enough for the journey, and how he would survive so far from his family," Sonam says. "But he got stronger as we crossed the ranges. And I began to see some of the stoniness of his grandfather the *gova* in the boy."

Sanduk studied the delicate way the yaks placed their feet on shifting stones and tried to imitate them. And he watched, but didn't dare to duplicate, the way his father walked calmly along the crumbling ledges, never leaning against a cliff face for comfort. Sanduk couldn't keep his fingertips from trailing along the stone walls, and he focused his eyes on his olive-green sneakers. If he let his gaze stumble out to the spray above the river, diving birds of prey demonstrated how far you could fall if you lost your purchase on solid ground.

They spent the first night in a cave his father often used while traveling with his caravans. Sanduk, who had never slept apart from his family, shook with fear after he heard Sonam begin snoring. At daylight, when Sanduk woke to see mist blowing past the cave's mouth, he discovered he'd wet the yak-hair blanket his father had wrapped around him. He feared what his father would do when he found out. "He could be very harsh, very strict," Ruit says. "But I think he understood what a leap it was for me to leave home. So he said nothing." Sonam draped the wet blanket across one of the yaks without a word and let it dry in the sun, an uncharacteristically tender gesture that calmed the boy.

They followed the caravan paths down to Sinwa, a hardscrabble settlement on a muddy bank above the Tamor where flimsy, drafty homes were built of timber and bamboo, and spent a warm night indoors. At Mitlung they left the Tamor, the river at the center of Sanduk's life, and began a sustained climb out of its valley up a steep ravine. Sanduk had finished his mother's corn cakes in the first few days, and on rest stops along the climb, leaning on the stone ledges porters had built to support their loads, he searched the bag for crumbs. Each taste, however tiny, of his mother's cooking made the distance he'd traveled from home feel less daunting.

Three thousand feet above his river, as they finally crested the ravine trail and emerged on a ridge that led to the district capital, Taplejung, Sanduk felt that his life was on the verge of irrevocable change. The storm that broke on their fourth afternoon of trekking, just as they approached town, pounded the point home, with thunderclaps that made the yaks twitch and strain at the leads threaded through their nose rings.

Taplejung, the largest settlement he'd ever seen, was overwhelming. Sheer stone staircases to the upper town ran with rainwater like treacherous man-made waterfalls. Many of the buildings were three, even four stories high. They were whitewashed, with trim freshly painted in bright blues and rhododendron reds and topped with strange tin roofs. More caravans than Sanduk could count stamped through the broad streets and squares with a discordant jangling of bells in competing keys. He had to press himself against the towns' wet walls several times to stay clear of the animals' horns, until his brown wool sweater was smudged with patches of white.

Many of Taplejung's people appeared as strange as the town. They were thinner than the Walunga, with darker skin and bright scarlet tikkas on their narrow foreheads. Passing their temples, he heard the brittle, unfamiliar sound of Hindu bells, ringing at a pitch higher than those dangling from the necks of their yaks.

Sanduk was amazed that, so far from home, his father seemed to know almost everyone they passed. Sonam shouted greetings to the Buddhist men at the head of several caravans, who stuck out their tongues politely, a sign of respect to a scion of the *gova*'s family. And when Sonam led his son into a tea shop to wait out the storm, the proprietor greeted Sonam by name and rushed to hang their wet garments by the fire to dry.

Sipping sweet milk tea from a chipped glass, Sanduk let his eyes rove, taking in unfamiliar machine-made products, foil packets of biscuits and sweets with strange foreign labels stacked in a glass case by the entrance. Across the muddy street, he saw shops stuffed with racks of multicolored machine-made clothing.

Looking at these shopkeepers' slim-faced children dressed in expensive clothes, lounging under eaves out of the rain, sucking on store-bought sweets, made him self-conscious, for the first time in his life, about the drab homespun garments his mother made for him. His sweater, steaming dry on a peg over the fire, looked like an animal pelt, especially with the mottled patches of whitewash stippling it like the hide of a spotted *dzo*. But Sanduk took some consolation in the fact that his father seemed perfectly at home, joking and exchanging news with the other customers about the condition of the trail and the most current price the paint and the machine-woven fabric they were carrying up from India would fetch in Tibet. Sanduk searched his bag, unsuccessfully, for one of his mother's last comforting crumbs and wondered if he'd ever feel at ease in the world outside Olangchungola.

When the rain stopped, Sonam stepped outside and addressed a slim man with corded muscles in a gruff, booming voice Sanduk had rarely heard; he realized his father was bargaining. They left their yaks in Taplejung, since they planned to descend nearly to the plains of India and the animals were prone to low-altitude sickness. They departed trailing a train of human porters, who carried Sonam's great swaying bundles of trading goods in bamboo baskets lashed to their foreheads.

Beyond the teahouses and shops of Taplejung, the route took them through wild high country, where hours might pass before they'd hear the bells of an oncoming caravan. To fill the time, Sonam told his son stories about the caravan trade. He said he wore his hair long because when he crossed the sun-seared passes into Tibet, the light reflecting off the snow was so harsh that a man could go blind if he wasn't able to cover his eyes.

He talked about the crowded cities on the plains of India, of sweltering marketplaces where he bargained for trade goods in snatches of half a dozen languages, of weather so hot the pavement steamed when you spilled water onto it and snow seemed as distant as a half-remembered dream. Sanduk couldn't form clear pictures of the places his father described, but he reveled in the opportunity to hear him speak at such length. At home, Sonam mostly sat quietly by the fire, sipping warm home-brewed *tongba* through a bamboo straw while the talk fluttered back and forth between Kasang and his aunts as they cooked and sewed and spun yak hair into yarn. But out here in the new world, the world his father had mastered, he drew comfort from Sonam's voice, and saw that this sort of conversation came to him as naturally while he traveled as the lowing of his yaks or the cries of birds calling from crag to crag.

After a week of trekking, an afternoon thunderstorm increased in intensity as dusk approached, stinging them with hail, and Sonam found a rude shelter against the base of an overhanging boulder. They were still high on a ridgeline, exposed to the wind, with no chance of keeping a cooking fire lit, but Sonam decided it was better to stop for the night than face the worst of the storm. He took off the gray felt cowboy-style hat he wore on the trail, pushed it down over his son's ears, and tightened the chin strap to secure it against the weather as the hail turned to snow.

They dined on hard kernels of cooked corn and a few precious strips of dried yak meat that Sonam had been saving for an emergency. He explained to his son the gravity of taking any animal's life and advised him, when living among the lowlanders of Darjeeling, to avoid eating small animals like birds and fish. "Every life counts against your karma," he said. "Better to use every scrap and strip of one large animal, like a yak, to feed many mouths than to have the death of all these little beings on your conscience for only a few bites each."

They walked through the wind and the snow the next morning, and

Sonam kept an eye on the boy as he strained to reach the crest of each pass, where lines of fraying prayer flags, strung between boulders scoured clean by the elements, crackled in the breeze, sending appeals through thin air up to the ears of any deity who might be listening. At the top of a fifteen-thousand-foot pass, Sonam searched for a substantial stone and heaved it onto a *chorten* piled at the apex of the rocky outcrop. "Let the mountain rise higher," he said as he added a few inches to its altitude.

From another such pass, Sonam pointed north toward the broad, five-peaked summit of Kangchenjunga, the world's third-highest mountain. It rose abruptly from shadowed foothills that surrounded it like kneeling supplicants, a divine white wave, forever cresting. "Remember," he told his son, "whether they fill your head with wisdom or foolishness at school in Darjeeling, never forget you are Walung, that no pass is too high for you to climb, that you come from country like *this.*"

On their thirteenth day after setting out from Olangchungola they crossed into India. Sanduk sensed an elemental change in the landscape. For two weeks they'd climbed crest after snow-covered crest, and marched through the waves of hard, dusty hills in between, an endless ocean of rock. Now the trails burrowed down through dense foliage, flecked with the pink and white blooms of giant rhododendrons. Sanduk drank in the comforting, homely scent. Beyond the blossoms, the air itself smelled unfamiliar—warmer, more moist earth than windscoured stone.

"I was seeing everything with wide new eyes," Ruit says. "It was only when I grew older that I understood what a cold, distant place it was where I'd been born. On that long walk you could really say we were coming down from the moon."

To European explorers hoping to survey the ranges surrounding Kangchenjunga, the region *had* once seemed as inaccessible as outer space. For much of its history, Nepal had been an isolated mountain kingdom, its borders firmly barred to Westerners. Nineteenth-century maps left the region where the Walung—one of Nepal's tiniest ethnic groups—lived and traded largely blank. In 1899, the English mountaineer Douglas W. Freshfield made the first successful circumnavigation of Kangchenjunga after several other Westerners, like the British botanist Joseph Dalton Hooker, had probed at the area before being turned away by the fragmented jurisdiction of local authorities and the limited utility of travel permits obtained at lower altitudes.

In the 1903 account of his journey, *Round Kangchenjunga*, Freshfield seems overwhelmed by the effort of describing the scale and majesty of the Kangchenjunga region. "I am, of course, conscious that my task is beyond me," he writes. "I must be content to do what I can, to record with all the emphasis I am capable of my conviction that nowhere else on the earth's surface can there be found, within so small a radius, a combination of tropical luxuriance, sylvan beauty, and mountain sublimity equal to that which meets the eyes . . . of the wanderer on the woodland paths beyond Darjiling."

To Sanduk, this luxuriance was as exotic as the ice-encrusted landscape of his homeland appeared to foreigners like Freshfield. He followed his father until they emerged, at sunset, from a tunnel of flowering trees into a vision so strange he had to tug at the sleeve of his father's fur-lined *chuba* and beg an explanation.

"Tea," Sonam said.

Late, low-angled sun lit the new world so that it pulsed with colors stronger than Sanduk had ever seen. Soft forms in the shape of eggs, with the breadth of boulders, in every conceivable shade of green poured downhill, thousands of them, more, far too many to count, spilling over the contours of the hills as if the foliage had transgressed against the laws of nature and flowed like water, seeking lower ground. These bushes seemed randomly spaced, until Sanduk noticed that they marched in deliberate, disorderly lines to the horizon. The plantation seemed too vast an undertaking to have been made by human hands.

"The Britishers planted these," Sonam said, plucking the tiniest leaf from the top of a shrub. He held it out on the tip of his callused finger for his son to inspect. It was palest green and barely the length of his fingernail. "They call these young leaves 'golden tips' and claim they are the tastiest sort of tea. I don't know about that, but for the price of a few sacks of these, you could buy a strong young yak."

Leaves the price of yaks. Plants streaming downhill like water. A world larger and more confusing than he'd allowed himself to consider. None of the rules he'd learned in Olangchungola applied. As darkness fell, even the stars seemed to change their behavior. Instead of appearing, one by one, at the top of the sky, as Sanduk watched, entire unfamiliar constellations flickered on at once, showering across the lower hills like sparks from a windblown fire.

"Until that moment," Ruit says, "I'd never seen an electric light."

He walked between the rows of tea bushes, behind his father, too confused to form the questions he wanted to ask, his fingers trailing along the golden tips, wondering what, other than a yak, they might be worth.

At full dark, they stepped onto level ground and the tea trail broadened into a track as wide as a dry riverbed. In the gloom just ahead, Ruit saw an unfamiliar structure raised up off the ground on large round, rubber supports that reminded him of something he'd once seen in a tattered Indian magazine. People sat on its low, wide roof. Sonam paid the porters and had them lift their bundles up to obliging hands. Then he grabbed his son under the arms and hoisted him up onto the roof as well. In the darkness, kind strangers helped settle him comfortably on sacks of bedding and barley, and his father heaved himself up at the boy's side. It seemed a crowded place to spend the night, but at least, after fifteen days of crossing the high passes, he was finally warm.

A small explosion—the engine starting—shook them, and then, so slowly he hardly noticed, then gathering speed, the shadowed world began sliding past. The elderly cargo truck approached a cluster of electric lights surrounding a tea shop, and Sanduk Ruit could see clearly that even though they were rolling uphill, no animals were pulling them along. He laughed aloud at the sensation of riding in his first motorized vehicle. And despite his fear of the unfathomable new life he found himself hurtling toward, he leaned back into his father's arms, raised his face into the balmy wind, and began to enjoy the ride.

CHAPTER 6

Stones on Your Chest

[The Bhoteea] are good-humoured and amiable-looking people, very
square and Mongolian in countenance . . . but all are begrimed with filth
and smoke . . . [so] that their natural hues are rarely to be recognized.
None had ever before seen an Englishman, and . . . they seemed infinitely
amused at my appearance and one jolly dame clapped her hands to her
sides, and laughed at my spectacles, till the hills echoed.
—Sir Joseph Dalton Hooker, *Himalayan Journals*, 1854

The first Western face Sanduk Ruit ever studied up close belonged to Father William Mackey, headmaster of the St. Robert's School in Darjeeling. "His skin was very, very light, like the color of cooked rice. He had large, round blue eyes, white hair, and shaggy eyebrows. I remember thinking he looked like a monkey," Ruit says, laughing, "and I wondered if all foreigners were so strange and ugly."

Darjeeling in 1961 was sliding into a state of genteel neglect. The British, who had finally succumbed to India's long struggle for independence, had abruptly abandoned control of the country in 1947. The hill station the colonial administration had built as its summer seat of government, to escape the broiling heat of the plains, was no longer a center of scurrying bureaucrats beholden to London, lunching over gin fizzes and clinging to the British class system at fancy dress balls. But the fading splendor of the hilltop town, the Tudor-style villas, and the lush lawns and gardens that had been planted to make lonely colonial officers and their wives feel closer to the English countryside than the dusty streets of Delhi were more than enough to awe seven-year-old Sanduk Ruit.

Sonam inspected the plain wooden dormitory his son would share with the other students and, satisfied to have installed him there, promised to look in when his travels allowed. With a curt, manly squeeze of Sanduk's shoulders, far different from his mother's clinging farewell, Sonam said good-bye.

"When my dad left me alone I really felt desperate, you know," Ruit says. "The electric lights and the buildings that looked like palaces made me feel funnily strange. For the first weeks I didn't say a thing, just tried to follow the others. I felt like a misfit. I felt this really is not my place." For most of his first year at school, Sanduk was acutely conscious of his outsider status. The other boys at St. Robert's were the sons of the local clerk and merchant class; their fathers had worked alongside the former British administration. They mocked Sanduk's country accent, his broad Tibetan features, and, most of all, his homespun clothes. "They called me 'Bhotia,' which simply means someone originally from Tibet," he says, and you can still hear an echo of the wounded boy in his voice. "But the real sense of the word to them was something like 'stupid, smelly hick from the mountains who rarely bathes.'"

Father Mackey was a Jesuit priest born and ordained in Montreal. He quickly mastered Nepali, the language most widely spoken across the foothills of the eastern Himalaya, after his posting, in 1946, to the mission in Darjeeling. When he noticed his newest student struggling, he became Sanduk's mentor in the manners of town life, and his protector from cruel classmates. Seeing how mercilessly the boys teased Ruit about his clothes, he purchased leather shoes, a pair of cut blue and maroon trousers, and a V-neck sweater for him, from his own modest salary. "There were some very fancy schools in Darjeeling," Ruit says. "My dad couldn't afford those. St. Robert's was just sort of middle-of-the-pack. But Father Mackey looked after me, and I don't know that I would have had a better education anywhere else."

During school holidays, when the other students returned home to their families, all the bunk beds but Sanduk's stood empty. The first Christmas break he spent forty-five days as the lone occupant of St. Robert's dormitory. Father Mackey looked in on him regularly, ate meals with him, steered him toward books in the school's well-stocked library that he thought likely to distract a lonely boy, and took him on long walks through the hilly streets of Darjeeling. They'd stroll through the Mall, the colonial architects' attempt to transplant a London high street seven thousand feet up into the Himalaya, or sit on a bench devouring the local specialty—cream rolls—in crowded Chowrasta Square. Mackey would pick out individuals among the masses of humanity moving past, teaching Sanduk to distinguish a Gurkha soldier (a long, curved kukri knife worn at his waist) from a South Indian tea picker (skin so sun-baked it seemed to absorb light) from a Bengali tourist up from Calcutta (arms full of shopping bags) from a Bhutanese businessman (dressed in a cotton plaid robe called a *gho*, knee socks, and polished dress shoes).

In 1959, two years before Sanduk trekked to school, another young Buddhist, disguised in the simple clothes of a commoner to elude Chinese sentries, had survived his own dramatic journey over high passes to India. The Fourteenth Dalai Lama had fled to escape the brutal Chinese occupation of Tibet. He now lived at the seat of the exiled Tibetan government in Dharmsala, which, like Darjeeling, was a hill station the British had built to escape the broiling plains.

By the fall of 1962, long-simmering border tensions between India and China threatened to boil over into war. Chinese troops advanced from Tibet, which Peking had begun referring to as simply a southern province of China. They crossed disputed borders and took up mountaintop fighting positions overlooking India. Prime Minister Jawaharlal Nehru responded by ordering his troops into position at altitudes of up to sixteen thousand feet in the eastern Himalaya.

On October 14, the *People's Daily* newspaper, an instrument of the Chinese state, issued the following warning in an editorial: "It is high time to shout to Mr. Nehru that the heroic Chinese troops, with the glorious tradition of resisting foreign aggression, can never be cleared by anyone from their own territory. If there are still some maniacs who are reckless enough to ignore our well-intentioned advice, well let them do so. History will pronounce the foolishness of using the lives of Indian troops as stakes in your gamble."

The following month, from his dormitory window at St. Robert's, eight-year-old Sanduk Ruit could hear the rolling thunderclaps of artillery and see flashes that lit the northern sky like heat lightning, as the superior Chinese forces advanced farther into India. Darjeeling authorities ordered a nightly blackout and curfew, fearing they could be the target of Chinese bombing raids. Sanduk lay in bed, telling himself to be brave but failing more often than not, imagining that every phantom nighttime noise was the roar of approaching bombers. And he longed for news about the safety of his family.

"That fall, I tried to keep my mind on my studies, but all we could talk about in Darjeeling was war," Ruit remembers. "And everyone was of the opinion that the Chinese were stronger, that they had more modern weapons and machineries. We felt they could rush down and sweep over us at any time."

But Ruit's most vivid memory from his five years at St. Robert's was a long, miserable Christmas break the winter he was nine and developed an abscess on his back. Father Mackey was out of the country, and Sanduk spent two weeks in a Darjeeling civil hospital without a single visitor, shaking with fever, frightened by the frequent injections, and numbed by pain that always seemed to peak in the middle of the night, when he'd lie with his eyes open in the dark ward, feeling so far from home, so exiled from intimacy, that he struggled to remember the faces of his family. "That was the lowest point of my life," Ruit says. "I felt like I was buried on the bottom of the earth. But that time made up a big part of what I am. I've really got some iron in my ass. I'm tougher and more stubborn than most people."

Also smarter.

Today, to remark that Sanduk Ruit is intelligent is as obvious as noting that the sun emits light and heat. But even as a boy learning to write Nepali, a language he'd mastered only in its spoken form, while simultaneously studying English, Ruit was an enthusiastic sponge for the education that hadn't been available in Olangchungola.

Sports helped him earn the respect of his peers. The St. Robert's campus possessed one of the rare flat expanses in the tilting region of Darjeeling. And on its small, dusty playing field, in full view of the mountain his father had instructed him never to forget, Sanduk earned a reputation as someone who wouldn't be pushed around. Exchanging elbows with older boys, shouldering them out of the way as he fired shots at the goal during scrappy games of soccer, Sanduk remembered Sonam's exhortation that he was Walung, that no path was too steep for him to climb.

On fine days between the monsoons, he could see Kangchenjunga's summit clearly from the St. Robert's campus. Through a trick of the atmosphere, its ice and stone staircases could seem achingly close. But those fifteen days of trekking had been imprinted on Sanduk; he knew precisely how far he was from the home where his father had been forced to pull him from the arms of his mother. And though he recalled how cold it could be in his family's house, it flickered in his imagination as the world's one source of dependable warmth.

The first time he returned, the steep trails and frigid passes he trekked over alongside Sonam's caravan seemed less formidable, made less of an impression than the raggedness of the travelers they passed and the poverty of the villages where they stopped for tea. Sanduk was pleased that his years in Darjeeling hadn't made him weak, that a growth spurt and fierce games of soccer had instead strengthened him. He prided himself on keeping up with the fast pace his father set, refusing his offers to rest or ride a yak. As he scrambled over boulders high above the Tamor, and got his first glimpse of the familiar blade of Throne of the Gods thrusting up at the end of his valley, he could think of nothing but his mother, and the last hours of the trek seemed interminable.

Three years after she'd reluctantly let go of him, Kasang crushed Sanduk in a hug, then stepped back to look at the way the world had changed him. He was taller; his face was broader and had hardened, his features now resembling those of her father the *gova*. He wore stout store-bought leather shoes and a machine-made sweater. And for a moment, on the veranda of her home, she felt shy in the presence of her own son, before wrapping him in another embrace and shooing him inside to the table, where she'd placed a plate of his favorite corn cakes and the silver cup of water she'd never allowed to stand empty throughout his absence.

His sister Yang La knelt by his side as he ate. Was it true, she wanted to know, her long braids swinging prettily as she peppered him with questions about Darjeeling, that there were fashionable foreign women, not nuns, who wore their hair as short as men did? She'd seen photos in a magazine that had traveled all the way to Olangchungola from India. Sanduk said he hadn't seen anyone like that, but he described the parade of every imaginable human type he'd watched passing through Chowrasta Square as he'd sat on a bench eating a cream roll.

"What's a *cream roll*, Sanduk *dai*?" she asked, and he described the sweet cream swirled inside a brittle pastry, like a lukewarm ice cream cone, well suited to the chilly climate of Darjeeling. Yang La was only two years younger, and they'd always been the closest of the six siblings, with an easy, teasing camaraderie. But Sanduk was pleased to note that she addressed him respectfully as "elder brother." He wriggled his toes in his leather dress shoes, conscious of how such a small symbol of status could make such a large impression in a place as remote as his home.

Some things in Olangchungola had remained the same. Broad prayer flags still hung from tall poles in the center of the village, shivering in the biting wind. The framed portraits of the king and queen of Nepal, Guru Rinpoche, and the Dalai Lama still hung over the family shrine. But fresh from the comforts of lowland life, he was struck by the harsh facts of existence at ten thousand feet. The village was wilder and shabbier than he remembered. Nearly everyone who greeted him seemed to have a cough or a chest infection. The Diki Chhyoling monastery, which had once seemed a grand palace at the top of the world, looked like a pile of rocks stacked on a hillside compared with the imposing colonial administration buildings and Gothic churches fitted out in carved-stone finery that formed the backdrop to his days in Darjeeling.

What Ruit doesn't remember is noticing the blind people who were surely there, struggling to navigate the steep paths of the village with walking sticks or the aid of a relative's arm. They were so common, so much a part of the landscape, even in Darjeeling, that he paid no special attention to them.

He did see that both his mother and father had obviously aged after only three years of his absence. Some of that could be ascribed to the beating inflicted on villagers who lived exposed to the elements. But Sanduk learned that other factors weighed down his family's well-being.

The stoicism of Sanduk's people, like so many who call the high villages of the Himalaya home, their uncomplaining acceptance of fate, is as much a part of their makeup as their broad Tibetan features. The village, Sanduk was told in a matter-of-fact manner, had been dealt several debilitating blows. The year before he'd returned, a flood from melting glaciers had torn through the Tamor valley, sweeping a dozen of Olangchungola's houses nearest the river's edge into the gorge but sparing their occupants, who'd had time to gather what they could while the river rose. Most worryingly, Sonam explained, trade with Tibet, the lifeblood of their culture, was threatened by events on the Tibetan side of the nearby border.

In the late 1950s, the anthropologist Christoph von Fürer-Haimendorf had visited Olangchungola while researching his book *Himalayan Traders*. He'd concluded that the trade route from Lhasa, Tibet, all the way to Calcutta via Olangchungola was the most profitable in the eastern Himalaya, surpassing the path through the Khumbu, the homeland of the Sherpas to the west. He'd been surprised to find that residents of Ruit's village cultivated hardly any crops, depending on profits from trade to purchase their food at lower altitudes.

In 1848, the first Westerner to visit the settlement, the botanist Sir Joseph Dalton Hooker, a colleague of Charles Darwin's, also found Olangchungola unusually prosperous. The settlement he referred to as "Wallanchoon" was, he wrote, "a populous village of large and good painted wooden houses, ornamented with hundreds of long poles and vertical flags, looking like the fleet of some foreign port; while a swarm of good-natured, intolerably dirty Tibetans, were ko[w]towing to me as I advanced."

A century later, free from the colonial condescension of Hooker's era, Fürer-Haimendorf found Ruit's people gracious hosts, and he admired the village, with its fluttering prayer flags and water-driven prayer wheels; he called it "a flourishing center of Buddhist culture."

But in the high villages of the Himalaya, fortunes can change as suddenly as the weather. The Chinese opened and closed their border posts unpredictably. And if the passes to Tibet were shut by barriers more formidable than snow, Olangchungola wouldn't remain a flourishing center of anything; its survival was, at best, uncertain. The *gova* called another family meeting and decreed that if the situation worsened, his offspring should disperse and move down to safer altitudes, where their livelihood wouldn't be at the mercy of shifting Chinese policies.

Back in Darjeeling, Sanduk was nearing the end of the 1966 fall semester when tensions between India and China flared up once again, in the form of brief but violent exchanges of artillery that he could hear pounding the hills north of St. Robert's. The solid figure of Sonam, in his battered gray cowboy hat, appeared in the doorway of Sanduk's dorm room just in time for the end of the term. Sanduk was so relieved to see his father that he almost ran into his arms like a child, but he caught himself, grasped his father's shoulder instead, and asked for news of the family. Sonam said everyone was well but that the unpredictability of the Chinese made life in Olangchungola unmanageable. He said while the rest of the family was preparing to move to property they owned at a lower altitude, he was taking his son to a new school someplace safer but almost unimaginably far away: the capital of their own country. "My dad was anxious that my schooling not be interrupted," Ruit says. "So we threw my few little things into a sack and left almost at once."

Sanduk left St. Robert's with passable English, a polished command of written Nepali, and a good stock of information about the world beyond the Himalaya—if not through experience, at least by exposure to worlds spun by the words of Jack London, Charles Dickens, and William Shakespeare.

Sanduk Ruit wouldn't be the only student from the far reaches of the Himalaya to benefit from the priest's passion for education. Before Ruit left, Father Mackey accepted an offer from the "Dragon King" of Bhutan to move to that most isolated mountain kingdom and reform its rudimentary education system. After learning that modern dentistry was not yet practiced in Bhutan, Father Mackey proved how thoroughly he planned to immerse himself in his new mission: He took the precaution of having all of his teeth pulled and getting fitted for dentures before departing.

Mackey spent the final thirty-two years of his life in Bhutan, where he became known as the father of its secular education system. With the enthusiastic support of successive generations of Bhutan's royal family, he helped transform a country with little more than a scattering of primary schools into a far more literate society, complete with an integrated system of primary, middle, and secondary schools. When he died, in 1995 at the age of eighty, he did so as a national hero in his adopted homeland.

Sonam paid for a ride on a transport vehicle traveling south. They sailed down, mile after mile, through the sea green swells of tea plantations, until the road became level and straight. As the truck rolled across a bridge straddling the calm, lake-like expanse that his Tamor River had become where the mountains met the plains, Sanduk felt something entirely new: heat. Heat of the prickling, probing, inescapable variety. Down at sea level, the sun, so welcome during its short transit across the shadowed river valleys at high altitude, became a foe.

Traveling west, along Nepal's southern border, passed off from truck to bus to British army jeeps packed with far more people than they'd been designed to carry, talking to his father to pass the hours in bus stations where the air was so hot and still that he felt his scalp crawling with sweat, Sanduk discovered another new enemy: swarms of relentless mosquitoes. Struggling to keep his skin covered, he learned that Sonam had decided to move their family down five thousand feet to Dhankuta, a trading hub in the foothills, where they owned a small parcel of land in a Hindu community called Hile, on the town's outskirts.

In the same terse way in which he'd related Olangchungola's troubles, Sonam declared that the caravan trade to Tibet was doomed and he planned to earn a living by letting customers come to him. Sanduk couldn't picture his father, so masterful at crossing mountain passes with his yaks or hearty Tibetan horses, living the sedentary life of a shopkeeper. But he was relieved that his mother and sisters would be living far from an armed border where obliteration could plunge from the sky, or floods could sweep away entire families while they slept.

Sanduk and his father arrived in Kathmandu on top of an overcrowded bus. He'd seen photographs of its gilded monuments and temples, and the intricate wood- and stone-carved façades of its Rana palaces in his schoolbooks. But when he climbed down from the bus on the eastern outskirts of the city, what he saw hardly resembled a royal capital.

The first wave of Olangchungola's refugees had arrived in the capital a few years earlier. Cousins of the Ruits' had launched a small carpet-manufacturing business. They'd also bought a disused gas station on the city's barren eastern fringe, with the aim of eventually returning it to service. Its pumps had been pried up and sold for scrap. Weeds and vines had burrowed through broken windows and choked the garages on the ground floor. But a small room on top of the station was snug enough for Sanduk and his father, after they swept it clean of rodent droppings, to install themselves while they searched for an acceptable boarding school.

They settled on Siddhartha Vanasthali, a vast high school of middling reputation with a tuition Sonam found tolerable. He bought Sanduk a used bicycle, two pairs of pants, and a blue-and-white-striped, short-sleeved dress shirt from street vendors, bargaining fiercely, counting out each rupee with reluctance. "I could see from my dad's face he was really not very happy at all about spending the money," Ruit says. "But he was so glad I hadn't missed any classes—I think that nearly made up for the expense of getting me sorted out."

Tenzing Ukyab, whose parents lent Sanduk the room, remembers his teenage cousin vividly from those days. "I'd see Sanduk bicycling to and fro, with heavy stacks of books," he recalls. "When we'd visit him, he'd be bent over those books, doing his homework by the light of a small flickering candle. And always, he was wearing that same striped shirt. He washed it and washed it until the color faded and all you could make out were slightly darker bits where the stripes had been. He was really struggling."

In Dhankuta, where Sonam opened a small shop, earning a living proved more difficult than he'd expected. He sold cloth, small necessities, and medicinal herbs. But so did most of the other merchants in the village. Competition was fierce and profit margins painfully slim. On school vacations, Sanduk would take a bus that dropped him at a trailhead, where he slept on pallets in a warehouse owned by one of his father's friends. If he left before sunrise, he could reach Dhankuta by dark, after a hard day of walking across two mountain passes and wading the shallows of the lower Tamor River.

During one visit, Sanduk learned that his youngest sister, Chundak, whom he remembered as little more than a small, swaddled creature carried on his mother's back, had developed a high fever and died, despite the efforts of the town's traditional healer to treat her. The depth of his family's grief was obvious to Sanduk, by the weight added to ordinary gestures, like the brooding way Sonam lit a butter lamp, or the trundling steps Kasang took toward him to refill his porcelain cup with tea. His parents told him about the loss of his youngest sister with the terse resignation that outsiders often misconstrue as callousness. He carried the weight of his family's loss with him back to Kathmandu.

Sanduk's daily life brightened considerably when his father sent Yang La to live with him and enrolled her in a girls' secondary school. "Yang La had become very pretty by then, and I always had to be on the lookout for rascals targeting her on the way home from school," Ruit says. He remembers that she was a capable student. But even more so, he recalls how happily she embraced the pop culture of Kathmandu. "When I think of my sister, when I visit her in my memories, she's always singing," Ruit says. "Yang La had a very nice voice. Very soft and clear. And she'd always be singing this or that new popular song as we walked along."

When he had a few rupees, Ruit would treat his sister to a matinee at a cinema on New Road, watching lavish Bollywood spectaculars or the Nepalese musicals that emulated the Indian films' intoxicating formula of romance, violence, class struggle, and choreography. Afterward, Yang La would reprise the love ballads and dance hits she'd heard as she swept the floor, washed clothes, or brewed tea to fortify her brother as he studied.

During her second year at school, Yang La started losing weight and her appetite. Sanduk sent word to Dhankuta about Yang La's declining health, and Sonam arrived to investigate. "My dad and I were really worried, and we walked all over Kathmandu trying to get doctors to see her. We were new in town, so it was difficult to get a reliable diagnosis," Ruit says. Finally, a doctor delivered the devastating news: Yang La was suffering from tuberculosis.

Sonam spent more than he could afford to send his daughter to a sanatorium in the hills, a day's walk from Kathmandu. Doctors put her on a course of conventional TB medications, and Sanduk was relieved, when he visited her, to see that she'd regained some of her weight. "We all thought she was getting better, and Dad decided it would be more healthful for her to move back with them in Dhankuta," Ruit says. "She worked in the shop, and for a year she seemed nearly fine. But then her condition dropped off a cliff."

Sonam rushed Yang La back to Kathmandu. "We ran from door to door, like refugees," Ruit says, "trying to find a doctor who could cure her." But the message they received at the crowded clinics they visited was crushingly, invariably the same: The drugs had stopped working. "They said we should take her home," Ruit says, "and make preparations for her death."

Ruit's voice, ordinarily so level when discussing even the most disheartening events, lowers to a melancholy croak when he talks about those days. "I remember feeling . . . incredible pressure. The whole time, as she got sicker, Yang La kept calling me 'elder brother' and begging me to find someone who could cure her. She looked up to me and believed I could help her. But I had no connections in Kathmandu and could do nothing. So we brought her back to Dhankuta to die."

The last time Sanduk visited Yang La at his parents' shop, his sister was lying on a mat behind the counter, too weak to sit up for any length of time but trying to be helpful, dragging herself upright to sell a bolt of cloth or a handful of herbs to a customer. "She had become nothing but bones, you know, but she was still beautiful," Ruit says. "She was wearing clean kurta pajamas and her hair was nicely done. And her voice, when she wasn't coughing, had become even more lovely. The last time I saw her, she held my hand and sang a famous Nepali song of romantic tragedy. *'Slowly putting stones on your chest,'* " Ruit sang softly, in a voice surprisingly tender for a man who could seem so gruff. " *'The stones are so heavy, but still you have to pretend to laugh. Your mind is very heavy, and yet you have to pretend to laugh.'* "

Sanduk was back in Kathmandu a week later, studying for his high school leaving exams, when he learned of Yang La's death. He had tests to take that would determine his future academic options, and he didn't travel to be with his family for the funeral. "She was cremated in a Buddhist ceremony in Hile, which was mostly a Hindu town, far from our real home," Ruit says. "I know that made my father very unhappy. It was very hard for him not having the support of his village at a time like that.

"I also struggled after her death," Ruit says. "I kept hearing the last song she sang. And I can tell you I felt something like the weight of stone on my chest, too. My whole family respected me and had hopes for my future. But in reality I was just a powerless student. I tried to understand where I had failed. Why did this have to happen? Somebody so young. When you talk about TB, it's not a very fatal disease. I know now that in richer countries, several effective new TB drugs had been widely available at that point, for seven or eight years."

As he sat in his room, straining to focus on his work, Sanduk put down his papers and laid his head on top of them. His parents had given birth to six children. Only three remained. The others had died of easily treatable conditions like fever, diarrhea, and tuberculosis.

"A fifty percent survival rate," Ruit says. "Unacceptable, unacceptable, unacceptable. The more I thought about it, the more I realized Yang La didn't have to die. None of my brothers and sisters had to die. They died because resources the rest of the world had were not available to us. And after a month or so of spinning round with my thoughts, suddenly I saw the path I had to follow. It was straight and clear; I realized I had to become a doctor. I had to become someone who could go out and get those resources. I'd been working hard, but I had to work harder. Real study began after that."

Sanduk was relentless. He targeted his grief, wedded it inseparably to his work. With Yang La's melodies still in mind even years later, as he prepared for the most important entrance exams of his life, was it really a surprise that this son of a salt trader, this casteless outsider from the wild Tibetan border, from a blank spot on a British colonial map, scored high enough, when pitted against all the students of the subcontinent, to earn a scholarship to Lucknow's prestigious King George Medical College?

Sanduk Ruit was no longer powerless. His feet were finally on that straight path, the clear course he'd chosen. He would put his faith and his sweat and his soul into exploring what wonders he could discover at the leading edge of science. There was no limit to the transformative powers he felt he should find there.

CHAPTER 7

Daylight in the Dark

Some of you may ask, what is the good of working so hard merely to collect a few facts which will bring no pleasure except to a few long-haired professors who love to collect such things? In answer to such question[s] I may venture a fairly safe prediction. History . . . has consistently taught us that scientific advances in basic understanding have sooner or later led to technical applications that have revolutionized our way of life. It seems to me improbable that this effort to get at the structure of matter should be an exception to this rule. What we all fervently hope, is that man will soon grow sufficiently adult to make good use of the powers that he acquires over nature.

—Enrico Fermi, the father of the atomic bomb, shortly before his death

The fireball that lit the night-dark sky over New Mexico seemed to usher in morning before daybreak was due. On July 16, 1945, at 5:29 A.M., during what was then known as Mountain War Time, John R. Lugo, piloting a U.S. Navy transport flying at ten thousand feet, thirty miles east of Albuquerque, was startled by the bright explosion. "What a ball of fire!" he told the *Albuquerque Journal*. "My first impression was, like, the sun was coming up in the south. . . . It was so bright it lit up the cockpit of the plane."

On the ground, in a bunker ten thousand yards from the blast, J. Robert Oppenheimer, the theoretical physicist who led the team of scientists gathered at the Trinity testing ground, had a prosaic initial reaction to the first successful detonation of an atomic bomb. "It worked," others in the bunker recalled him saying. But as the explosion lit the mountains ringing the Jornada del Muerto, and a mushroom

cloud billowed more than seven miles above the blast site, Oppenheimer later famously said, a phrase from the *Bhagavad Gita*, the Hindu
holy book, flashed through his mind: "Now I am become death, the
destroyer of worlds."

Enrico Fermi, the physicist most responsible for the scientific
breakthrough that made the bomb possible, was, as always, consumed
by practicalities. During the explosion, he huddled with Julius Tabin
and two other young scientists at the test base camp, ten miles from the
blast site. Seconds after Fermi, Tabin, and the others watched the blin-
dingly bright explosion through sheets of dark welding glass, they
stood and observed the forces they'd set in motion. Fermi threw a
handful of paper he'd torn from his notebook into the air as the shock
wave rolled toward them. From the distance the confetti flew, he calculated that the yield of the explosion was equal to at least ten kilotons
of TNT. It later proved to be nearly twice that powerful.

The physicist Philip Morrison, another scientist at base camp that
morning, recalled not only the bright light of the explosion but the
sensation of feeling the heat of the sun on his face ten minutes before
the real sun rose. In interviews after the test at Trinity, he referred to
the unforgettable day that he saw two separate sunrises.

After they watched a mushroom cloud form, then drift away over
the desert, three young scientists from Fermi's team moved in to collect evidence. Herbert Anderson, the most senior of the three, rode in
a specially shielded tank to collect core samples from the periphery of
the crater. He was followed by Darragh Nagle, who traveled a third of
the way in. Then Julius Tabin climbed into the retrofitted M4 Sherman. As the tank commander put the vehicle into gear, Tabin struggled
to control his nerves. He had volunteered to be the first scientist to
examine the center of the blast site, and there was no guarantee he'd
come back alive. The tank had been lined with lead to reduce his exposure to radiation, but it couldn't be pressure-sealed to provide reliable
protection.

"I was twenty-four and single, so I said 'I'll do it,'" Tabin remembers. "You had to be a little crazy to go out there. But there's tremen-

dous strength in young people. I believed what I was doing was important enough to take the risk."

Tabin had followed his mentor Fermi from the University of Chicago to Los Alamos, New Mexico. Fermi, Italian by birth, had won the 1938 Nobel Prize in physics for his groundbreaking experiments detailing the structure and behavior of the atom. As World War II approached, he fled Italy for America, to protect his wife, Laura, who was Jewish, from the catastrophe he saw coming when Mussolini followed the example of his fascist ally Hitler and enacted anti-Jewish laws.

At first Fermi's team worked in a secret laboratory under the University of Chicago's football stadium. They were the sharpened point at the tip of the Manhattan Project, the vast secret collaboration between the Allied nations' finest scientific minds, trying to develop atomic weapons before the Nazis could construct their own. Fermi's team built "Chicago Pile-1," a rudimentary nuclear reactor, on a squash court under the stands of Stagg Field. And there they kindled humankind's first atomic flame, setting off a nuclear chain reaction and proving the atomic bomb to be no longer a theoretical device but a weapon that might be used to bring the war to a swift conclusion. Further research with a reactor was considered too dangerous to conduct in a city, and, after earning a PhD in physics, Julius Tabin joined Fermi, helping him run tests on another reactor the Manhattan Project had built, this one at Argonne, a classified facility surrounded by a forest preserve southwest of Chicago.

Finally, Fermi's team was sent to New Mexico, where they set up a laboratory dedicated to weaponizing their discovery. Some scientists feared the power of an atomic detonation could set the entire planet's atmosphere on fire and lead to the destruction of life on earth. Fermi's team calculated that the yield would be larger than any man-made explosion that had preceded it but that it posed no danger, other than radioactive fallout, to the planet as a whole.

"We built a new reactor at Los Alamos," Julius Tabin says. His primary assignment was to calculate how much fissionable material it would take to construct a viable atomic device. "And with Fermi, we developed a system for measuring how much energy the bomb was going to emit, how many kilotons. I knew it was going to be big, but boy," Tabin says, "was it even bigger than I imagined!"

Crouched inside his Sherman tank, rolling toward the center of the blast site, Tabin blocked out the faces of his parents and elder brother and tried to control his fear by focusing on the importance of the task at hand. Two months earlier, the U.S. Army had detonated a hundred-ton block of TNT, near the spot where the atomic device they all referred to as "the gadget" would soon be tested. At the time, it was the largest conventional explosion in history. On his training run that day, Tabin had traveled in the tank, through the crater the TNT had created, and he'd been temporarily stranded in dust eight feet deep as the M4's treads spun and spun, before they found enough purchase to escape.

Heading toward the center of a far more formidable crater, Tabin worried that his tank might not make it through. If simple TNT had created dust deep enough to stop an M4, what might he be churning toward after an atomic explosion? "It *was* a bit of a shaky time for me," he remembers. "If we got stuck out there, there would be no one to help us. And we knew that if you stepped out into that radiation for even a second, you'd be fried."

The Sherman tank rolled on with unsettling ease. Unlike the dust created by conventional explosives, the heat of the atomic blast had fused the desert sand into glass. Pebble-sized pellets were thrown miles into the air and rained down by the thousands, creating what appeared to be a lake of pale green glass. At the center of that liquid-looking waterless landscape, Tabin took a breath, held it, and opened a small trapdoor on the underside of the tank. He lowered a drilling device, gathered core samples of the material at the center of the crater, and closed the door as quickly as he could.

"We'd set up a mobile lab to measure the radioactivity of the samples I brought back," Tabin says. "When I climbed out of the tank and walked inside, every instrument in that room went crazy. I probably took more radiation than any person ever had."

The following month, on August 6, 1945, the first atomic bomb was detonated, over Hiroshima. Three days later, a second device was dropped on Nagasaki. On September 2, Japan surrendered unconditionally, ending World War II as rapidly as the architects of the atomic bomb had hoped. The military thanked Tabin for his service, and required him to sign a release saying he wouldn't hold the U.S. government responsible for whatever happened to him in the future. Military doctors told him they couldn't predict what he'd face after exposure to so much radiation. Tabin wondered what sort of life he'd be able to lead, and whether he'd ever be able to father children.

Enrico Fermi died less than a decade later, at age fifty-three, from stomach cancer he attributed to the radiation he absorbed during his days working on the Manhattan Project. "He believed the work he did was important, the risk was worth it, and he died perfectly reconciled to his fate," writes his biographer James Cronin. Two other members of Fermi's team also died of cancer within the decade.

But Julius Tabin continued to confound expectations. "I did feel tired for a while, afterwards," Tabin says, "but it wasn't so bad." Nine years later, he and his new wife, Johanna, gave birth to their first son, Clifford. Two and a half years after that, on July 3, 1956, the Tabins' second son entered the world, a compact, energetic bundle they named Geoffrey. "Cliff and Geoff were both delights, but they were different sorts of children—you could see that right away," Julius told me a few weeks before celebrating his ninetieth birthday. "Cliff was calm and introspective. But from the moment Geoff was born, he was in perpetual motion. There was no quiet time with that kid; he always had sixteen things going on at once. No one else in the family had that kind of energy. I don't know where he got it."

It's tempting to look to science fiction, toward a comic book kind of explanation for the appearance of a Geoff Tabin, to compare the massive dose of radiation his father received when he opened the trapdoor in the Sherman tank to creation myths like Spider-Man's. In the cartoon's case, superpowers were conferred on Peter Parker when he was bitten by a radioactive spider. But Tabin credits something far more mundane for his overachievement: doggedness, an obsessive focus on self-improvement. "With tennis or climbing I was never the most talented," he says. "I was just willing to hit a few hundred more balls than anyone else. Or stay out until after dark, until I'd climbed twelve pitches, when most people would leave after four or five."

Cliff remembers how difficult it could be to concentrate in his bedroom down the hall from Geoff, in the large, comfortable brick house two blocks from Lake Michigan where they grew up; Glencoe, a northern suburb of Chicago, had such a large Jewish community that it was sometimes derisively referred to as Glen-Cohen. As a young boy, Geoff took up the harmonica and attempted, loudly and obsessively, to master it. "Whenever Geoff would start something, you couldn't get him to stop," Cliff says. "I remember he decided he had to hit a Ping-Pong ball against the wall in his bedroom a thousand times without missing. He'd get to three hundred, or four hundred, miss, and start over, again and again. I'd be trying to read and—*pok, pok, pok*—the ball would just keep coming, driving me crazy."

By age ten, when Geoff began regularly beating much older boys in tennis tournaments, he was spending hours practicing topspin drives against the garage door. "He wouldn't hear you if he was focused on something, whether it was tennis or his homework," remembers his mother, Johanna. "I'd call him for dinner a dozen times, but the only way I could get him to come was to take the racquet or the book out of his hand." By the time Geoff left for his freshman year at Yale, he had won several statewide junior tennis championships, and the garage door was a wreck, dented and scuffed in so many spots it had to be replaced.

For most of the Tabins, achievement seemed to come as easily as setting a course and conquering it. After Los Alamos, Julius found work teaching physics at MIT while simultaneously earning a degree at Harvard Law School. After graduation, he began a long and lucrative career as a patent attorney, representing clients in the atomic industry whose scientific breakthroughs he was so well equipped to understand. But Julius never left pure science behind. One of his many achievements was developing a mirror device astronauts placed on the lunar surface. It was able to reflect back a laser aimed from earth with such precision that by timing the beam's travel, scientists could measure the distance to the moon within inches.

Julius married Johanna in 1950, after he moved back to Chicago. Al Teton, a friend of both Julius's older brother, Seymour, and Johanna's family, engineered the encounter. "Teton said, 'There's someone I want you to meet. He's not very tall, but he's otherwise perfect for you,'" Johanna remembers. "And he was. I walked into a room and saw Julius for the first time. He was laughing at something my father was saying, and I thought, 'He's not exactly handsome, but he has the most wonderful face I've ever seen.'"

As a newlywed, Johanna completed her postdoctoral fellowship in psychoanalysis with Sigmund Freud's daughter Anna, a founder of modern child psychiatry, and soon set up a busy private practice. When I spoke with her at age eighty-two, after nearly sixty years of marriage, she was still counseling patients most days, while Julius continued to show up for work at the oldest law firm in Chicago, where he'd served as a partner for half a century. "I've never been interested in retiring," Johanna says. "A lot of people in my field burn out. But I've always believed that every individual is utterly fascinating and unique. There's no limit to what you can learn from people if you observe them closely enough."

Parents as successful as Julius and Johanna Tabin can cast intimidating shadows. "But we never pressured Cliff or Geoff to study or follow in our footsteps," Julius says. "I told the boys, 'Don't worry about getting straight A's. You should be learning and enjoying the process.' We tried not to interfere with the people they were going to become."

Their grandmother took the opposite approach. She was determined to steer both boys toward meaningful lives. Johanna's mother, Sara Krout, had been born in Latvia, and she was one of the few female Latvians in medical school when World War I broke out. She fled to America after surviving an aerial bombardment during which she saw a mother and the infant in her arms killed by shrapnel. In Chicago, where American medical schools wouldn't accept the credits she'd earned in Latvia, she switched to studying dentistry, then opened one of the first female-run practices in Illinois.

She would often take Fridays off to spend with her grandsons, creating art projects and science experiments for them. "Our grandmother Sara was a really strong woman," Cliff says. "She was a huge influence on us."

"I remember her talking to me about my future," Geoff says. "She'd speak about the suffering she'd seen in Europe, and argue about how important it was to choose a career that offered the opportunity to help people."

Despite the frequent noise and vibrations emanating from the bedroom down the hall, Cliff left for college with sufficient powers of concentration to become a gifted and groundbreaking research scientist. He is currently the chairman of genetics at Harvard Medical School. His lab's leading-edge research into how instructions, written in genes, direct the human body's growth and shape may one day help people debilitated by injuries and disease regenerate limbs and regrow complex organs like the heart.

After Geoff left for New Haven, in 1974, he was careful to complete all of Yale's required premed courses, considering medical school a likely path if careers in climbing or professional tennis didn't pan out. As the captain of Yale's tennis team, as well as its number one singles player, Tabin took tennis very seriously. But the fact that he was only five foot eight made playing professionally unlikely and spared him from spending every moment honing his game. As would be the case for the rest of his life, Tabin was tugged in multiple directions. Julius had taken the boys hiking and skiing as soon as they could walk. His second son was a natural athlete and excelled at all manner of physical activity. At age twelve, he won a yo-yo championship the Duncan company staged in Chicago. At fifteen, he got his first taste of rock climbing, on a trip to Devil's Lake, Wisconsin. And while at Yale, he began slipping away with climbing partners to attempt technical ice and rock routes in the Hudson Valley's Shawangunks and New Hampshire's White Mountains, driving overnight back to New Haven and arriving in time to stroll into his morning classes, bleary-eyed and unwashed, with bloody abrasions, but able to marshal enough energy to excel in his academic work.

"I really had only the fuzziest idea about my future in those days," Tabin says. "I had a vague idea of working as a mountain guide. I liked science, and in an abstract way, I remembered my grandmother's advice and thought of medicine as a way to help people. But above all, I began to think of myself as a climber."

At Yale he devoured the literature of climbing and exploration. He was drawn to adventurers like Heinrich Harrer, the Austrian alpinist who escaped an Allied prison camp in India during World War II, crossed the passes to Tibet, and became a tutor to the young Dalai Lama. Or Sir Richard Francis Burton, the rogue British explorer, scholar, and erotically omnivorous translator of the *Arabian Nights* and the *Kama Sutra*, who, among dozens of other swashbuckling achievements, added Arabic and Pashtun to the twenty-seven other languages he was said to speak fluently, disguised himself as an Afghan doctor, and, risking death if he was unmasked as an infidel, snuck into the holy Muslim cities of Mecca and Medina.

"I guess if you had to sum it up," Tabin says, "my heroes weren't the people who asked, 'Why?' They were the ones who asked, '*Why not?*'"

After graduation, Tabin was awarded a Marshall Scholarship to study philosophy for two years at Oxford University. The summer before classes began, he moved to England and played in several European professional tennis tournaments. Though he won a few matches, his results were disheartening. "I was really fast in those days. I could run down shots anywhere on the court," Tabin says. "But when you're playing against a fit Swedish player who's six foot four—and there were a lot of guys like that—the difference in strength was just too much."

When he arrived at University College for the beginning of the fall term, Tabin continued playing tennis recreationally, but his mind was focused on mountains. Fortunately, Oxford's academic calendar offered ample opportunities for escape. "I was used to Yale, where most of my time was structured," Tabin says. "But at Oxford, we'd have eight weeks of classes, then a six-week break. That meant twenty-eight weeks a year of paid vacation. 'Work' meant reading philosophy, then getting together with a tutor and arguing for two hours a week while we sipped tiny cups of sherry. It was paradise, and I had all the time I wanted to run away and climb."

On Tabin's first day at Oxford, in University College's common room, he spotted a tall, thin man dressed in rugged outdoor clothing, pacing impatiently. "Does anybody else here climb?" he asked. "My gear is all packed in my car, and I want to go." After four years of single-mindedly studying biology at the University of Pennsylvania, Bob Shapiro had also won a scholarship to Oxford, where he was reveling in the freedom he had to read philosophy and psychology, subjects he'd missed during his premed college career. Shapiro viewed his time at Oxford as a pleasant interlude during which he could indulge his passions, before buckling back down to pursue a career in neuroscience.

"It's one of the great good fortunes of my life that Geoff and I were both at University College at the same time," Shapiro says. Tabin had met a kindred spirit, a peer who would become his climbing partner, confidant, and lifelong friend. Like Tabin, Shapiro was addicted to the literature of mountaineering and exploration. Like Tabin, he was not merely an armchair adventurer but someone willing to take risks in the real world. They left the next day to climb the sea cliffs of Cornwall.

In a quaint country inn where they stopped to dine on the way back to Oxford, Tabin called out loudly for two cold beers before they'd even been seated. While the waiter bent to take their order, Shapiro noticed that Tabin had lifted a heavy silver fork from the spotless white tablecloth and was using one of its tines to scrape dirt from his fingernails.

"My first impression of Geoff Tabin was that he was very young and very oblivious to cultural norms and expectations," Shapiro says. "I mean, this was a *real* restaurant, someplace *nice*. I thought, 'How is this guy going to survive in a place obsessed with manners?'"

The Oxford social calendar is crammed with formal events, each requiring a strict dress code. "I think Geoff just saw it all as a series of costume parties," Shapiro says. "He had a white polyester tuxedo with wide lapels, the kind you'd rent for a high school prom, and whether the occasion called for white tie, black tie, dinner jackets, or tails, Geoff would show up wearing that same tux with tennis shoes. There are people who can't stand Geoff because of this sort of thing, who consider him a clown. But to really know him is to utterly forgive anything like that."

Soon Shapiro and Tabin were slipping away to places where the only code that mattered was the "brotherhood of the rope," the reliance on your climbing partner to protect you. They ticked off classic climbs across the British Isles and dashed off for weekends in the Alps, where they'd repeat ascents of famous climbing routes over the course of a few sleepless days and nights. "We were ideally matched as climbers," Shapiro says. "I'd do the planning and worrying. Geoff would charge in blithely with his 'damn the torpedoes' approach. We complemented each other's weaknesses. I gave him a little injection of common sense, and he helped me screw up my courage. And of course we both shared the pleasure of torturing our Jewish mothers with our climbing obsession."

During the fall of his second year at Oxford, Shapiro read Felice Benuzzi's *No Picnic on Mount Kenya*, the true story of Italian climbers who escaped a British POW camp during World War II to climb Mount Kenya, Africa's second-tallest and most technically challenging mountain. Benuzzi's team fashioned crampons and ice axes out of scavenged scrap metal and, even in their weakened state after years of imprisonment, nearly managed to reach the summit before a storm and depleted provisions drove them back down to captivity.

"To me, it's the greatest mountaineering book ever written," Shapiro says. Benuzzi planned his escape for the sheer joy of challenging an unknown mountain, knowing that the price he'd pay for his temporary freedom was to be recaptured and locked in solitary confinement after he descended. Shapiro pressed Tabin to read the book, then proposed that they attempt Mount Kenya over their Christmas break. They left for Africa on a cold December day at term's end.

Benuzzi's first glimpse of the summit, from captivity, so overwhelmed him that he immediately began to plot his escape. He describes the moment when he saw "an ethereal mountain emerging from a tossing sea of clouds framed between two dark barracks—a massive blue-black tooth of sheer rock inlaid with azure glaciers, austere, yet floating fairy-like on the near horizon. I stood gazing until the vision disappeared among the shifting cloud banks. For hours afterward I remained spell-bound. I had definitely fallen in love."

For route planning, Felice Benuzzi had only the distant view of the peak he could see on clear days from his barracks window, a crude map he'd copied from another prisoner's book on the customs and folklore of the region, and a label from a can of Kenylon brand preserved meat that featured a detailed and, he hoped, accurate drawing of the south side of the mountain, the side he couldn't see from camp. Shapiro, too, had fallen for Mount Kenya from afar. But he reached base camp, after months of study, with an encyclopedic knowledge of the historical first ascents and common routes to the summit and surrounding peaks. Tabin arrived only slightly better informed than Benuzzi. "All I really knew about Mount Kenya when Bob and I set up our tent," he says, "is that it was huge and there was no easy way to the top."

Tabin and Shapiro tried the traditional route to the summit first and were discouraged to find that they were climbing too slowly to reach it before their energy and supplies would both be depleted. They spent a bitterly cold night on Nelion, the lower of Mount Kenya's twin summits. When daylight arrived, the view was obscured by swirling, powdery snow, and they headed back to base camp, dejected. They wondered what kind of *Übermenschen* would be able to complete such a hard technical climb at altitude.

After a few days of acclimatization, they felt stronger and attempted another classic path to the summit, the more difficult "Ice-Window Route." After a thousand feet of maneuvering up a steep ice-and-rock ascent, they entered the eerie cave that gives the route its name. Scrambling up through a sloping forest of sixty-foot icicles, they reached the rear of the cave and found a wall of blue ice more than a foot thick blocking their progress.

They were the first climbers to attempt the route that season, and they set to work with their ice axes, hacking toward the brightness they could see beyond. Finally, they climbed out the narrow window they'd fashioned, clung to the nearly vertical headwall of the Diamond Couloir with their crampons, and were rewarded with a frightening and spectacular view. Below them, ice cliffs fell away for two hundred vertical feet. And above, the pinnacle of Batian, the tip of the rocky tooth that had lured Benuzzi through barbed wire, sparkled in fine weather, beckoning them on.

This time, they'd come equipped with sleeping bags, stoves, and extra food and clothing and slept in an alpine hut built for mountaineers that Shapiro had circled on his map. They reached the summit of Batian in bright equatorial sunshine the following morning, elated, and snapped celebratory photos. "Reaching the highest point on Mount Kenya led to a strong sense of accomplishment," Tabin says, "and a powerful realization that mere mortals could safely do tough technical climbing at altitude."

Back at base camp, Tabin and Shapiro buzzed around on an adrenaline high. "Following established routes in a guidebook was great fun," Tabin says. "But I began to understand the thrill of climbing into the unknown, the excitement that making your own way up a big mountain could provide." Tabin and Shapiro decided to attempt the sort of high-risk, technical route that had made the heroes of their mountaineering books famous, the type of climb that only a week earlier they'd believed was beyond their ability. The Diamond Buttress was considered the toughest hard-rock route on the mountain and had been climbed only three times before.

Tabin and Shapiro set off at sunrise.

"We could both sense something profound had changed," Tabin says. "We were climbing as easily and confidently as if we were down at sea level." Tabin led the way up the first two pitches. They were "free-climbing," threading their rope through hardware Tabin placed in the rock for protection in case either of them fell, but relying only on their hands and feet to ascend the daunting sunbaked face. Some toeholds were only the width of a quarter.

Shapiro suggested that since they were making such good progress, they attempt to free-climb the entire Diamond Buttress, something no one had ever accomplished. "On the third pitch," Tabin says, "I found myself a hundred and thirty feet above Bob with nowhere to go. I was hanging by a single finger from a crack and could see no holds above me. After ten minutes my arm was shaking and stretched to its limit. My mind started seizing up." Tabin eased his bruised finger out of the crack and down-climbed twenty-five feet; there he met Shapiro on his way up. Tabin told him he couldn't sense any way to safely proceed. So with the symbiosis of perfectly compatible partners, Shapiro summoned up his courage and led the next section. He set off on a long traverse to their right, tiptoeing with the sticky rubber edges of his climbing shoes along a ledge only a few inches wide. "This is pretty thin stuff!" he yelled to Tabin. "But I think we can do it!" Tabin followed, trying not to look down at the sheer drop to a glacier five hundred feet below.

They reached a ladderlike series of handholds and hauled themselves up the buttress's final pitch to a wide ledge, big enough for both of them to lay out their sleeping bags. They decided to spend the night there and celebrate.

"When we reached the ledge," Tabin says, "It looked as comfortable as a five-star hotel. I collapsed and let out a whoop of joy. I couldn't believe we'd achieved the sort of thing that until then I'd only ascribed to mythical creatures, to the climbers I'd idolized. I realized that you never know what your true limits are until you test them. I learned that the most difficult obstacles to overcome, in mountaineering as in life, are mental."

Gaston Rébuffat was one of the mythical figures who loomed unusually large in Tabin's imagination. In his book *Starlight and Storm*, he explains why such moments are so precious to mountaineers. "In this modern age," Rébuffat writes, "very little remains that is real. Night has been banished, so have the cold, the wind and the stars. They have all been neutralized: the rhythm of life itself is obscured. . . . What a strange encounter then is that between man and the high places of his planet! Up there he is surrounded by the silence of forgetfulness. If there is a slope of snow steep as a glass window, he climbs it, leaving behind him a strange trail. If there is a rock perfect as an obelisk, he defies gravity and proves that he can get up anywhere."

Tabin had come to Oxford to study philosophy. But the most meaningful philosophical discovery he made during those two years dawned on him not among sherry-sipping, pipe-smoking professors but during a spectacular clear night, connected, as if by electrical cables, to the life force climbers like Rébuffat sought, on a ledge protruding from a snow peak in equatorial Africa, sprawled beneath a blanket of stars.

CHAPTER 8

A Bit of Sport

*Our ignorance proved an insuperable handicap from the point of
view of material achievement; but from the spiritual point of view, which
is of far greater importance to the true mountaineer, it was in the
nature of a gift from God. Every step led to new discoveries, and we were
continually in a state of amazed admiration and gratitude. It was
as though we were living at the beginning of time, before men
had begun to give names to things.*
—Felice Benuzzi, No Picnic on Mount Kenya

Ith his last term at Oxford winding down, Tabin planned to
enroll at Harvard Medical School. He'd been accepted before
he'd left Yale and had deferred admission twice, reapplying successfully both times. But Harvard's administrators had made it clear that
they would look unfavorably on any further delay. Tabin felt conflicted,
since he still harbored dreams of working as a mountain guide. He
made plans to move to Boston in the fall, figuring his path would become clear once classes started. But before he left the tea party circuit
behind, he was introduced to an indelible fixture in Oxford society
named David Kirke, who offered him a glimpse of another brand of
adventure to be found far from academia.

One morning at 3:00 A.M., a nearly sober Kirke pounded on Tabin's
door. "Geoff," he slurred, "do come to America and have a bit of sport
with us."

"I can't," Tabin said. "I have a tutorial at eleven and exams coming up."

"Pitch it!" Kirke commanded. "We're going to jump off the highest bridge in the world. We need you to fix the harnesses and handle the safety angle. I will pick up all of your expenses. The flight leaves Heathrow in eight hours. What do you say?"

"I thought," Tabin says, "'Will I regret this more if I do it, or if I don't?'"

Tabin told Kirke he was in.

David Kirke was the founder of the "Dangerous Sports Club." Most afternoons, Tabin says, he could be found lunching on omelets and ale at a pub called the Bear. Afterward, he installed himself in his favorite gentlemen's club, perusing newspapers and downing single-malt scotch. With his beer drinker's paunch, gray-flecked beard, and receding curls, Kirke didn't look like a typical adrenaline junkie. But, inarguably, he was.

Tabin says that Kirke, a former journalist, had discovered that he liked making news far better than writing about people he found less fascinating than himself. Tabin was so taken with Kirke that he was happy to oblige. He wrote a profile of Kirke that was published in *Playboy* called "The World's Most Daring Sportsman." In the piece, Tabin detailed how Kirke began concocting outlandish sporting events, and inviting sponsorship and media coverage. In the summer of 1977, Tabin wrote, with no serious climbing experience to speak of, Kirke hauled himself up the Matterhorn. The following month, he launched a kayak down the Landquart River in Switzerland, surviving one of Europe's most fearsome stretches of whitewater as a novice.

During his drinking sessions, Kirke and the other members of the club designed an official club tie (black with silver wheelchairs) and competed to invent the most original and artistic ways to risk death or dismemberment. They participated in the running of the bulls, in Pamplona, on skateboards. They snuck onto bobsled runs in the Alps and slid down them at preposterously high speeds on blocks of ice fitted with saddles.

Kirke's first major splash in the media came when he convinced the BBC to film a documentary about members of the Dangerous Sports Club climbing Kilimanjaro and sailing off the summit on hang gliders. Kirke, the least fit-looking member of the group by far, took pride in his ability to stride straight to the top of the nineteen-thousand-foot peak, while his younger and stronger clubmates wheezed and suffered from altitude sickness. "Kirke had portrayed himself as a champion hang glider to BBC producers," Tabin says. "But actually, he'd never bothered to master the basics of the sport."

As the cameras rolled, Alan Weston, the only experienced hang glider pilot in the club, crashed on takeoff, destroying his glider and injuring his ankle. Two of the other club members abandoned their plans to jump as they struggled with altitude sickness. That left Kirke to salvage the club's reputation. He launched himself off Kilimanjaro's summit, wobbled, and smacked his wingtip against the side of the mountain, then rose on an updraft before power-diving out of control, and out of sight. "The film crew captured twelve seconds of the Kirke posterior disappearing into a bank of clouds," Tabin says. "It was a disaster for the BBC, but made Kirke into a media darling." He flew on through the clouds and mist, without a compass or altimeter, eventually gliding in for a gentle landing on a coffee plantation twenty-five miles away.

"You could call Kirke the ultimate dilettante, and say that he was deranged to take such outrageous risks," Tabin says. "But there was a psychological toughness to him I couldn't help admiring. He believes he will survive, and through sheer force of will, he does."

After returning from Christmas break and his climb of Mount Kenya, Tabin met Kirke. During their expedition, Tabin and Shapiro had read Heinrich Harrer's *I Come from the Stone Age*, his account of climbing Carstensz Pyramid, in New Guinea, the highest peak in Oceania, accompanied by Dani tribesmen. They were trying to finance an expedition of their own to Carstensz.

Tabin told Kirke about the potential trip to New Guinea. "If you go," Kirke suggested, "you must try the Vanuatuan vine jump." Kirke, while casting about for ever more original ways to cheat death, had fastened on the coming-of-age ritual common to New Guinea and other Pacific island cultures, wherein adolescent boys climbed to the top of a palm tree, or a tower specially built for the purpose, tied a vine around their ankles, and dove from as high as one hundred feet, headfirst toward the ground. If the vine held, islanders believed, and the boys' foreheads just grazed the forest floor, they would prove their mettle as men, and ensure a successful yam or taro harvest.

Kirke told Tabin he wanted to re-create the ritual in Britain and over many pints of beer they discussed how it could be done, deciding to substitute bridges for tall trees and bungee cords for vines. With improvised climbing harnesses and lengthy bungee cords Kirke's associates "borrowed" from a British naval base, Kirke prepared his vine jump. On April Fool's Day 1979, Kirke and three other club members tied their cords to the 245-foot Clifton Bridge in Bristol, England, and dove off.

Encouraged that no one had died, Kirke cast around for a more dramatic venue. He chose what, at the time, was the world's highest suspension bridge, the 955-foot Royal Gorge, near Cañon City, Colorado. Kirke arranged for ABC's *That's Incredible!* to fund and televise the leap he'd convinced Tabin to leave Oxford for and take with him.

On March 6, 1980, Tabin and a dozen other Oxonians drove through a Colorado snowstorm in a convoy led by a wildly fishtailing white Cadillac convertible. They arrived to see cameramen arrayed around the bridge, an ABC helicopter circling overhead, and, more ominously, an ambulance parked nearby. They were pleased to find the piano they'd rented for the official accompanist they'd flown in from Oxford set up next to the railing where they planned to take the plunge.

Just before 3:00 P.M., Kirke passed around several bottles of champagne, fortifying his team. Then the five jumpers were all made to sign releases absolving bridge authorities of responsibility in the event of their deaths. "Kirke's hand trembled as he held the pen," Tabin says. "None of us had ever seen him show any sign of fear before, and we were all a bit unnerved."

Finally, with the camera helicopter hovering overhead, the rotor blades drowning out the piano and ruffling Kirke's black tails, the Dangerous Sports Club members steadied themselves for their most hazardous stunt to date. Tabin, clad in his well-used white tux, climbed onto the railing alongside his fellow aerialists. Kirke, of course, stood in the center. "Nearly a thousand feet below, the Arkansas River looked like a thread," Tabin says. The canyon narrowed from a width of eight hundred feet to only sixty as it reached the river. "From where we stood," Tabin recalls, "it looked like the canyon walls were only inches apart."

Tabin had knotted all the cords securely, triple-checking each man's harness, especially Kirke's, which was longer than the other jumpers', since he hoped to rebound just shy of smashing into the Arkansas River. But no one knew exactly how far the cords would stretch, whether the jumpers would pass out from g-forces, or if the wind whipping through the gorge would blow them off course. "I worried that if we hit the granite walls," Tabin says, "we'd end up as strawberry jam smeared on rock."

Kirke raised his hand, counted to three, and calmly stepped out into the air. "We all followed him," Tabin says. "My mind screamed, 'Error!' My testicles retreated up into the safety of my body, and I was like a cartoon figure, desperately trying to walk back to the bridge. Then I dropped. My mind stopped as I free-fell. I came to a gentle stop four hundred feet down while Kirke was still falling; then I was catapulted violently up, out of control. I was elated. My knots had held! I could see all my teammates falling and rising, and I was so relieved none of us had become strawberry jam that I made sure to enjoy my last few bounces by doing somersaults."

Finally, Tabin came to rest, hanging at the end of his cord, waving to the helicopter's camera, trying to ignore the tight harness cutting off the supply of blood to his legs. He was suspended below the bridge and above the river, swaying gently between canyon walls. He'd answered the query he'd put to himself the morning Kirke had issued his invitation; he definitely would have regretted missing the experience, the voltage that pulsed through him as his body transmitted euphoric messages to his brain that he had survived.

But as he dangled, poised between earth and sky, reflexively scanning the granite walls of the canyon for climbing routes, Geoff Tabin couldn't help pondering another question. Could he really abandon a life of adventures like these? Would he ever be able to stop swerving and embed himself in the grinding regularity required to succeed at

Harvard Medical School? While the Oxonians remaining on the bridge celebrated with champagne toasts, then struggled with the problem of how, exactly, to haul the jumpers up, he had more time than he wanted to wonder.

Before enrolling in medical school, Tabin managed to squeeze in one more adventure. "Bob did some research and discovered trust funds for "strenuous holidays" that were artifacts from a time when it was considered a sacred duty for Oxford gentlemen to go off and 'civilize' people in 'primitive' parts of the world," Tabin says. He and Shapiro applied for a grant from the "A. C. Irvine Travel Fund," which partially paid for their attempt to climb Carstensz Pyramid. Because of the expense of reaching such a remote mountain, they were accompanied by Sam Moses, a writer for *Sports Illustrated*, which had agreed to pick up the remaining cost of their expedition in exchange for publishing a piece about the trip.

Moses initially found Tabin too bizarre to take seriously. Before he'd left Oxford, a girlfriend of Tabin's had painted his toenails bright red and blue, and they were still decorated that way when a sandal-wearing Tabin first met Moses in New Guinea. "Despite [Tabin's] intellectual credentials, it seemed to me there were some missing steps in Geoff's way of reasoning; his conclusions appeared out of kilter with the evidence; his arithmetic somehow off. I resolved to keep up my guard [with him]," Moses said early in the thirty-page feature he wrote, which ran in two consecutive issues.

Carstensz Pyramid is one of the Seven Summits, and the least frequently climbed, because of its extreme inaccessibility. The most technically challenging thing about climbing it is the ten-day trek to the base camp, through the double- and triple-canopy jungle inhabited by the Dani, a tribe of former headhunters.

To reach Carstensz, the team had to trek forty-four miles through a maze of game trails from the landing strip where a small plane had deposited them. Shapiro had worried that they wouldn't be able to hire enough porters to carry their climbing and camping gear, but the Dani turned the trip into a community outing, and entire families divided the loads into small bundles and set out together. Old men joined the procession for a few miles at a time to exchange gossip. Women wearing *yums* from their foreheads, net bags woven from reeds and adorned with colorful orchids, carried either heavy loads of sweet potatoes in their bags or babies swaddled in leaves and moss. And hour after hour, accompanied by the counterpoint of hornbills and birds of paradise, the Dani sang.

"Every day I grew more amazed by our companions," Tabin says. "We had brought hundreds of pounds of high-tech gear, but they found everything they needed in the forest." The men traveled naked except for their *kotekas*, the jutting tusklike gourds they wore to cover their penises. If it rained, they whipped together pandanus-leaf ponchos. If they were hungry, they ate the sweet potatoes they carried, foraged for roots or bugs, or caught a bat, which they'd roast over a fire built by striking flints onto handfuls of moss. Then they shared out tiny portions, so that everyone got a mouthful.

During the ten days of trekking, the Americans' greatest difficulty proved to be staying on top of the logs the Dani confidently strode across, rather than wading through the muddy jungle floor. Moses describes how frightening the logs could be. But "Geoff, in blue boxer trunks, a preppie gray wool crewneck sweater and galoshes, and a *yum* full of potatoes hanging down his back . . . Geoff would amble blithely and eagerly onto even the slimiest log; it wouldn't have surprised me," Moses wrote, "if he had taken off his galoshes and gone barefoot, like the Dani, just for fun."

Carstensz Pyramid rises two vertical miles from the jungle floor to a height of 16,023 feet, an ominous gray shark fin surfacing from a sea of trees. Tabin, Shapiro, and Moses were only the sixth party to successfully climb to Carstensz's summit. Tabin led most of the way as they forged a new route to the top. For the summit photo, all three posed naked, except for the long, curving *kotekas* they'd borrowed from the Dani. Today, that photo is framed and proudly displayed in the Tabin home.

Toward the end of his article, Moses admitted that he misjudged

Tabin when he first met him. Tabin might be "cheerfully oblivious to society's norms," he wrote, but he would certainly "have [him] as an expedition partner again."

For Tabin, the climb felt anticlimactic after the experience of traveling with a tribe that lived much as they had since the Stone Age. "The real adventure had been the privilege of spending time with the Dani," Tabin says. "Watching them, I realized just how much we had sacrificed in the name of 'civilization.'"

Two weeks later, Tabin found himself in a lecture hall at Harvard University. Despite his long-held fear of stepping onto the conveyor belt of conformity, when he enrolled, in the fall of 1980, he was surprised by how thrilled he was to be studying medicine. "There was a lot of grunt memorization and basic anatomy to learn, of course," Tabin says, "but the faculty was incredible. Every week we'd listen to someone lecture who was pushing the boundaries of their field."

For Tabin, the number of career paths open to him seemed infinite. Specialties and subspecialties began to branch and fork in his imagination like the lavishly detailed charts of the human nervous system that sprawled across the pages of his textbooks. Tabin says he had little sense of which specialty to pursue. "Vaguely, in the back of my head, was a desire to connect the idea of helping people my grandmother had instilled in me with travel and adventure," he says. "But I had only the fuzziest notion of how that might work."

Meanwhile, to keep the needle of his fun-o-meter from flatlining, Tabin gathered a collection of climbing partners in Cambridge, and when he had time, he'd try to solve the problem of a pitch or two of challenging rock. Six weeks after classes started, he was bouldering, climbing a small outcropping without a rope, just outside of Boston at Hammond Pond, a small body of water behind a Bloomingdale's department store. A piece of rock he was using as a handhold broke off while he was on an overhanging ledge with his feet hooked up over his head. "The last thing I remember was torpedoing straight down," he says.

He fell fifteen feet headfirst, knocking himself unconscious and breaking his left arm. Tabin's climbing partner and classmate, Hansell Stedman, ran to Tabin and realized he had stopped breathing. Stedman remembers the moment vividly. He says he had the sensation of scanning all of the medical texts he'd studied to date and blacking out the sections, as if with a Magic Marker, that weren't applicable. When he was certain of the correct course of action, he gave Tabin mouth-to-nose resuscitation, carried him several hundred yards, and flagged down a passing driver, who rushed them to the nearest hospital.

Tabin remained in a coma for thirty-six hours, and when he emerged from it, the first thing he saw was the face of a doctor swimming into focus by his bed; then he heard his alarming words. "The doctor told me, 'You are the luckiest sonofabitch I've ever seen,'" Tabin remembers. "'If your friend hadn't done everything exactly right, you'd be dead.'" Tabin left the hospital after a week and returned to Harvard.

"The irony that Geoff, who'd survived so many dangerous mountain climbs, had nearly died on a boulder behind a Bloomingdale's was not lost on our classmates," Stedman says.

When I asked about his near-death experience, Tabin was characteristically unruffled. "There've been so many times I could have been killed climbing that it felt like just another close call, and it certainly wasn't going to stop me from doing what I loved. As you can imagine, my mother saw it a little differently."

Sam Moses published his *Sports Illustrated* story that March, and it fashioned Tabin as the energetic hero of the Carstensz expedition. "Geoff was up there on the leading end of the rope," Moses wrote, "the 'sharp end,' as climbers call it, often unprotected, 800 feet off the ground, standing on loose little clumps of grass and clinging to a wall of rock while icy water dribbled down his sleeves to his armpits." The article put Tabin on the climbing community's radar.

At the end of the semester, as he was studying for his pharmacology exam, he received a phone call from a San Francisco neuroscientist named Lou Reichardt, one of the world's most celebrated high-altitude mountaineers and the first person to summit K2, the planet's second-highest peak, without the use of supplemental oxygen. Reichardt said he was leading an expedition to the last unclimbed face of Everest. He explained that they had a full complement of members but asked Tabin if he was willing to serve as the team's first alternate, in case any of them weren't able to go.

"I couldn't believe Lou would consider me," Tabin says. "He was one of my heroes, and I'd have been thrilled just to meet him. But a chance to attempt the last unclimbed face of Everest!" Tabin could hear himself breathing into the phone as he took stock. He knew in his gut he wasn't experienced enough for such a challenging technical climb at that altitude. After his accident, he was in the worst physical shape of his life. He told Reichardt he was honored even to be considered and promised to be ready to leave at a moment's notice.

A week after the expedition left for Tibet, Tabin received word that one of the climbers had broken his ankle, and he began jamming gear into duffel bags. From the San Francisco airport, Tabin sent a scrawled postcard to the medical school's dean of students, saying he was off to climb Everest and requesting that the university hold his place. He knew that leaving Harvard suddenly to spend months on an expedition might permanently derail his medical career. He didn't hesitate, and boarded a plane bound for Asia.

The Himalaya may be at their most impressive when seen from the north. Unscreened by the range's southern foothills, and thrusting starkly up from the Tibetan plain, the mountains that would come to define Geoff Tabin's life overwhelmed him as he walked toward them, accompanied by a yak caravan loaded with the expedition's supplies. "I thought I knew a bit about mountains," Tabin says. "But nothing I'd ever seen prepared me for the grandeur of the highest Himalayan peaks."

For the first few days of the week-long trek to base camp, Tabin was so deliriously happy to be on his way to Everest that his sunburned face hurt from grinning. The Tibetan yak herders sang as they walked, accompanied by the lulling chimes of their animals' bells. Here it was, in three dimensions, the world he'd read about in books since boyhood, the ultimate test that he'd fantasized about while climbing lesser peaks. Around each bend in the trail, new vistas appeared, each more improbable than the last. The snowfields and summits of Makalu, Chomolonzo, Lhotse, and Everest revealed themselves in stages, glittering ice cathedrals that rose from the dry brown plateau with the eccentric clarity of dreams. "It was the greatest hike of my life," Tabin says. "Most of the way I felt like I was soaring ten feet off the ground."

Two days from base camp, a tall, elderly man who looked remarkably like Sir Edmund Hillary strolled unsteadily toward them, his head wrapped in bloody bandages. He squinted as he tried to focus his pale blue eyes on Tabin. "Are you driving the bus?" Tabin thought he heard him say.

Tabin was tempted to blame the inexplicable vision on the altitude, but Jim Morrissey, the man accompanying New Zealand's most famous citizen, confirmed that it was, in fact, the great man. Hillary had trekked to base camp with most of the other expedition members several weeks earlier and was suffering from cerebral edema, a swelling of the fluid around the brain caused by high altitude. Morrissey, a Californian cardiologist, was rushing Hillary down to the relative safety of lower altitude. But while they'd been crossing a seventeen-thousand-foot pass on their return trip, Hillary had been knocked off the trail by a yak caravan, and had slammed his head against a rock.

"Jim was terrified that our expedition could become famous for killing the world's greatest living mountaineer," Tabin says, "so he was in a hurry to keep moving and I only had a moment to spend with Hillary." Morrissey said he'd be back in a few days, and Hillary summoned the lucidity, before stumbling away, to clap his hand on Tabin's shoulder and wish him luck.

Unfortunately, the image of a bloodied Edmund Hillary augured the low morale Tabin found infecting base camp. The first night he shared a tent with John Roskelley, who'd completed so many technically challenging first ascents that many in the media had anointed him the greatest mountaineer on earth. Tabin climbed into the tent and unrolled his sleeping bag. "I was so happy to be there," he says. "There was so much I hoped to learn from John. I had a thousand questions I wanted to ask."

But before Tabin could make a single inquiry, Roskelley sat up and stared at Tabin bleakly. "This face is suicide," Roskelley said. "If you climb on this route, in these conditions, you're going to die." Then he rolled over and went to sleep.

The Kangshung Face has often had that kind of effect on a climber contemplating it from below. In 1921, after becoming the first foreign mountaineer to receive permission from the Thirteenth Dalai Lama to attempt Everest from the Tibetan side, the Englishman George Mallory—famous for answering "Because it's there" when asked why he wanted to climb Everest—arrived to survey the Kangshung Face. "Other men, less wise, might attempt this way if they would, but, emphatically, it was not for us," he recorded in his journal, before dying during his attempt to climb Everest from the Nepalese side.

Rising after an understandably sleepless night, Tabin gulped strong coffee and assessed the situation. The team had broken into factions, arguing about which route to attempt. Roskelley's faction wanted to entirely avoid the Kangshung Face, which he considered too avalanche-prone, and try a different route along a ridge to their north. The other group, led by the Colorado climber George Lowe, pushed for a route straight up the five-thousand-foot buttress of vertical rock and ice that stood between base camp and easier climbing on upper snow ridges. Lou Reichardt ignored the controversy and led by example, carrying heavy double loads to the high camps they'd established, doing the hard, tedious work of caching supplies partway up the mountain so the team could prepare for whatever probes the climbers made toward the summit.

"I was shocked to see my heroes bickering and confused about how to proceed," Tabin says. "If Sir Edmund Hillary had altitude sickness and an elite mountaineer like John Roskelley felt that the conditions on the Kangshung Face made it too dangerous to climb, I wondered what business I had being here. Base camp, at seventeen thousand feet, was as high as I'd ever been."

A week later, Roskelley made an impassioned plea to his friend Kim Momb. "Come off the mountain if you want to live," he radioed while Momb was fixing ropes high on the Kangshung Face. "I owe it to your family to bring you home alive!" Momb and Roskelley left the next day.

Tabin, who'd had a week to acclimate, tried to put the drama out of his mind. "I realized what a privilege it was to be in that place, and I thought I might never make it back, so let's see if I can do this." He was feeling strong enough to try to help the remaining climbers push a route farther up the center of the Kangshung Face. "I was amazed by the climbing they'd already accomplished," Tabin says. "I'd never done anything that difficult." Tabin pushed upward, helping to carry loads and fix ropes, nearly to the top of the buttress, gratified to learn that he was capable of tough technical climbing at Himalayan altitude.

Arguments and injuries drove most of the team away. Six weeks after base camp had been set up, there were only four climbers willing to continue: Reichardt, Lowe, Tabin, and the team doctor, Dan Reid, a diminutive cardiac surgeon who favored kilts and had a frenetic energy rivaling Tabin's. They took inventory of their options. They had no Sherpas to support them, and only limited supplies remained. According to Tabin, Reid half-jokingly suggested that they all sign a "death pact" and make a frantic dash for the summit, agreeing that if anyone became sick or injured on the way up, the others would abandon him. "I stared at 'Death-Pact Dan,'" Tabin says, "and realized the expedition was over."

CHAPTER 9

The Problem of Her Eyes

Only our eyes had met. The lips had still not spoken. The days that we're apart, I know not where she has gone. The sun crowns the snow peak. The lowland lies in darkness. I tune my mind to her. I lay my pillow down, pointing my head toward where I hope she'll be. I wish my soul would run, to wherever she has gone.

Nepalese poet Madhav Ghimire, "Aaja Bholi," as translated by Dr. Singha Basnyat

There was the problem of her eyes. Eyes were rarely a problem for Ruit nowadays. He could diagnose a youthful cataract from across an examination room, before a patient even sat down at his slit lamp. Astigmatisms, abrasions, the telltale pressure bulge of glaucoma—all these Ruit could detect with almost mystical insight, faster and more accurately than any of his peers. But her eyes were a problem he couldn't solve.

Her name was Nanda. Nothing had passed between them but the proper synchronicity of a surgeon and an excellent scrub nurse. She'd anticipate the instrument he'd need, and just as he'd turn to ask for it, there it would be, in her slim, steady hand. Her dark eyes, framed in the narrow band between her surgical mask and cap, were wide, and clear, and calm. When he turned from a patient on his operating table in the Nepal Eye Hospital and looked into them, searching for a spark, any indication that she felt the way he did, he found nothing but professional attentiveness. And that made him anything but calm.

Of course he'd made the usual inquiries. What he'd learned was daunting. She was Newari, a daughter of the original residents of Kathmandu, masters of wood carving and stonemasonry who had built the cultural heart of the capital. The temples and palaces of central Kathmandu, Patan, and Bhaktapur were her heritage, as surely as the boulderscape of Olangchungola was his. Her father was not wealthy, but she had been born into an upper stratum of class-conscious Kathmandu society. An even more formidable obstacle than caste stood between Ruit and his aspirations: Her family was Hindu.

He finished his case, and as Nanda waited for him to lean back on his stool so she could bandage the patient's eye, Ruit hunched forward, staring into space, summoning his courage. He'd already asked her to have tea with him, somewhere away from the hospital, several times, and each time she'd rebuffed him with a simple "no thank you," her eyes as unreadable as ever.

"*Thik cha?*" she asked. "All is well, Dr. Ruit?"

"Please, Nanda. *Please*. Won't you go out someplace with me when we're finished here?"

She lowered her lashes modestly, and he took her silence for assent.

What was happening to him? Where was his focus? For more than a decade since Yang La's death, he had hewed to the path that had been revealed to him. There had been a few diversions. At King George he'd joined the basketball team. And though he stood only five foot seven, he played "pivot," as the center position was known locally, because he was broad and powerful enough to bull his way toward the basket against taller players. He had dated a bit, without much emotional consequence. There might have been a bit too much whiskey in Delhi, at the All India Institute, the country's top medical school, where he'd been accepted, after blazing through King George, to specialize in ophthalmology, too many late nights drunkenly speculating about the future with his classmates. But Ruit understood that, in Asia, raw knowledge without the social connections to put it to use would lead nowhere. So he'd added a few rupees to the hat passed to purchase local spirits.

Despite the occasional bleary morning after, he became all business at All India. The school had the finest facilities in a nation of nearly a billion souls, and he was drawn to the new technologies on offer in their well-equipped research labs, especially the emerging field of microsurgery. After graduating from King George Medical College with his general medical degree, he'd been assigned as a medical officer on a team of cartographers mapping Nepal's northern border. He kept the surveyors safe from altitude sickness and treated their sprained ankles, strained limbs, and other minor ailments. Ruit spent months trekking from Everest eastward to Sikkim, to villages that reminded him more and more of home as he approached the upper Tamor River. And he did what he could with his limited medical kit for local people wherever they camped, far from the resources of the capital. What he discovered shocked and enraged him.

"I found all manner of malnutrition and infectious disease, of course," Ruit says. But what amazed him was the staggering extent of preventable blindness he'd taken for granted as a boy. "It was everywhere! In every village I'd find people blinded by cataracts living like animals, actually worse than animals, because even *dzo* are taken out for fresh air and can rely on being fed. But these people, thousands and thousands of them, were stranded in the darkness of their huts. I asked people why they didn't seek treatment. They talked about the distance to hospitals. But really the essential was this: resignation to fate. They said, 'Your hair grows white, your eyes grow white, and then you die.' I knew this was nonsense, that when you've lost your vision in such steep places like the mountains of Nepal, blindness takes away ninety percent of the meaning of life. I knew cataract surgery could give them their humanity back."

By the time Ruit reached Olangchungola, he was dismayed to see how impoverished it had become. A third of the houses had been washed away by floods. New roads from Kathmandu to Lhasa had slowed the busy stream of trade between the people of the Tamor valley and Tibet to a trickle. It seemed there was no one left in the village but destitute people.

As he trekked away from the community his father had worked so hard to help him escape, he felt a detailed vision of his future coming into focus. Every complex sort of medical care was needed by those who lived at the margins of Nepalese society. But restoring sight was relatively simple. He spun the prayer wheels flanking the central lane of Olangchungola as he set out, perhaps for the last time, away from the place where he'd been born. He injured both arms and survived, chanting the *pujas* his father had taught him, asking for the blessings of Guru Rinpoche and of the spirits of the earth and air, preparing for the climb forming clearly in his head, no matter how steep.

In Delhi, at All India, Ruit lived and breathed the study of ophthalmology. He haunted the laboratory where the rhesus monkeys he used to hone his surgical techniques were kept. "I would be there so often, at such oddly hours, that I'd have to give the night watchman some baksheesh, a few rupees or cigarettes, to let me in," he says.

The microsurgical treatment of cataract disease was a far more subtle and technically challenging way to cure blindness than the crude technique still common in the developing world during the 1980s. But Ruit was determined to master it. Learning to operate under a microscope was difficult. He had to move his hands very slowly and delicately, but magnified by the lenses, subtle movements appeared jerky and exaggerated. Reconciling his brain to deal with this disjunction took patience and repetition.

Ruit's research required that he blind dozens of living creatures, monkeys who could look up at him with such moist, humanlike eyes that his hands shook, at first, before he began to operate. "I knew how my dad would feel about me causing these animals suffering," Ruit says, "particularly a creature like a monkey that we venerate in our culture. But I'd become different. I'd feel troubled at first, but as soon as I picked up my instruments, I thought about nothing else but improving my technique."

The distance he'd traveled from the Buddhist certainties of his boyhood could now be measured in lives taken, not only miles trekked through mountains. Despite Sonam's solemn request that he eat only large animals, life in a British-style boarding school had swept away such distinctions. He had come to eat unthinkingly, to fuel his studies. But he'd never forgotten Sonam's advice to remember that he was Walung. He carried that knowledge always, near his belly, like the silver bird-shaped belt buckle his mother still wore.

And now he'd just asked a Hindu woman to tea.

They strolled through Durbar Square. Around them, the carnival atmosphere of the old city center whirled. Emaciated sadhus marched by in loincloths, clutching their trident staffs as tightly as the vows they'd made to renounce the material world. Holy wanderers squatted on the terraces of multitiered temples, chanting praise to Lord Shiva, or snoring as they sprawled on warm paving stones, inches from the bare feet of street children who darted between them, playing tag or untangling kite string by winding it around temple pillars carved with acrobatic images of erotic couplings. Tikka-paste and marigold vendors held out their wares, admonishing passersby to consider parting with a measly rupee or two, so their karma could benefit from the draping of a statue of Krishna with flowers or the smearing of a stone god's forehead with a daub of crimson.

Ruit walked on in awkward silence, his tongue stilled by a city that hadn't seemed as foreign, as fundamentally Hindu to him, since he'd arrived as a teenager fresh from the mountains. He was aware of the way men's eyes followed Nanda, who looked even lovelier out of hospital scrubs than he had imagined. And he felt their eyes on him, too, calculating what a Tibetan type was doing beside this beautiful Newari woman in a pale blue sari that rippled like water as she walked. Ruit realized that his plan to lead Nanda to a table at a sidewalk tea shop would expose her to more of this scrutiny, so he pushed open the door of the first sanctuary he spotted, a dim, narrow Chinese restaurant he wasn't sure he could afford, because it catered to tourists. It was too early for dinner, and he was relieved to see that they were the only customers.

At first, as they sipped sugary black tea and picked at a plate of fried vegetable rolls, Ruit talked in jolts and starts. But he detected a flicker of warmth in Nanda's eyes, now that they were alone, and this encouraged him. Suddenly, the plans he'd been nurturing for the future came pouring out. He explained that when he'd graduated at the top of his class from the All India Institute, he'd had his choice of lucrative jobs in Europe and America, that there had even been an offer to serve as physician to the sultan of Oman, with a cook, a home, and a driver of his own. Instead, he'd made a promise, not only to the memory of Yang La but to the underserved majority of the Nepalese people, and, he told Nanda, he intended to keep it.

Turning down profitable work like the job in Oman meant that Ruit lived in a bachelor's studio apartment near the Nepal Eye Hospital, where he'd been hired in 1985, and his junior surgeon's salary left him just enough to put out plates of biscuits and brew large, weak pots of tea for the staff who often gathered at his apartment in the evening to discuss the country's political dysfunction. The subject they circled back to frequently was their frustration with Nepal's medical caste system, in which few but members of the royal family and other VIPs received high-quality care.

Ruit told Nanda that he'd urged his colleagues to adopt microsurgery for removing cataracts, and that they recognized his skills and ambition but the established surgeons clung to their expertise: the older procedure called "intracapsular" surgery. The process involved filleting a patient's eyeball nearly in half, extracting the diseased lens whole, sewing the eye back together, and prescribing glasses with thick lenses that the patient would then have to wear for the rest of his or her life. Recovery from such an invasive surgery required that patients spend a week flat on their backs, their heads immobilized between sandbags so their wounds wouldn't burst.

Intracapsular surgery, he said, left patients with, at best, a narrow tunnel of vision, which was nearly useless to people trying to navigate steep mountain trails. And he confided to Nanda that when he'd argued, at a tense meeting with senior staff, that it was the hospital's duty to send medical teams to rural areas, to treat patients who weren't able to travel to Kathmandu or pay surgical fees, he was reminded of his junior status in the institutional hierarchy and bluntly instructed to stop making waves.

The waiter asked if they wanted to order more food. Ruit declined, with the air, he hoped, not of someone who couldn't afford another overpriced dish but of a man too busy to be interrupted. Nanda hadn't said much, but he felt sure she was listening carefully.

"Have you had enough to eat?" Ruit asked, and Nanda nodded. He let his mind swim from these shallow conversational depths toward the solid shore of the question he really wanted to ask.

Sitting cozily in a booth beside her, in a quiet tea shop he had managed to find on Kanthi Path that offered shelter from prying eyes, Ruit asked Nanda to marry him for the first time. The moment felt right. But after he gathered the courage to propose, she seemed not to have heard his question. So he repeated it. Nanda flatly refused, saying that the communities they came from were too different for it to work.

The second time, Ruit brought her back to the Chinese restaurant near Durbar Square where they'd gone on their first date. He ordered tea, a plate of egg rolls, and an extravagant dish of Hakka noodles and tried again. This time she fended him off, laughing, as if he'd just told a mildly amusing joke.

"I began to feel really desperate," Ruit says. "Nanda was beautiful, and I know I'm not so handsome, but I felt sure we were right for each other. I could see she had a very straight character. When you fall in love, you like everything about your darling—her hairstyle, the way she walks. The way she works. I felt I could watch Nanda work forever. I wanted to give her time and let the feeling come from her side. I tried to throw myself at my own work even harder, but I worried, when I had lonely time to myself, that all the love was coming from my side only, and she might marry some other joker."

One morning, after Ruit's third and fourth unsuccessful attempts to change Nanda's mind about marriage, he was dispatched, as one of the Nepal Eye Hospital's junior surgeons, to pick up an important foreign doctor at the airport.

Since Ruit's return to Nepal from the All India Institute, foreign doctors had been his lifeline to advances in cataract surgery. The Dutch doctor Jan Kok was a frequent visitor to Nepal and brought Ruit news of advances in artificial intraocular lenses. Dick Litwin, a bearded Berkeley ophthalmologist who looked more like one of the backpackers who wandered the Thamel District in a hash haze than a leading-edge eye surgeon, performed one of the first IOL implantations Ruit ever witnessed. "In the mid-eighties," Litwin says, "lens design was changing so fast that perfectly good year-old IOLs were being thrown away in America. So I cultivated lens salesmen and brought duffel bags of obsolete but perfectly good IOLs to Nepal."

Litwin remembers teaching IOL implantation surgery to junior staff at the Nepal Eye Hospital. "When I walked in the OR, all the surgeons stepped away from their tables and asked, very obsequiously, 'Dr. Litwin, will you finish my case?' All except one." So Litwin bent over to watch Ruit struggling, then succeeding at implanting an artificial lens. "I was struck by both his determination and his skill, so I invited him to lunch."

Litwin chose an Indian restaurant far too expensive for Ruit to frequent. And while they talked, between bites of their samosas and curries, Litwin became even more fascinated by his lunch companion. "It was obvious from the moment I met him that Sanduk was fearless, that he had a vision for changing health care in his country," says Litwin, now a member of the HCP's advisory board. "Well, maybe not completely fearless, because he was pretty anxious about our tab. He let me buy lunch, but he insisted on paying for our taxi back to the hospital. I was very impressed by that, and by him, so whenever I returned to Kathamandu, I always looked in on Sanduk and left him supplies."

The domestic arrivals area at Tribhuvan consisted of a chain-link fence, which flexed and buckled as it held back the scrum of touts, taxi drivers, baggage wallahs, and guesthouse booking agents, all competing to be the first to lay a proprietary hand on the passengers debarking from small Royal Nepal prop planes and trying to squeeze through a narrow gate.

Ruit jogged over to two tall Caucasian men in suits and ties who were wrestling with baggage wallahs, trying to regain control of their suitcases. "Dr. Hollows?" he asked.

"Over here, mate!" shouted a short, sturdily built man in a rumpled bush coat, clutching a pipe between his teeth and carrying a battered leather shoulder bag. He smiled warmly, under an untrimmed hedge of gray hair and eyebrows so shaggy it was a wonder he could see past them well enough to perform surgery, and held out his hand.

"From the first minute I met Fred I felt we were brothers," Ruit says. "Some foreign VIPs would treat Nepalese like we were just there to carry their baggage. And here was one of the most famous doctors in the world with no air about him at all."

Fred Hollows tended to provoke strong reactions wherever he went. He had become infamous throughout Australia by publicizing the inferior quality of health care available to the nation's aboriginal population. After conducting a series of research trips to the outback in the 1970s, Hollows concluded that, in terms of health care, Australians lived in two separate countries. The cities of coastal Australia provided first-class, first-world care to their residents; but in the largely aboriginal interior, third-world care was the best citizens could expect to receive, if any medical facilities existed at all. Once he had the data to back up his charges, he went public. Loudly. And Hollows used the press to call out politicians who resisted changing the status quo, shaming them into addressing the crisis in aboriginal health care.

"Fred had a soft corner for communism," Ruit says. "He really believed all humans deserved equal care. And if the high and mighty told him to be quiet, he'd just curse at them louder."

When Ruit picked him up at the airport, Hollows had just returned from surveying eye care in Nepal's rural western districts for the World Health Organization. He concluded, and Ruit agreed, that rates of preventable blindness in rural Nepal were among the highest in the world. On their trip into Kathmandu, the two men discovered that they were both driven by the same passion: taking action to transform conditions they considered morally unacceptable.

At the Nepal Eye Hospital, after Hollows observed Ruit operating, he knew he'd met not just a talented peer but "a soul-mate," as Hollows wrote in his autobiography. "Sandook," Hollows said, mispronouncing Ruit's name as he always would thereafter, "we've got to organize getting you over to Oz and trained up in all the latest tricks of modern cataract surgery."

"If I'm ever free, of course I'd like to come," Ruit said, wondering when his scheduled hours at the hospital, unscheduled attempts to win Nanda's heart, and the years he faced of trying to transform his country's eye-care system would ever allow him the time required to take such a trip.

In the village of Gurmu, in the mid-hills to the northwest of Kathmandu, Kamisya Tamang sat in the doorway of her small stone hut. Since her eyes had begun to fail her, the boundary of her daily life had contracted, year after year. At first, she had still been able to join the others at the village loom, until her vision became too unreliable for her to thread the shuttle through the strands of yarn and the other women scolded her for ruining the shawls they hoped to sell. For nearly a year after that she was able to step carefully down the steep, rocky path to the village water tap, if she felt her way with the flat bottoms of her bare feet, which had become more reliable at sensing the contours of the ground than her eyes.

Now her world had shrunk to the dimensions of her hut of stacked stones, to an eight-by-ten-foot rectangle of packed dirt and, on days when it wasn't raining, the stone slab outside her low doorway, where she could squat and listen to village life going on without her.

Kamisya's husband, Baajyo, worked as a porter, and he was gone for months at a time, walking barefoot with his heavy woven basket wherever loads needed to be carried. Kamisya had given birth to a daughter once, while she was still able to see. The vision of the child's small red face, clenched like a fist, had filled Kamisya with hope, and relief that she'd no longer be alone when Baajyo was away. But the infant girl had developed a fever and died after only fifteen days, as so many of the newly born in Gurmu did, where only half of the children survived to see their first birthday. With the nearest clinic three hard days of walking away, what could be done?

Kamisya's father had died so long ago that the precise cause escaped her. Her mother's second husband had died from an untreated pain in his stomach, and after that, Kamisya's mother lived with her in-laws, more a maid, now that he was gone, than a member of the family. She visited Kamisya when she had time between her duties cleaning, cooking, and working in the family's barley and potato fields. She brought Kamisya what little her household could spare: kindling and rice and dried lentils so her daughter could cook dal, and greens and potatoes when they were in season. She also tried to keep the five-gallon plastic gas can where Kamisya stored her water filled, but often her chores kept her away.

"You can live without food for some time," Kamisya says. "But when my water ran out, I was really in trouble. I would sit in the door of my house, calling out in fear for someone to take my container to the village tap."

Kamisya would squat on her stone slab, listening to the sound of other womens' laughter from the loom, or the cries of children at play drifting up to her home, and weep. "All my eyes were good for was making water," she says. "And life became very sour for me."

Finally, during a sleepless night, Kamisya considered how to kill herself. Cutting her wrists with the dull knives she used to prepare food would be slow, painful, and unlikely to do the job. She could set fire to her home, but only the straw mat where she slept and the wood beams would burn, and her courage might fail her when she sensed the flames approaching. So she decided to run off the edge of the ravine. There'd be no surviving the fall to the river rocks far below.

Stealthily, as if the entire village could hear her thoughts, she clutched her walking stick and stepped outside of the home she hadn't left for months. It had been years since she'd been able to see the river gorge, but the sound of the wind gusting through the ravine was unmistakable for ears that had become as sensitive as Kamisya's.

She quickened her step, putting one bare foot in front of the other, navigating toward the wind that would release her. She had always striven to be kind to others, had tried her best to raise a family. Kamisya felt sure that her next incarnation would be better—she would be freed from this darkness. She could sense she was nearing the ravine, could feel the roaring void in front of her and ran toward it, paying no mind to the thorny scrub that pierced her feet, just as something slammed into her from the side, knocking the breath from her lungs, holding her down and pinning her to this life.

It was her mother, who'd come with cooked dal and a basket of greens for Kamisya's breakfast. She had seen what her daughter planned to do, and old and weak as she was, the advantage of her eyesight had enabled her to catch Kamisya before she reached the edge. The two women lay on the ground, out of breath, holding on to each other. "Stay," her mother said, "stay. We'll think of something."

When Baajyo returned from a month's work, carrying building materials along the mid-hill trails, he had a fistful of rupee notes tucked into his woolen vest, and, after hearing about his wife's attempt at suicide, he developed a plan. He'd listened to a radio program one evening that had talked about a doctor in Kathmandu who was restoring sight to the blind. "We'll take you to Kathmandu by bus," he told Kamisya. "We'll have him make your eyes."

Baajyo lowered his wife into the bamboo basket he hauled to earn his living. With her feet hanging out behind him and her head propped up against a board he'd placed to steady it, they set out, her weight supported by a thick woven strap he wore across his forehead. The journey to the road was a short trip by Baajyo's standards, and a simple matter for him. His wife, who was small to begin with and had lost much of her weight since losing her sight, was far lighter than his usual loads of cement, cases of soft drinks, or corrugated tin roofing.

After a few turns down the twisting road, Kamisya vomited. Baajyo cleaned her up as well as he could and spoke to her gently, saying there was nothing to fear, that they should enjoy the ride and see how easily some people were able to travel, and they settled in for the trip to Kathmandu.

In his examination room at the Nepal Eye Hospital, Ruit saw Kamisya arrive gripping Baajyo's arm. Tenderly he took in her torn and weather-faded clothes. "The doctor sahib spoke to me so kindly," Kamisya remembers, but she was afraid of what he was going to do to her. There were rumors. Many village people believed that doctors like

Ruit plucked out their patients' eyes before putting in new ones. But Ruit explained very clearly what Kamisya could expect and told her she wouldn't have to pay for her surgery.

"She was only forty years old, and had early onset of fully mature cataracts," Ruit remembers. "A perfect candidate for the kind of surgery I could provide."

"Don't worry, *didi,*" he told Kamisya. "It's a simple procedure. I'm going to make two cuts in your eyes, take away the small pieces that are giving you problems, and put in something called intraocular lenses."

"What is that, Doctor *dai?*"

"In fact, it's an in-built spectacle," Ruit told her. "A few days after the surgery, you should be able to see perfectly well." Three days later, with two precious IOLs inserted where Kamisya's diseased lenses had blocked the light, and her wounds sewn shut with sutures, Ruit gently removed the gauze swaddling Kamisya's head and peeled off her bandages.

Recounting her story, Kamisya pauses, searching for words able to convey the sense she felt of complete release from her captivity, of the difference between living in darkness and living in light. "The first thing I could see was the doctor's face," Kamisya says. "He didn't look anything like the city person I imagined. He looked like he might have come from the hills above Gurmu. But I didn't think about that for long. This man had made my eyes! I was too excited to find out what they could see to think about anything else. I looked out the window, and I was able to make out little birds flying by. Birds! Then he held up fingers for me to count, and I could see them as clearly as I can see your nose," a sixty-year-old Kamisya told me, on a visit two decades later to Tilganga.

She wore a cardigan sweater with a faded T-shirt underneath that said HAPPY BIRTHDAY TO ME. I doubted she had chosen it for the message in a language she couldn't understand. It had probably come to her as flotsam, a first-world castoff, as did so many of the clothes worn by Nepal's poor. But I couldn't help feeling it was perfectly appropriate, that every day after not jumping to her death in Gurmu was a kind of birthday for Kamisya Tamang.

Kamisya said she made a point of visiting Ruit and bringing him some small token of thanks—some fresh eggs or potatoes from her field—when she returned to Kathmandu to sell weavings and shop for necessities. "It's not enough, I know," she said. "I bring the doctor *sahib* only simple things. Yet he has given me back my life."

Preparing her instruments for surgery early one morning, Nanda was brisk and efficient, as usual. She laid out scalpels, clamps, and cotton balls in neat rows. She checked that bottles of IV fluids were full and snapped the necks off glass ampoules of sterile eye wash, lining them up on her stainless steel tray. Ruit studied her, admired her, and planned to wait, professionally, to broach the subject after their work was done. But he couldn't help himself. "Damn it, Nanda," he said. "I've had lot of time to think, and I need you to be my wife! I can't live without you!"

Nanda lowered her head, continued arranging the items on her tray.

Ruit grabbed one of the glass ampoules. He raked its jagged spout across the palm of his left hand, the instrument that made his life's work possible, drawing a deep gash that filled with blood.

Nanda had been consumed for months by the difficulties they'd face, the break with tradition, the banishment from her family if she were to marry Ruit. "But when Sanduk sliced his hand," she says, "I realized how much he loved me. And I knew we'd be all right."

"Do you think it will work?" she asked.

"We'll make it work," Ruit said, grinning despite the pain, grinning even while his efficient scrub nurse blotted away his blood and poured antiseptic into his open wound, which foamed and burned with delicious vigor, like his plans for their future.

They were married two days later, in a civil ceremony attended by eight of their friends. "I thought, 'While the fire is hot, hit it,'" Ruit says. They hid the news from their families and celebrated at the

Shangri-La Hotel's restaurant, with the entire wedding party fitting comfortably around a single table, exchanging toasts, and returned to spend the night in their separate homes.

"Ever since I met Nanda, I knew I wanted to marry her," Ruit says. "But she made me work so hard to wear her down I hadn't thought much about what we would do if she said yes." Ruit's apartment was too small for the two of them, and Nanda still lived in her parents' home in the Newari neighborhood of Patan. Their families would be furious when they learned the truth, and unlikely to help them find a place to live or contribute to the cost of assembling a household. It dawned on Ruit that marrying Nanda might make him a refugee once again, unable to care properly for his wife if they were both torn from the web of family connections and support they'd need to start a life together in Kathmandu.

While he sought out a more permanent solution, Ruit arranged funding from a Dutch NGO for the two of them to travel to Amsterdam and study for two months with an old friend, the ophthalmologist Jan Kok. But Ruit knew he was just buying time. Nanda left for Holland without telling her family that she'd married. Frantically, her parents telephoned her friends and employers until they discovered the truth, which they found shocking enough to shun her.

Kok helped Ruit tame the Dutch telephone system enough to put in a call to Australia. He heard Hollows's raspy voice on the other end of the crackling line.

"Fred," he said. "It's Sanduk, from Nepal. I got married."

"That's great," Hollows said. "Congratulations."

"What I mean," Ruit said, conscious of the handfuls of Dutch guilders swirling down the drain every moment he lingered on the expensive international call, "is that now we have no place where we can live together. Were you serious about inviting me to Australia? There'd be two of us coming now."

"Well, shit," Hollows said, as casually as if he were inviting them over for a beer. "Then I'd better send you two tickets."

CHAPTER 10

The Eighth Summit

*Just as a white summer cloud, in harmony with heaven and earth, freely
floats in the blue sky from horizon to horizon, following the breath of the
atmosphere—in the same way the pilgrim abandons himself to the breath
of the greater life that . . . leads him beyond the farthest horizons to an aim
which is already present within him, though yet hidden from his sight.*
—Lama Anagarika Govinda, *The Way of the White Clouds*

"How did I get back into Harvard? Begging, basically. I told them I'd been bad," Tabin says, "and I promised to be better."

After his unsuccessful expedition, Tabin returned to find he was out of medical school. He met with Dr. Daniel D. Federman, the dean he'd sent the postcard to from San Francisco, to plead his case. "For some reason, the dean wasn't as excited about Everest as I was," Tabin says. Tabin tried to explain how rare the opportunity he had been offered was. It was *the last unclimbed face of the world's tallest mountain*!

"Yes, and some of our students like to visit the beach during their holidays," Federman said. "But they return when it's time to work." Tabin promised that if he was allowed back in, he'd devote himself unstintingly to his studies. "If you pull anything like this again," Federman said, relenting, "don't count on coming back."

By his third year of medical school, Tabin had restricted his climbing to weekend trips in Vermont or New Hampshire; when he needed a quick fix, he'd scale the stone embankment next to his local train station, drawing amused comments from commuters who watched his progress until their trains arrived. Most important, Tabin was excelling academically, and he worked hard to regain the faculty's faith that he was dedicated to a career in medicine.

Until the phone call came from Death-Pact Dan.

Dan Reid told Tabin that they'd obtained another permit to attempt the Kangshung Face in the fall. He said that *National Geographic* had signed on to be their principal sponsor and six climbers were already on board. "Let's go get on top of that bastard!" he said.

The language Tabin used when he went to meet with his faculty adviser, to ask for another leave of absence, was considerably more polite. As Tabin recalls, the response from Dr. Michael Wiedman, an ophthalmologist on Harvard's faculty, was not. "You, young man, have to be the most mentally deficient student ever admitted to Harvard Medical School," he said. "This august institution would never permit you to leave simply to climb a mountain. But, as I'm sure you're aware, Harvard has a long and illustrious tradition of sending its students out in the world to do medical research. You're planning on traveling to Tibet to conduct 'field research,'" he said, winking at Tabin. "Right?"

Wiedman shared Tabin's enthusiasm for mountains. He had once trekked to Everest base camp and was interested in high altitude's effect on the eye. It was difficult to gather data from extreme heights, and Wiedman saw the expedition as an ideal research opportunity; Tabin could assist him by examining the eyes of his team members as their climb progressed. Wiedman was curious whether any evidence of retinal hemorrhaging Tabin might observe could predict whether climbers would later suffer cerebral or pulmonary edema, the flooding of the skull or lungs with fluid that endangered many mountaineers. He gave Tabin basic training in the use of an ophthalmoscope, so he could examine and photograph his teammates' eyes at altitude, and his blessing to pursue the dream of conquering Everest's most intimidating face.

The next fall, Tabin arrived in base camp wearing two hats: those of climber and of ocular researcher. Dan Reid wore even more. He arrived as the team doctor, as an aspiring summiteer, and as a fully kitted-out representative of his Scottish heritage. He'd brought a formal kilt to wear whenever he wasn't actually climbing and had also embroidered the phrase THE LITTLE ENGINE THAT COULD on all of his gear.

This time Tabin arrived in peak physical condition. To test his stamina, he says, he sprinted across New Hampshire's Presidential Range in four hours, a route that often takes hikers two days. He jogged the five miles between his apartment and Harvard twice every school day, detouring to sprint up and down the steps of the football stadium. He climbed every weekend. He ran the Boston Marathon and had so much energy left after crossing the finish line that he drove to New Hampshire and completed a five-pitch climb later that afternoon.

Tabin arrived at base camp prepared and confident. Older masters he'd clicked with on his previous trip, like George Lowe and Lou Reichardt, had returned. Jim Morrissey, the cardiologist who had escorted Sir Edmund Hillary to safety, led the expedition. "Jim was the perfect leader for this kind of trip," Tabin says. "He had vast experience, lots of common sense, and because he was primarily a doctor, he didn't have a climbing ego that would clash with the rest of the team."

But when Tabin saw the younger professional climbers wandering around base camp, shirtless, he felt his confidence waver. "Kim Momb, Carl Tobin, Carlos Buhler, and Dave Cheesmond did nothing but climb full-time, and they looked like miniature versions of the Incredible Hulk," Tabin says. "In my daily life I was used to feeling pretty invincible, but at Everest I realized I was the weakest member of the group."

Relations among the members of the 1983 team proved to be far more harmonious than those of the 1981 expedition. Reichardt once again took the lead, carrying enormous loads. Base camp manager John Boyle arrived with a novel plan to cut down much of the grunt work that had demoralized members of the earlier expedition. Knowing they were climbing from the east, where they would once again be unsupported by native load carriers, Boyle had brought an important ally: a rocket launcher. By firing off a rocket tied to rope from a high point on the Kangshung Face, he hoped to attach the rope to yachting pulleys and a generator, then haul their supplies up into place. The first two launch attempts fizzled. But their last rocket cleared the Kangshung's rock outcroppings, and they were able to ferry hundreds of pounds of rope, fuel, and food up the mountain, saving the climbers dozens of trips.

Tabin's main task was still hauling gear. They had named one narrow ice chute that accessed the top of the face the Bowling Alley, because every day, when it was warmed by the sun, bowling-ball-sized chunks of ice and rock ricocheted down its length. "I raced up it every time as fast as I could, like a scared rabbit," Tabin says.

After depositing one load, Tabin was rappelling down the Bowling Alley when he heard a roar above him. A house-sized block of rock had broken off and was accelerating directly toward the spot where he hung in the center of the chute, as helpless as a bowling pin. "It hit and shattered one hundred feet above me," Tabin says, "and car-sized chunks rained down all around me. I curled up as small as I could and prepared to die." Tabin remembers how blank his mind became as he calmly watched three large pieces scream by within five feet of him, leaving him dangling unscathed, while the acrid gunpowder scent of shattered rock drifted through thin air.

On October 8, after six weeks of labor, the men had their tents and gear positioned at 25,900 feet and a window of perfect weather. Morrissey divided the climbers into three summit teams. The strongest—Reichardt, Momb, and Buhler—would make the first attempt. They set out at 4:00 A.M. By noon, their Chinese interpreter had radioed from base camp to say that he'd spotted climbers ascending the summit ridge through his telescope. In the background, Tabin could clearly hear Tibetans chanting mantras for their success. At 2:45 P.M., Momb's voice crackled over the radio. "We're on top of this fucker!" he said, openly weeping. The three walked the final steps to the summit together, where they spent thirty minutes enjoying the view from the top of the world in air calm enough that they could have lit a candle.

The second party—George Lowe, Dr. Dan Reid, and Jay Cassell—summited the next day. The strongest, Lowe, sped to the top by 10:00 A.M, turned around, and warned Reid and Cassell, whom he met while they were still on their way up, to descend if the weather worsened. Lowe hurried to lower altitude but turned his headlamp on and left it hanging inside a tent for his teammates. Reid and Cassell didn't reach the summit until nearly 4:00 P.M., and more than four hours later, they were still stumbling through darkness and blowing snow. They were arguing about whether they'd descended past their high camp when they spotted the light Lowe had left for them, just beneath the spot where they stood. They collapsed into the tent. Lowe's forethought almost certainly saved their lives.

The window of fine weather had iced over and frozen shut. On October 10, high winds and two feet of new snow meant Tabin had to turn around. "It was agony," he says. "I was elated that we'd succeeded in solving a face many considered impossible. But I'd been waiting my turn for two days. Ever since I'd read Rébuffat's *Starlight and Storm,* I'd taken his mantra to heart: I prefer dreams to memories. And I dreamed of standing on top of the world. Now the weather wasn't going to give me that chance." Morrissey radioed the group remaining at their high camp that their only job now was to get everyone safely off the mountain.

Descending through the Bowling Alley, Tabin slipped, his heavy pack spun him upside down, and he couldn't right himself. As he hung there, helpless, spindrift avalanches swept down the chute, filling his mouth and nose, and he feared he was going to drown. Then the indefatigable Dr. Dan, barely recovered from his summit climb, came to his rescue. "Dan Reid labored back up ropes he'd already descended, untangled me, and saved my life," Tabin says.

"We weren't the strongest group of American climbers you could have put together that year," Jim Morrissey told me, still a confident, commanding presence in his mid-sixties, wearing a blue blazer and a crimson tie embossed with a logo of the Khangshung Face.

"But we were the best *team,*" Lou Reichardt said, finishing Jim's thought before stuffing a seared tuna hors d'oeuvre into his mouth. I was with surviving members of the expedition, who'd met for a reunion in San Francisco.

On the top floor of a skyscraper at dusk, they looked past the tip of a man-made mountain, the Transamerica Pyramid, toward Alcatraz, and raised their glasses to departed friends, including Dr. Dan Reid. He had fallen to his death in 1991, along with his wife, Barbara, on Mount Kenya, the mountain where Tabin had first discovered his ability to climb tough technical routes at altitude. Nearly thirty years after making the first ascent of the Kangshung Face, this tight-knit group of fit middle-aged men still seemed mildly shocked that they'd made it. In the years since their first ascent, no one else had repeated their route.

Tabin survived his headfirst fall while bouldering, his two leaves of absence, and his two brushes with death in the Bowling Alley to graduate from Harvard Medical School in 1985. The high-altitude ocular data he collected on Everest became the basis of several papers he published with Professor Wiedman. But Tabin wasn't planning a career in ophthalmology. He figured the best way to combine his interests in outdoor adventure and medicine was to become an orthopedic surgeon, perhaps eventually establishing a practice in a mountain town.

While his classmates had been preparing single-mindedly for specialized careers, Tabin had alienated the medical establishment with his serial escapes to the mountains. "The way they saw it, I was an unreliable loose cannon," he says. His applications for residencies in orthopedic surgery were all rejected.

Tabin enrolled as a general surgical resident at the University of Colorado. His disappointment was tempered by his proximity to his favorite climbing partner from Everest, George Lowe, who offered an escape hatch from the grind of hospital rounds. Lowe would collect Tabin after his overnight shifts in the emergency room, feed him thermoses of strong coffee, and fly him in his single-engine plane to sandstone pinnacles in the deserts of eastern Utah. The Aspen mountaineer Neal Beidleman would often join them on these outings.

In the clarifying desert light, Tabin was able, for a few hours at a time, to empty his head of the gunshot and knife wounds he'd treated the night before by narrowing his concerns to the precise placement of fingertips and toes on sunbaked rock.

Beth Peterson, a second-year resident in Denver, remembers how distinct Tabin's bearing was from that of the other doctors. "Geoff was always bubbling with energy and wit and focused like a laser beam on his patients. His joyfulness and ability to completely inhabit the present is unique among humans, not just first-year residents. I was wowed by him."

One evening, as they were leaving the hospital in a dense snowstorm, she mentioned that she needed a ride. "I'm taking you to dinner," Tabin said, inhabiting the moment in a matter of seconds. Their romantic relationship would last six years.

Peterson had run away, briefly, from the medical establishment herself. She'd come to Denver fresh from a year she'd spent in a bungalow without electricity or running water among the rice paddies of central Bali on a Henry Luce scholarship. "Officially, I was researching public health in Indonesia. But really," she says, "I just needed a break before deciding if I wanted to dedicate my life to becoming a surgeon." Once word spread that she was a doctor, however, Peterson was besieged by patients, who lined up outside her door every morning. She enjoyed ministering to the unpredictable problems her patients brought to her so thoroughly that she returned to America to begin her residency.

Tabin adored Peterson and Denver's proximity to mountains. But after his first year in Denver, he snapped at the opportunity to transfer to a prestigious orthopedic residency at the Michael Reese Hospital, at the University of Chicago. He and Peterson continued dating long-distance, while he tried to devote himself to his chosen specialty. "Geoff was not only a risk taker physically, but his social behavior was risky as well," Peterson says. "Even though he only wanted what was good for his patients, he could be blinded by his sense that everyone should be enjoying themselves all the time. And he seemed unaware that a lot of forces in adult life drag you down. You could already sense that he wasn't going to fit in a formal medical community."

Tabin was nearly booted out of Reese when his antics in the emergency room were reported to the head nurse. The mother of a six-year-old boy with an injured arm had brought her son to Tabin for treatment. She seemed unusually devout, praying fervently for her son's arm to heal. "So I just sort of went with the flow," Tabin says. He examined the boy's arm and recognized that he was suffering a dislocation common among young children called "radial head subluxation."

"The cool thing," Tabin explains, "was it was an injury you can cure simply by pulling on the arm and popping the bones back into place." Tabin put the booming theatrics of a faith healer into his voice as he sat his patient in his mother's lap and swept his hands dramatically over the entranced boy's arm. "Sweet Lord Jesus!" he chanted. "We need a miracle! I'm imploring you to help this boy heal!" he shouted, grabbing the boy by the wrist and tugging his elbow joint firmly into place until he heard the telltale pop that indicated the procedure had been successful. The child was distracted by Tabin's theatrics and laughed, flexing his healed arm happily. "Praise Jesus!" Tabin hollered. "But let's confirm the miracle by X-ray."

Summoned to the chairman of orthopedics' office the next day, Tabin was contrite, promising to curtail faith healing in the future, but he was genuinely baffled that such a satisfying and successful interaction with a patient could be grounds for his dismissal. As he progressed through his residency, Tabin became increasingly concerned that he'd chosen the wrong career. "It was nice to be near my parents in Chicago, but I missed the mountains," he says. "I wasn't finding the work all that fulfilling, and, for the first time in my life, I wasn't where I wanted to be, or even on a path toward someplace I could imagine being genuinely happy."

Tabin put out feelers, itching once again for adventure, inquiring whether any of his climbing buddies knew of an expedition that needed his medical skills. In the summer of 1988, halfway through his residency, the invitation to serve as team doctor for a group trying to put the first American woman on the summit of Everest came just in the nick of time, as Tabin saw it. His colleagues at the hospital viewed his plan to rush back to the Himalaya somewhat differently. "They told me I was crazy, that if I walked out on an orthopedics residency I'd be blackballed from medicine for life."

Tabin called Beth Peterson and asked her advice.

"I was Geoff's best friend the whole time he wavered between medicine and mountaineering," she says. "Of all the people I've known, Geoff has listened most carefully to his inner voices. I knew he'd already made up his mind, so I told him to follow his heart."

The Lhotse Face is an immense snowfield that rises nearly four thousand feet toward the summit ridge of Everest. Tabin trudged up it, setting his crampons carefully into sun-warmed snow the consistency of Styrofoam. He paused to check his pulse and says he was delighted to learn that even though he was climbing above twenty thousand feet, his heart rate barely exceeded his resting pulse at sea level. After six and a half hours, Tabin joined his potential summit partner, Nima Tashi Sherpa, in his tent just after 2:00 P.M.

Two days earlier, Tabin's teammate Stacy Allison had reached the summit, quickly achieving the expedition's goal. "Like Dr. Dan, who was supposed to be a team physician but insisted on climbing, I'd argued I was of more use to the team if I stayed high on the mountain, where they were most likely to need urgent medical care. That was true," Tabin says, "but I also knew it meant I was more likely to get a shot at the summit."

Tabin crawled into a small tent at the high camp he'd leave later that night to make his summit bid, feeling strong but unbearably thirsty. Nima Tashi handed him a bowl of noodle soup, flecked with hot chilies, which Tabin devoured; then Nima served him seconds. "I felt fantastic but tired," Tabin says. "I asked Nima if he'd melt snow so we'd have water for our summit attempt while I slept for three hours; then I'd do the same while he rested."

Tabin woke and glanced at his watch, which said 11:00 P.M., then at Nima Tashi. "Why didn't you wake me?" Tabin asked.

"It's okay," the Sherpa said, grinning, and handed Tabin a thermos full of hot tea.

"The Sherpa belong to the Nyingmapa sect of Tibetan Buddhism," Tabin says. "They believe in delaying nirvana for themselves until everyone on earth is able to achieve happiness. I can't think of more delightful companions to be with on a big mountain. Nima had sacrificed his own sleep so I could have seven blissful hours of uninterrupted rest."

They melted more water and set out at 2:00 A.M. The batteries in Tabin's headlamp died just as a full moon rose over the horizon, spotlighting Everest's highest ramparts as brightly as if it were day. Tabin climbed confidently along a two-foot-wide ridge, avoiding the fixed ropes so he could move faster. Beyond a fragile cornice running along the eastern edge, twelve thousand feet of empty air separated him from the camp where he'd twice attempted to reach this ridge from Tibet. "After all this time," Tabin says, "I knew I was going to make it, to fulfill a lifelong dream. The feeling was indescribable."

The summit of Everest was a rectangular platform of ice, six by three feet across. "The size of a small desk," Tabin says. He climbed on top of it just after 10:00 A.M., stamped his crampons into the ice, and leaned into the wind, savoring the view. He saw the burned-looking brown Tibetan plateau he had trekked across years earlier on his way to the Kangshung Face, saw how it dropped away and vanished beyond the curvature of the earth. He saw morning sun lick like flames at the peaks of five of the world's eight highest mountains. "For fifteen minutes, until Nima Tashi arrived," Tabin says, "I was the highest person on earth."

Trekking back toward Kathmandu, Tabin enjoyed the same floating sensation he'd had on his first memorable hike to Everest from Tibet. His career in high-powered American medicine had once again gone off the rails, so after celebrating in Kathmandu with his teammates, he decided to linger in Nepal. He volunteered to work at a small medical clinic Sir Edmund Hillary had built in the mountain village of Phaplu, on one of the less-traveled trekking routes in the Khumbu. Tabin made himself useful, and he found some satisfaction setting broken bones and treating respiratory infections. "But there was just so much sickness and poverty and need," he says, "and I felt frustrated by how little I could do to change it."

While he was practicing general medicine, Tabin met a group of Dutch eye surgeons conducting cataract surgery in a nearby village. "I introduced myself and asked if I could watch what they were doing," he says. He saw the doctors examine a silver-haired Sherpa woman named Dolma, whose milky cataracts were large enough to be diagnosed even by a doctor with no training in ophthalmology. For three years, her vision had been limited to discerning between light and dark. Tabin had visited his summit partner Nima Tashi's family on his way down from Everest. He was familiar with how difficult conditions were, even for the sighted, in Sherpa villages. "I thought about the narrow stone trails we'd been walking on, the swaying bridges I'd had to cross, and couldn't imagine how a blind person could survive in a place like this."

Tabin observed Dolma's cataract surgery. And the next afternoon he saw the doctors remove her bandages. "The day before, she hadn't even been able to detect a hand waving in front of her face," Tabin says. "I watched her see the faces of her grandchildren clearly for the first time. And as I looked at the tears of joy running down her face, I knew exactly what it was I wanted to do with my life. I wanted to restore sight. But ophthalmology is one of the most competitive specialties in medicine, and I knew with my checkered history, I didn't have a prayer of getting admitted to another residency."

For the next few years, Tabin set his dream aside and focused on mountaineering. He wrote an outdoor adventure column for *Penthouse* magazine called "View from the Top." He swerved far from his medical career and cobbled together work as a climbing guide, leading paying customers to the top of Antarctica's Mount Vinson, Alaska's Denali, Argentina's Mount Aconcagua, and Tanzania's Kilimanjaro.

In 1985, Dick Bass, the founder of the Snowbird ski resort, became the first person to climb the highest mountain on each of the seven continents. Since Tabin had already reached the top of the most remote, Carstensz Pyramid, and climbed six of the seven peaks, he decided he'd like to join the exclusive club Bass had founded.

He organized a trip to the Caucasus Mountains of western Russia during the summer solstice of 1990 and invited four favorite clients he'd guided to come celebrate with him at the top of the highest point in Europe, an 18,510-foot dormant volcano named Mount Elbrus. On June 22, 1990, in a stiff wind, Geoff Tabin stood atop Elbrus, at the peak of his climbing career, the fourth person ever to complete the Seven Summits.

The comedown from such a monumental achievement can be disorienting, even depressing. Tabin tried to embrace his career as a rogue, a refugee from medicine's linear predictability. He even carried business cards he'd had printed that read, GEOFF TABIN: BUM. Climbing the Seven Summits had been the adventure of several lifetimes. It should have been more than enough for his only orbit through life. But Tabin kept picturing the ecstatic face of the no-longer-blind Sherpa woman named Dolma and realized he wanted to help others like her more than he wanted to climb any mountain. He couldn't help wondering if there wasn't an eighth summit he might aim for, an achievement not of an individual nature but of a more universal, more meaningful sort. It had to be out there, past the horizon, beyond the curvature of his dormant career in medicine, someplace he could happily stand with his feet firmly grounded.

Beth Peterson, meanwhile, had hewed to her chosen career track and moved back to her native North Carolina to train in plastic surgery. "Whenever I saw Geoff, I encouraged him to climb and guide because I knew that made him happy," she says. "But when I realized he was feeling remorseful about possibly being out of medicine forever, I kept my eyes open for possibilities."

In the winter of 1991, at Utah's Snowbird ski resort, where Dick Bass had invited Peterson and Tabin, his fellow Seven Summiteer, for a ski vacation, Peterson was riding a chairlift toward the ski area's high alpine terrain when she struck up a conversation with a man who said he was at Snowbird for an ophthalmology conference. Her seatmate, in fact, was Arthur Geltzer, a retinal surgeon who taught at Brown University's medical school.

"My boyfriend graduated from Harvard," she told him. "He wants to get into ophthalmology, but he's led such an unconventional life I don't think anyone would admit him."

"Tell me more," Geltzer said.

"Well, he actually did some research on high altitude's effect on the retina for Harvard Medical School. He's a brilliant doctor. But really," she said laughing, "he's just a bum. All he does is climb mountains."

Geltzer said he was particularly interested in the effect of high altitude on the eye and told Peterson that he'd read several fascinating papers about retinal hemorrhaging at altitude predicting edema that had been written by Dr. Mike Wiedman at Harvard.

Peterson sensed the machinery of fate spinning combinations until they clicked, unlocking a bolt. She put her shoulder to the door and pushed. "Geoff did all the field research for Dr. Wiedman's papers. While he was climbing Everest," she said. "You should meet him."

"I suppose it wouldn't hurt to have a drink," Geltzer said.

No matter how far he traveled from the world's highest peaks, regardless of how single-minded he tried to be about medicine, the mountains always seemed to seek Tabin out. Brown University, where Tabin began his ophthalmic residency on July 1, 1991, was located in Providence, Rhode Island; the highest point in the state was only 812 feet above sea level. And for much of his first year, Tabin felt a long way from the Himalaya. But the distance evaporated in the instant it took him to tear open the letter from his Everest summit partner, which arrived during his second year of study.

"Dr. Geoff, I've had a great misfortune," Nima Tashi wrote, the anguish evident in his language. "I've broken the wrists of both legs!" He explained that he'd narrowly survived a fall while carrying a triple load of kerosene down a snowy pass during a storm and it had taken him several painful weeks of travel before he was able to see a doctor. The Nepalese surgeons he consulted said there was nothing they could do to repair his legs.

Tabin split the cost of Nima Tashi's plane ticket to Rhode Island with one of his climbing partners, Pete Athans, who had been in Nepal at the time of the accident. And Tabin shared his apartment in Providence with the Sherpa while he recuperated from lengthy operations Tabin arranged for him with his friend Ken Kamler, an orthopedic surgeon. Kamler was able to reassemble one of Nima Tashi's ankles but had to fuse the other, since it was so badly shattered that repairing it wasn't possible. Trying to be helpful after he was once again able to walk, Nima Tashi insisted on accompanying Tabin on his clinical rounds and carrying his medical bags. "Patients would ask, 'Who's he?'" Tabin remembers. "I'd just say, 'That's my Sherpa' and continue treating them without mentioning him again, as if all ophthalmologists were issued one, like a stethoscope or slit lamp."

Tabin felt as committed to ophthalmology as he'd been conflicted about his adventures in other medical specialties. At Brown he decided to pursue a competitive fellowship in corneal surgery. His commitment to the woman who'd supported him during his wanderings through the medical wilderness was less absolute. Beth Peterson finished her training in her chosen specialty—pediatric plastic surgery—and moved to Spokane, Washington, where she opened a successful private practice. "Why didn't Geoff and I end up together? I'm not sure I know the answer to that," Peterson says. "Geoff was really there when he was there. When we were apart, he was more committed to living in the moment. It made me sad. But I understood."

At Brown, in his mid-thirties, Tabin spent more than a year romantically entangled with an undergraduate tennis prodigy named Anna Sloan, though he never formally broke off his relationship with Peterson. Sloan and Tabin moved in together after Nima Tashi returned to Nepal, and Tabin says he was blindsided when she abruptly broke up with him days after her graduation. "You're a great guy, Geoff," she told him, "but I just don't see what sort of future we could have together. I don't know that you could really be there for anyone."

"I was really wounded, and it took me a while to shake it off," Tabin says. But pressed to explain how he'd drifted from Peterson to Sloan, and then on to the next series of women he dated, Tabin is uncharacteristically at a loss for words. Being able to restore sight, as he'd seen the Dutch doctors do, was a goal he trained obsessively to reach, and reaching it came at a cost: the self-absorption Anna Sloan wasn't willing to accept.

Tabin learned that he would be admitted to train in his chosen specialty, as a corneal fellow, at Johns Hopkins. But at an American Academy of Ophthalmology meeting Tabin attended in the spring of 1994, before moving to Baltimore, he met Hugh Taylor, who had accompanied Fred Hollows on his research trips to Australia's outback and had helped gather the data that had proved that Australia's aboriginal population received third-world-quality medical care. Tabin was anxious to impress a man of Taylor's stature, especially one who'd managed to forge a career as both a respected academic and an agent of social change, the kind of career Tabin longed to create for himself.

There is a certain type of sly, knowing smile that creeps onto a person's face when you first ask about their history with Geoff Tabin. It was there on the face of the dignified sixty-year-old academic in gold-rimmed glasses when I brought up the subject of his former corneal fellow during a visit to Melbourne's Royal Victorian Eye and Ear Hospital. "You know, the only time I was ever thrown out of a topless bar was in the company of Geoff Tabin," Taylor said, laughing. "When I met him in America, I was drawn to his passion," he added. "And he didn't shy away from promoting the part of himself that he thought would interest me most. Geoff front-loaded our conversation by telling me that he'd published lots of articles, and mentioned he'd climbed a few mountains. I later found out that most of the publishing he'd done wasn't medical but adventure pieces he'd written for *Penthouse* magazine. And those few mountains he mentioned were the toughest and highest in the world."

Taylor had helped found Johns Hopkins's Dana Center for Preventive Ophthalmology, and he'd taught there for more than a decade before returning to Australia. He told Tabin that, in his opinion, the cornea program he currently ran at the University of Melbourne was the finest in the world. Taylor invited Tabin, on the spot, to join him as one of only two fellows he accepted each year.

"Don't you want to see my transcripts?" Tabin asked.

"If you're good enough for Hopkins, you're good enough for me," Taylor replied. "Whaddya say? Want to come work with me down under?"

CHAPTER 11

If You Can Dream

Many politicians and anthropologists, it seems to me, deal in and accentuate the differences between people. I think it's more helpful, and it certainly behooves a doctor, to emphasize our common humanity—even if some people don't like to be reminded of their kinship with others.
—Fred Hollows

"We've got a guest, newly arrived to Australia," Fred Hollows said, propping his elbows on his oversized kitchen table. "He may be an ace in the operating room, but can he hold his liquor?" Hollows, as usual, was surrounded by the crowd of drinkers, artists, civil rights activists, and opposition politicians who often lingered at his home into the night or lived for a time in his mansion's many rooms. "Bottoms up, fella. Save that long, serious face for the hospital and finish your whiskey!"

Ruit drained half his glass and put it down delicately on the table, hoping no one noticed how drunk he was. But he needn't have worried. He was the most sober person in Farnham House's chaotic kitchen. Fred Hollows squinted disapprovingly at Ruit's shot glass and refilled it. "I said bottoms up, Sandook!" Hollows roared. "No half measures here!" Ruit picked up the glass, eased it to his lips, and disposed of the whiskey in a single gulp.

The applause woke Farnham House's resident poet, Max Williams, who'd been snoring with his head down on the kitchen table next to an ashtray overflowing with Hollows's spent pipe tobacco. He rubbed his eyes, refilled his glass, and, after lubricating his throat, recited a fragment of his favorite Kipling, which, he said, had kept his spirit from breaking during the years he'd languished in prison, after his previous, unprofitable career as a burglar and petty thief:

> If you can keep your head when all about you
> Are losing theirs and blaming it on you;
> If you can trust yourself when all men doubt you,
> But make allowance for their doubting too . . .
>
> If you can dream—and not make dreams your master;
> If you can think—and not make thoughts your aim;
> If you can meet with Triumph and Disaster
> And treat those two impostors just the same;
> If you can bear to hear the truth you've spoken
> Twisted by knaves to make a trap for fools,
> Or watch the things you gave your life to, broken,
> And stoop and build 'em up with worn-out tools . . .
>
> If you can talk with crowds and keep your virtue,
> Or walk with kings—nor lose the common touch,
> If neither foes nor loving friends can hurt you,
> If all men count with you, but none too much;
> If you can fill the unforgiving minute
> With sixty seconds' worth of distance run—
> Yours is the Earth and everything that's in it,
> And—which is more—you'll be a Man, my son!

"Mightn't you men turn the volume down a notch?" said Gabi Hollows, leaning in from the dark sunporch where she'd been sitting under a lamp, reading the same sentence of a novel over and over as the din from the kitchen escalated. "We have a gentlewoman fresh from Nepal sleeping in the next room who's not used to your lack of manners."

Farnham House stood on a bluff in Sydney's leafy Randwick suburb, a short walk from the Prince of Wales Hospital, where Hollows ran the Department of Ophthalmology, and to one of the city's most freewheeling public spaces, Coogee Beach. Before arriving in Australia, neither Ruit nor Nanda had ever seen the ocean, except from the window of a plane.

The first day they arrived, Gabi strolled down to the sea with her guests, anxious to show off her city and witness the mountain people's first exposure to white sand and warm blue water. "Sanduk stuck his toes in a bit," Gabi remembers, "and Nanda was far too modest to go for a swim. They glanced at the ocean like they'd seen it every day. But what really shocked them was the sight of two women kissing, just down the beach. Not the sort of thing you'd see in Nepal, I imagine."

Freedom. It was both a shock and a blessing to the Ruits when they arrived in 1987 to spend a year in one of the world's most spirited cities. "In Kathmandu," Nanda says, "especially in those days, you were always thinking about caste and religion, and you were conscious of everyone's eyes on you at all times. At Fred and Gabi's, we were free from all of that. Once we adjusted, it was like the honeymoon we never had."

Farnham House had a history as unconventional as Hollows's own. Since the construction of the sprawling sandstone mansion in the 1850s, it had been a brothel, a boardinghouse, and a convent for the order of the Sisters of Loreto. When Hollows bought it, it was a wreck; the once grand residence was divided into seven flats containing eleven refrigerators. The tin roof leaked badly, and the grounds were overgrown with brambles.

Hollows went to work tearing down the partitions, removing the refrigerators, patching the roof, and restoring the house to a state of disorderly grandeur. He left the frescoes nuns had painted in the hallways and filled the rooms with books and the furniture he built in his basement workshop. But he had no interest in turning Farnham House into anything like a normal home. Hollows distrusted the institution of the nuclear family, and he felt that small families tended to tear each other apart. He conceived of his home as an alternative, a place where a large, revolving cast of characters would keep life interesting and tension to a minimum.

As a student in New Zealand, Hollows attended Bible college and was considering seminary school when he got a summer job as an orderly at a mental hospital. "Before that, I had assumed that life outside of the church . . . was the slippery path to perdition," he wrote in the autobiography he produced with Peter Cornis. "I'd had a proper job done on me, and I'd gone along with it. Working in that place for a couple of months completely changed my life." Hollows was strongly influenced by the other attendants. They were "rough, knockabout blokes . . . some who'd been in the war. But they were . . . kind and gentle. I never saw one of them display any spleen or antagonism towards the inmates, no matter what the provocation. It was amazing. Those men were good and religion had nothing to do with it. I found out what secular goodness was."

Hollows returned to college determined to embrace earthly life and pursue a career in medicine. "Sex, alcohol and secular goodness are pretty keen instruments," he wrote, "and they surgically removed my Christianity, leaving no scars."

After training in the United Kingdom as an ophthalmologist, Hollows headed back beneath the equator, for a job as a professor at Sydney's University of New South Wales. He performed surgery and instructed ophthalmic residents at the university's Prince of Wales Hospital. But it was the work he did outside the hospital walls that made him one of the most famous people in Australia. Living in Sydney, Hollows knew in a vague way that there was a basic "disequity," as he put it, between the lives of white Australians and those of the native aboriginal population. When he began traveling the interior of the continent, to conduct a national survey on the scope of the eye disease trachoma among aborigines, his goals in life took another turn.

Trachoma is an infection of the mucous membrane lining the eyelid. It's caused primarily by unsanitary living conditions and is easily treated. If trachoma is allowed to progress to the stage where it leaves lasting scars on the cornea, it causes blindness. At nearly every stop in the outback, Hollows found entire communities suffering from advanced trachoma.

Hollows thought that he'd seen every eye condition in existence. When he started examining patients in aboriginal settlements, "it was like something out of the medical history books," he wrote, "eye diseases of a kind and degree that hadn't been seen in Western society for generations! The neglect this implied, the suffering and wasted quality of [human lives] was appalling."

Hugh Taylor was one of Hollows's lieutenants on the survey, and has since become one of the world's leading academic ophthalmologists. "I was led astray at an early age by Fred, and I've been astray ever since," Taylor told me over cups of bracingly strong espresso at his Melbourne office, sitting in front of a wall of framed photos of a younger, sunburned version of himself. In one, he and Hollows sit on the tailgate of a Range Rover streaked with bright red dust, smoking their pipes meditatively. "When it rained in the outback it was like trying to drive through chocolate mousse. But the biggest obstacle to our work was the attitude of the white cattle station managers. I came across aboriginal patients who were called Spider, or Airplane, or Potato Chip, by drunk station managers who were too lazy to learn their real names. You have to remember that aborigines were only granted Australian citizenship in 1967, and these men seemed to think they were worth less than their livestock. I remember one big, tough white bloke walking over to us as we were beginning to examine aboriginal patients, and saying, 'I've got cows that could use your help. Why waste your time on our niggers?' But what we found—some communities with trachoma follicles in eighty percent of the aboriginal children—caused a scandal that changed the country."

Fanning the flames of outrage, Hollows championed the creation of a national aboriginal health service, the most important improvement to aboriginal living conditions in Australia's history. Dry data about the prevalence of eye disease wasn't about to capture the nation's attention, so Hollows held press conferences after he returned home, publicity stunts aimed at shaming Australian politicians. "Fred liked getting up the noses of people, especially powerful people," Taylor said.

At his press conferences, Hollows gave the kind of crisp, angry reports from the field that were guaranteed to capture headlines. He recalled one of the first visits to an aboriginal settlement that got his blood pumping about disequity. "I examined a hundred and fifty black fellows sitting by Watti Creek and found the amount of eye disease you'd need to look at about a million and a half whites to discover," he said. *So what are you going to do about it? Are you willing to live in an Australia where much of the population is forced to live like dogs?* were the unspoken questions that hung in the air after each of his public appearances.

The political establishment tried to mollify Hollows by offering him the nation's highest honor, the Order of Australia, for his work. He turned it down. "My God," he wrote in his autobiography, and in letters he sent to Australia's leading politicians, "this is not the time to be accepting accolades for pointing out problems in Aboriginal health." It was time, in other words, to take action to fix them.

Among the medical workers accompanying Hollows to the outback was a striking orthoptist, a specialist in visual disorders that primarily affect children, named Gabi O'Sullivan. Hollows was immediately attracted to her. "Gabi must have examined two hundred people that day, and she was as soothing and agreeable to the two hundredth as she had been to the first. I noticed something else: Gabi's tone of voice, manner and body language didn't change, whether she was dealing with the station manager or the oldest, most withered Aborigine in the camp. That kind of innate goodness is rare," Hollows wrote. Rare enough that Hollows felt extraordinarily lucky when Gabi agreed to marry him.

The naturally shy Nanda was also lucky to have Gabi as her host. As perhaps the most talkative citizen of Sydney, the aptly named Gabi set Nanda at ease, smoothing over hiccups in her emerging English and filling any uncomfortable lulls in the conversation with lighthearted chatter. "Gabi was so kind you can't imagine," Nanda says. "She knew Sanduk and I couldn't afford to do much in a city as expensive as Sydney. So she was always slipping us pocket money and changing the subject when I tried to thank her."

Ruit was less interested in sightseeing than in exploring a first-world medical facility. He seized the opportunity to work with the latest technology at the Prince of Wales Hospital. "From my side, I don't think I needed training so much as real access to resources," Ruit says.

Hugh Taylor agrees. "It was obvious from the moment you watched him that Ruit was going to be a superstar," he remembers. The cases Ruit treated at the Prince of Wales were much less challenging than those he saw in Nepal, but having an unlimited supply of intraocular lenses, and first-rate microscopes, he was free to experiment. He streamlined his technique, hoping to return home having perfected a simplified form of the surgery, appropriate to practice in the villages of Nepal, where resources would be scarce.

After Ruit returned to Nepal, he used and taught many of the Prince of Wales Hospital's surgical techniques. But when Hollows flew to Nepal and looked in on Ruit's progress, he was amazed to learn that Ruit had improved and refined so many of Hollows's own methods for operating on cataracts that the Prince of Wales Hospital adopted his improvements and renamed their style of cataract surgery the "Nepal technique."

"Spending a year in Australia was a wonderful way for Nanda and me to really fall in love, from both sides," Ruit says. "We had time to talk and talk and talk. But Nepal was our home. Nanda said our battle-field had to be there, and I agreed. All the while we were in Sydney I thought about what to do when we returned. My duties at the Prince of Wales were not too taxing, and I had time to plot and plan how I wanted to change eye care in Nepal. Being away, it became clear to me that I had to break off on my own when I got back and start my own center. So what was my plan? I was a mosquito, buzzing in Fred and Gabi's ears the whole time we were there, asking for help to make that happen."

Before he left, Ruit and Gabi founded a modest organization dedicated to raising funds to support Ruit's dream. They named it the Nepal Eye Program Australia. Ruit and Tim Macartney-Snape, who, with his climbing partner, Greg Mortimer, had been the first Australians to summit Everest, spoke at a small fund-raiser they organized. And at the end of the evening, Ruit had $500 of seed money to establish NEPA in Nepal.

After a year of intoxicating freedom at Farnham House, the Ruits returned home with a duffel bag full of intraocular lenses and microsurgical instruments, Hollows's parting gift. Sonam, who was the first family member to accept his son's mixed marriage, left his shopkeeper's life in Dhankuta and bought a narrow lot in central Kathmandu. He built a three-story structure, leased out the ground floor to a camera and copy shop called Archie's Photo, and moved his family in. Sonam and Kasang lived on the top floor; Ruit and a pregnant Nanda moved into the one-bedroom flat one floor below.

It was a dank, depressing place, with little natural light and limited ventilation. When they cracked open the small windows, the fetid scent of the Bagmati River seeped into the crowded rooms from across the street, mingling with the fumes drifting upstairs from film-processing chemicals. But it was a home of their own. And in July 1989, after Nanda gave birth to their first child, a boy named Sagar, which means "ocean of happiness" in Sanskrit, Ruit's relatives began to visit.

Nanda's family was slower to accept the mixed marriage. A few of her relatives arrived, bearing sweets and baby clothes, but Nanda's parents continued to keep their distance. Nepal's calendar, especially among the Newari, is a kaleidoscope of religious festivals. Being married to a Bhotia meant that Nanda wasn't comfortable celebrating them publicly. Late at night, while a dozing Sagar breathed softly beside them in the bed they all shared, Ruit told Nanda that he was sorry she had to miss so many holidays on his account.

"We're our own festival," she said, kissing her husband passionately, and putting both him and his concerns to sleep.

Satisfied patients are an eye surgeon's best form of advertising, and Ruit's patients were more satisfied than most. While Ruit continued asking Hollows for help establishing an independent eye center, Ruit returned to his position at the Nepal Eye Hospital. Word of his skill spread beyond Kathmandu, and patients began asking for him by name.

One day a handsome young Buddhist monk arrived, accompanying three older monks in matching crimson robes who all suffered from severe cataracts. They had traveled for several days, from Kalimpong, in northern India, and the young monk politely requested that Ruit perform the surgeries. Ruit removed their bandages the following morning, gratified to see that all three monks' eyes appeared clear and free from complications.

Unlike most of his patients, who were often overcome with emotion after their sight was restored, the monks simply smiled, as if noting no difference between the internal world of darkness where they'd been residing and the bright material world to which they'd returned. The young monk bowed to Ruit and led the older men away. Every few months from that point on, small groups of blind monks arrived at the hospital, always accompanied by the handsome young monk, and always requesting Ruit by name. Ruit resolved to ask the young monk more about himself, but he was always too busy between surgery and his clinical work to find the time. One morning, while Ruit was still at the Nepal Eye Hospital, the young monk arrived alone, with a request that the doctor join him and some friends for dinner.

The taxi driver sped through Kathmandu at rush hour, threading skillfully through bullock carts, cycle-rickshaws, and cows that diverted traffic with lordly indifference. They parked in front of a gated colonial-style mansion, in the wealthy Buddhist enclave of Boudha. The number on the gate matched the address the monk had written down for him, but that couldn't be right, Ruit thought.

A servant in formal livery swung the filigreed iron gate open, and an elderly lama in scarlet robes whom Ruit recognized as one of his former patients led him through a set of grand wooden doors carved with designs of dragons, and into the home. The lama, whom the young monk had brought to Ruit with very mature cataracts, wore no glasses and stepped nimbly up a long marble staircase, leading him to a reception room thrumming with conversation.

"His Eminence the Jamgon Kongtrul will see you now," the lama said.

Ruit took a moment to find his bearings. The large room was filled with high-ranking lamas from Nepal and India. Kathmandu businessmen in dark suits and women in jeweled saris and *chubas* stood talking to them, stooped reverently, or waited their turn in line to receive a blessing. On a raised wooden dais at the end of the room, the handsome young monk sat cross-legged, wearing a tall sunflower-colored cap that curved forward like the beak of a bird and embroidered robes of bloodred and unblemished gold. Ruit picked his way toward him through the crowd, conscious of the short-sleeved work shirt he'd worn to what was obviously a dressy affair. He was led to the front of the line.

"Excuse the formality, Dr. Ruit," the Jamgon Kongtrul said, grasping the doctor's hand warmly in both of his. "You know how it is."

Ruit hadn't known. The polite clean-cut monk, who'd humbly shepherded so many patients onto Ruit's operating table, was the Third Jamgon Kongtrul, one of the paramount leaders of Tibetan Buddhism. Ruit knew his story as well as he knew the history of the Walunga, and he imagined how delighted his father, Sonam, would be to see him in such a high lama's presence. The Walunga had migrated over the mountains from central Tibet hundreds of years earlier. The Jamgon Kongtrul had arrived later. Born in 1954, he'd been spirited out of central Tibet by his supporters in 1959, as had the Dalai Lama. He lived in a monastery built for him by his disciples, in northeastern India, where he was renowned for his encyclopedic knowledge of Buddhist scripture, as well as his charitable works. He was also building a monastic retreat called Pullahari in the hills outside of Kathmandu.

A businessman in a sober suit coughed behind Ruit, impatient for his audience. "When all this hubbub dies down, sit next to me at dinner," the Jamgon Kongtrul said, releasing Ruit's hand. "We have a lot to talk about."

In Nepal, more than 90 percent of the population subsists on two meals of rice and dal a day, garnished, perhaps, with a bit of meat or whatever boiled vegetables are available. Ruit was part of that group. But what waited for him this evening, on a long, starched saffron-colored tablecloth in the home of a wealthy donor, could only be called a feast. There were plates of onion, pumpkin, and lotus root *pakoras*, fried in batter as light as clouds. Uniformed servers placed steaming curries and biryanis of cauliflower, potatoes, peas, almonds, and golden currants in a row of silvery chafing dishes.

"Please, Doctor," the Jamgon Kongtrul said from his seat at the head of the table, ladling cauliflower curry onto Ruit's plate. He sat on a plush cushion that elevated his head above the other diners', but otherwise he wore his authority with humility. Only after Ruit had taken a mouthful did he begin to speak in earnest: "I asked you to come here tonight because we've been watching you for some time. You've not only restored sight to many of my monks, but I've noticed you treat your patients with true compassion. You've done so much for us already. Will you allow me to ask for more?"

"Of course," Ruit said.

"I've heard about the hospital you hope to build, how it will serve people in far-flung areas. I'd like to help you reach patients near my home. And in Tibet, too. The need is very great. Are you willing to travel so far?

"Very willing," Ruit said.

He returned to Nanda that evening in a daze, with a painfully full belly, an invitation to conduct cataract surgery for the needy in Kalimpong, near the lama's home, and the profound gratitude of one of the Buddhist leaders he respected most. There had been days since Ruit had formed his plan to leave the Nepal Eye Hospital and found his own facility when the risks he would take by breaking with his country's medical establishment worried him, days when pinpricks of doubt pierced the surface of his certainty. This wasn't one of them.

Ruit began recruiting like-minded medical personnel to his cause. He thought about patients like Kamisya Tamang, about the distance they had to travel to reach his operating table, and became more determined than ever to set out and serve them where they lived. He gathered the young ophthalmic technicians, nurses, and orderlies he judged to be the hospital's brightest and most dedicated staff, including Nabin Rai, an ambitious ophthalmic technician who had completed a degree in economics before changing fields, and a Brahman scrub nurse named Beena Sharma. He brewed an extra-large batch of tea and set out a plate of expensive Indian-made butter biscuits to sweeten the recruitment he planned to attempt. After the group had arranged themselves in a circle on the floor of his apartment, he called the meeting to order.

"I know all of you have good jobs," he said, "and good jobs in Nepal aren't easy to find. Now I'm going to ask you to put your careers little bit at risk. I asked you here because all of you really seem to care about your patients. But the hospital won't allow us to help the people who need our services most, those who are too poor to come to Kathmandu."

Then Ruit laid out his plan to begin conducting surgical camps in Nepal's underserved rural areas and, eventually, build his own hospital. Enough funds had accrued in NEPA's coffers by then that Ruit had been able to purchase surgical supplies and a portable Konan brand surgical microscope that cost $5,000. With these and the IOLs he'd received from Fred Hollows and other foreign doctors, Ruit would try to provide hospital-quality care to Nepalese in the countryside.

"At the hospital, it was an open secret we were planning to break away," says Beena Sharma. "People asked me, 'You are a Brahman, but your boss will be a Bhotia. How will this work?' I told them, 'Never mind that—I have a social obligation.' I wasn't concerned with caste or money," Sharma says. "I just knew Dr. Ruit would take us to a higher place."

During a long holiday weekend when they would have extra time off, Ruit declared his intention to travel north to the mid-hills, where they would attempt to provide modern cataract surgeries to Tamang people in the farming village of Tepani. "If they can't get to us, it's our duty to go to them," Ruit told his recruits. "I can't guarantee you won't find yourself in some shit with your bosses, but I can see clearly this is the correct path, and I'm asking you to come with me."

Their departure was delayed by their search for a four-wheel-drive vehicle they could afford to rent; in the end, they settled on an aged, sunburst-orange Volkswagen bus that was at least large enough to hold the team and their supplies. The vehicle was crowded with gear, and members of the team took turns riding on the roof.

Sixty miles north of Kathmandu, the VW strained to climb an ungraded dirt road that wound up into the hills. Ruit clutched the roof rack as they swayed over deep ruts, managing barely five miles of progress per hour. They'd planned to arrive just after noon, but it was dark by the time they reached the trailhead to Tepani. Ruit had dispatched an ophthalmic technician to prepare the village for their arrival. Sonam came from a Sherpa family who lived in the hills beyond Tepani, and he knew the area well. He had already screened potential patients and arranged for Ruit's team to operate in the single-room village school.

Sonam had also arranged for seven porters to meet them at the base of the trail. The team found only five thin, surly men, smoking in the dark. The porters insisted that the trail to Tepani was dangerous, that it skirted a deep river gorge, and argued that they shouldn't leave until morning. "In Nepal, porters are often expert cheats," Ruit says. "I presumed they were trying to negotiate and ignored them, pushing everyone to pack up and leave that night." The team choked down a meal of uncooked instant noodles, not wanting to lose the time it would take to make a fire, and set off for Tepani. They had two flashlights for fifteen people. The porters walked ahead with the one that functioned reasonably well. "We had one weak torch for the rest of us," Ruit says. "We couldn't see a thing. We just put our feet down wherever the torchlight went."

To their left they could sense a void and hear a constant roar of either wind or water. "The climb was steep, and we had a lot of young, juicy boys and girls with us," Ruit says. "They'd not seen much difficulty in life, so I had to figure out how to push them, isn't it?" After an hour, when he began to hear grumbling, Ruit deployed his secret weapon. "Sonam was a talented musical boy," Ruit says. "His singing was really palatable to everyone, so I told him we needed to hear the most romantic songs he knew."

"You should not be so cold to me when I'm trying to romance you," Sonam

sang, luring the line of trekkers uphill like a snake charmer with the sinuous allure of his voice. *"Let's talk about love and affection before too long. You are like the rhododendrons on the hillside. Your beautiful colors draw my eyes."*

Ruit couldn't help thinking of Nanda. He'd asked her to stop working after Sagar had been born. Nanda hadn't been happy about it. She'd protested, arguing that if he was going to wage a war, she should be by his side, joining the fight. Despite his maverick approach to eye care, Ruit could be quite conventional socially. He'd insisted that her place was now with Sagar and the rest of the children they hoped to have. Still, marching uphill, away from the home they'd made, he realized how rarely they'd been apart and just how much he missed her. She really was the rhododendron on his hillside, he thought, lost in the romantic spell Sonam had cast in the darkness.

The spell was broken by a fetid scent drifting down the trail that caused him to scrunch up his face in distaste. "Who ever is making such a stench?" Beena Sharma asked in her refined Brahman accent. "If you can't control yourself, move to the back. There's not enough air to breathe up here anyway!" They were still laughing and singing when they arrived in Tepani, just after midnight.

Examining the classroom where they planned to operate the next morning, Ruit was dismayed by the challenge of making it into a sanitary space. He looked at the muddy floor, the cobwebs, and the pile of roughly cut lumber the villagers had gathered for them to cobble together an operating table. Ruit thought of the immaculate Australian operating rooms he'd worked in, and laughed when he imagined the horror a doctor like Fred Hollows would feel if he had to perform surgery in such a place.

His team shared a quick breakfast of boiled ramen noodles. Then, for the next three days, they paused only to eat and sleep. He was gratified to see that the staff he'd chosen proved as energetic as he'd expected. They transformed the filthy classroom into a suitable operating theater, banishing rodent droppings and spiderwebs, nailing surgical drapes over the frames of open windows to keep flies from the patients' eyes, and hanging plastic sheets from the ceiling so dirt and insects couldn't drop from the thatched roof onto the unsteady operating table they hammered together.

Ruit operated over the course of two twelve-hour days, with each case averaging nearly forty minutes. It was hard to keep the room dark enough for the Konan's low-powered lamp, so staff members took turns holding flashlights over the patients so Ruit could see clearly enough to remove the cataracts, slide the artificial lenses into place, and stitch the wounds closed. He was optimistic that the work they were doing, even under such challenging conditions, was solid.

Their last morning in Tepani, Ruit assembled the patients outside. "There was one boy I was really worried about," Ruit says. "He'd come with his mother, but she paid him no attention. He just squatted on the ground, curled up with his head between his legs." The boy wore torn and filthy clothes. And when Ruit asked about him, his mother said they'd stopped sending him to school five years earlier, when he lost his sight. "I hate to say this about my own son," she said. "But it's like living with a stone. He can't work the fields or feed himself. He does nothing but sit by himself. He's just a mouth with no hands."

Ruit removed the boy's bandages anxiously. He knew that the child's quality of life was at stake. Before surgery, when he'd examined him with a penlight, the boy's retinas had flashed red, indicating that they were equipped to process visual information if Ruit removed the opacity that blocked light from reaching the backs of his eyes. He was relieved, after he unrolled the bandages, to see that the boy's eyes looked untraumatized, and Ruit asked, in his slowest and clearest voice, if he could hear him.

"The problem is not with my ears," the boy said.

"Then let's see if your eyes are working," Ruit said. "How many fingers am I holding up?"

"How should I know? Didn't my mother tell you I'm too stupid to count?"

Secretly pleased by the boy's defiance, Ruit moved on to his next patient. "But I kept an eye on him while I was working," Ruit says. "And every time I looked over, it was like watching one of those fast-motion movies of a plant growing. He uncurled. Then stood up straight. Then held his head high. He bloomed like a flower right in front of my eyes. I know his mother saw it, too. She looked at him as if he'd just grown a second head or a third eye. And I knew now he had at least a fighting chance. That we had brought little bit of brightness back into the boy's life."

Tepani is set between huge rock outcroppings, at the edge of a ra-vine dropping down to the Melamchi River. Ruit asked an elderly man he'd operated on if he could see well enough to walk. The man climbed up a curving path to a ledge above the village, then stepped off the trail and picked his way confidently down a treacherous slope of scree until he stood, grinning, face-to-face with Ruit.

"What a moment that was!" Ruit remembers. "With everyone cheering like we'd all performed a magic trick. Can you imagine what it was like to be blind in a place like that? Now dozens of Tamang farmers could return to working their fields, rather than sitting at home all day, burdening their families. For three days we'd pushed ourselves to the edge. But seeing what we'd accomplished, we were so happy we felt like we could fly back to Kathmandu."

They packed quickly and trekked back down the trail they'd climbed by torchlight. "When we started walking, we were alarmed to see what we had come up in the dark," Ruit says. For more than two miles they descended along a ledge less than two feet wide. Hundreds of feet be-neath them, the white water of the Melamchi rushed around boulders that had fallen from the heights. "We walked carefully along that ledge, just hanging there in space, looking down at a very angry river far, far below," Ruit says. "I think we all realized we could have ended up down there like those boulders, and I said to the team, 'I think the patients pulled us up. They didn't let us slip down. They needed us and wouldn't let us fall.'"

Riding back toward Kathmandu on the VW's roof, Ruit felt he'd proved something important: It *was* possible to bring the best modern medical care to people in remote areas. You just had to dedicate yourself to traveling a more precipitous path.

Ruit spent several weeks prior to a Kathmandu conference of the International Agency for the Prevention of Blindness refining and fretting over a speech he was due to give. Fred Hollows, who by that time had become a globally known figure in ophthalmology, was flying in for the event, and he and Ruit planned to give a presentation on the viability of bringing high-quality cataract surgery camps to rural areas not only in Nepal but across Asia.

"Jesus, Sandook, you can't do that out in the bush! Think about the infection rates!" Hollows had said when Ruit had first told him he was operating in rural areas. But Ruit had taken his team to several other remote villages since his return to Nepal, and had replicated the success they'd had carrying a mobile surgical theater up the crumbling trail to Tepani. He'd sent Nabin Rai to follow up in these villages, studying the condition of the patients. Rai documented that the quality of the surgery Ruit had done in Tepani and other villages was virtually indistinguishable from the excellent results he regularly achieved in the controlled environment of his hospital.

The data persuaded Hollows that Ruit had made a major breakthrough. And he came to Nepal to say so to his peers and to suggest that they follow Ruit's lead. Hollows and Ruit presented their findings at the conference, held in a meeting room at Kathmandu's historic Yak and Yeti hotel. Leading ophthalmologists and public health policy makers listened to them argue for a fundamental reorientation of the way the world medical community fought cataract disease. They said that providing the latest technology, and the best possible care, to blind patients in the most remote rural areas was not only morally imperative but practically feasible because of the procedures Ruit had been perfecting in the field.

"At the time," Hugh Taylor says, "most of the powerful forces in international eye care were still advocating quick and dirty intracap surgery for people in the developing world, then handing out a pair of glasses. They didn't like the waves this upstart from the back of nowhere was making, and they were prepared to knock Ruit down a peg or two."

As Ruit was presenting data on the low infection rates he'd achieved in facilities like school buildings and army posts converted into temporary operating theaters, an Indian ophthalmologist, one of the world's most respected authorities on providing eye care to the poor, interrupted in a loud, belittling voice.

"I've done my level best to listen and keep my mouth shut," he said. "But this is nonsense! There are millions, from Pakistan to Peking, who need our services, and what you're talking about is simply too costly. Can we kindly turn our attention to more serious matters?"

A high-ranking American public health official stood and applauded his Indian colleague. "You're wasting our time," he told Ruit. "Our resources are not infinite. It's only logical to make do with techniques that have been proven in the field."

Ruit, so firmly in command of his daily life, had always been uncomfortable making formal speeches. Gripping the podium, he told himself to keep his voice calm, to concentrate on making his case with the data he'd ridden on top of buses and climbed canyons in the darkness to collect. But his face reddened at these condescending foreigners dismissing the vision he believed in with absolute certainty: that people trying to survive the rocky footpaths and rigors of existence in mountain villages deserved excellent eyesight at least as much as wealthy citizens of the developed world who lived in comparative ease. He felt his blood pounding in his temples.

"Would you let your own mother or father be operated on with a technique twenty years out of date?" Ruit asked. "Are you saying these millions, the poor, deserve less than you or I? Are you saying," he continued, recalling the good, the impoverished, the underserved people of Olangchungola, "that they are children of a lesser god?"

Fred Hollows patted his friend on the shoulder and reached for the microphone. His face had turned a shade of pink that rivaled Ruit's. "You," he sputtered. "You *people*. You're the *pus* in the *pimples* on the *arseholes* of everything that's wrong with the field of medicine."

He threw his arm over Ruit's shoulder. "Come on, Sandook," he said. "Let's get the hell out of here, have a whiskey, and figure out how to do it ourselves." He led Ruit off the podium, out the door, and onto a stool at the Yak and Yeti's wood-paneled bar.

Many plots—some successful, too many catastrophic—had been hatched in the bar of the Yak and Yeti. Edmund Hillary and the explorers who'd followed in his large footsteps had haunted the cozy carved-wood sanctuary for decades. Tabin had sat on one of these stools a few years earlier, plotting logistics for his third, and successful, attempt on Everest. Now Ruit and Hollows were laying the framework for another type of assault.

"You know, it all boils down to the cost of lenses," Ruit said. "We can't keep depending on donations." At the time, the artificial-lens industry was dominated by American and European corporations, who fixed their prices and charged as much as $150 for a single first-rate IOL.

"I've been giving that problem thought for some time," Hollows said. "We could build a lens factory right here in Kathmandu. Christ, all you'd need to do is throw up a shed and get to work."

"I can promise you, no one would work harder at this than we Nepalese," Ruit said, excited. "We could produce lenses for a tiny, tiny fraction of the cost and sell them to countries across Asia. Imagine the impacts that would have!"

"It wouldn't be cheap, but I don't see why it couldn't be done if we twist the right arms," Hollows said, sliding a glass of scotch down the bar toward his friend. "If you can't work with them . . ." he said, raising his own glass.

"Knock them on their ass and teach them to do better!" Ruit said, giggling happily, as they sealed the new Australian-Nepalese partnership with a bracing sip of liquid from Scotland.

CHAPTER 12

Stream of Sesame Seeds

*We are, all of us, pilgrims who struggle along different
paths toward the same destination.*
—Antoine de Saint-Exupéry

One day, while bicycling his usual circuit through the hills of Sydney, Fred Hollows felt short of breath. He had been an enthusiastic mountain climber in his youth and had led an active life of trekking and cycling ever since. He'd always considered himself a "scrappy little bugger," because he usually seemed to have enough stamina on reserve for any physical task, so he knew immediately that something had to be wrong. He had a CAT scan performed, and the results were grim. Hollows had a large, cancerous tumor on one kidney, and secondary tumors had spread to both of his lungs. "It was a very sad time for us," Hollows told his biographer, Peter Corris. "But we made certain resolutions, principally, that we weren't going to pussy-foot around pretending things weren't as they are."

As Hollows's reputation had grown, so had his ambition for battling blindness around the world. He'd traveled widely, teaching modern surgical techniques in dozens of developing countries, and the more he'd traveled, the more firmly he'd become convinced that he and Ruit were right: Developed countries controlled the artificial lens business and kept the prices artificially high. He'd decided to champion the construction of factories producing low-cost lenses not only in Nepal but in Eritrea and Vietnam as well.

Hollows had his cancerous kidney removed and radioactive iridium rods inserted into his lungs, to slow the growth of his smaller tumors. He resolved to dedicate whatever time he had left to turn his dream of lens factories for the third world into reality. Though he'd always had a prickly relationship with the country's leaders, he'd become a folk hero to ordinary Australians, and news of his cancer led to an outpouring of accolades and public support. In 1990, he received several humanitarian awards and was once again offered the Order of Australia; this time he accepted, knowing the publicity it would lend his cause. He was also named the 1990 Australian of the Year, a position that involved a lengthy speaking tour and extensive media coverage.

Hollows turned his lectures into fund-raisers and gave interviews from his hospital bed when he wasn't well enough to travel, determined to surf the wave of publicity as long as possible. "The big goals, the establishment of lens factories . . . keep me going," Hollows told his biographer. And the awards "have given me a platform to speak out about the things that most concern me . . . the responsibility we, as privileged citizens of First-World countries, bear to the people of the Third World."

Ruit traveled with Hollows on several of his international teaching trips. Hollows was especially eager to visit and teach in Vietnam, but he suffered a relapse just before he was due to leave and was hospitalized. When his doctors told him he was too weak to make the trip, Hollows, defiant to the end, pulled out the breathing tube they'd inserted in his trachea and demanded to have his lung function measured, to see if he was capable of surviving the flight to Hanoi. When the doctors told him he had a chance of returning home from Vietnam alive, he left the following week. Ruit accompanied him.

"In Vietnam it was really still the Iron Gate era," Ruit says. They were welcomed in an official state ceremony by General Vo Nguyen Giap, the elderly architect of his nation's defeat of both the French and the American armies, a visit that delighted Hollows and Ruit, whose sympathies were always allied with the world's underdogs. At hospitals in Hanoi and Hue, Ruit took the surgical tools from the hands of his friend and mentor, and took the lead in demonstrating modern surgical techniques to doctors. Hollows wore an oxygen mask, tired easily, and was too ill to do more than admire the masterful surgeon Ruit had become.

Back in Kathmandu, Ruit strolled the length of the vacant lot, lost in thought. He paced every inch of the property, drawing and revising the blueprints in his imagination. The waiting area would be important. Too many medical facilities in Nepal crowded patients into airless rooms. So an open courtyard, shielded from the sun but surrounded by plants—a garden he would tend. The examination rooms should be nearby, so blind patients needn't be led far from benches where they could wait comfortably, cooled by breezes. Most critically, the lens laboratory would stand near the entrance gate, advertising the advanced technology he had brought to Nepal, trumpeting the improvement in eye care he intended to provide.

Lying on his deathbed, at home in Farnham House in early February 1993, Hollows learned that the project in Vietnam was plagued by red tape. But he took solace in the fact that they'd raised enough money to build the lens factories in Eritrea and Nepal, and that the Australian government had committed matching funds to see that they were finished.

Fred Hollows died on February 10, 1993. Michael Amendolia, a young photographer for Australia's News Limited newspapers, who had accompanied Hollows and Ruit to Vietnam, visited Hollows frequently during the last months of his life. Amendolia was so moved by Hollows's dignity and lack of self-pity that he shot hardly any images during the time he spent at Farnham House. "It was just such a privilege to be there that I didn't want to poke a camera in Fred's face. Not that he would have minded," Amendolia says. "Fred's dying was a very public event, and there was no solemnity allowed. There were always twenty or thirty people out on the terrace, drinking and carrying on, while one or two at a time came inside and shared a quiet word or a laugh with Fred. His behavior at the end cemented his status as a national hero. He had the courage to leverage his dying to make a difference."

Nearly two decades later, Gabi Hollows pointed out the spot where her husband's life came to an end, a large drawing room cluttered with messy piles of books, too many framed awards to fit on the walls, and the heavy, hand-lathed wood furniture Fred built in such quantities that it made the enormous room seem paradoxically small. Though it looked frozen in time, Farnham House hadn't become a museum. Far from it. Fred and Gabi Hollows's college-aged children, as well as assorted houseguests, inhabited the rooms. The home was still crowded with an unpredictable assortment of diners during meals. But the presence of the departed doctor clung to the walls, like smoke from his omnipresent pipe.

"You know what one of the last things Fred said before he died was?" Gabi asked, sitting at the heart of Farnham House, her scuffed kitchen table. "I'll tell you," she continued, without waiting for a reply. "He said, 'You know, if all I've achieved is launching Ruit, then my life's been a success, because I know he'll change the world.'"

"Fred gave orders to the end," says Rex Shore, a British citizen who'd fled Europe for a more adventurous life in Australia. He'd worked for sixteen years as an ambulance driver and paramedic in Sydney before arthritis made lifting patients too painful. Shore had met Hollows in Sydney and had found the doctor's disregard for convention refreshing.

"I've never been very good at following rules," Shore says. He found England "too organized and ritualistic" for his taste. Before his injury, he'd reveled in Australia's freedom, skydiving, shooting, and sailing his way through the hours between his shifts in the ambulance. Shore took advantage of Australia's proximity to Asia to travel widely when he took time off. On a trekking vacation in Nepal, he'd fallen in love with the country and had bonded with his porter, Prakash Sherpa. He'd returned frequently to visit Prakash's family.

During his time in Kathmandu, Shore had been introduced to Ruit by a common Sherpa friend. He was struck by the dream Hollows and Ruit shared of bringing high-quality eye care to the world's poor, whatever the obstacles. "They really were soul mates in that way,"

Shore says. He offered his skills as a fluent English speaker to help Ruit communicate with the diplomatic community, whose help, and funds, Ruit sought to make the hospital he envisioned a reality.

That's how Rex Shore found himself spending his days weaving through Kathmandu's unpredictable traffic on a black Bajaj motorcycle, with a modest salary as a representative of the Nepal Eye Program Australia, traveling to meetings with government officials. "Everything was quite ad hoc in those days and we just got on with things," Shore says. I thought Oz was adventurous at first, but compared to Kathmandu, it was predictable and boring. Nepal was the Wild, Wild West."

Hollows had also helped Ruit gain a powerful ally when he pressed Les Douglas, Australia's ambassador to Nepal, to help Ruit any way he could. "You should support this man," Douglas remembers Hollows saying. "He knows what he wants to achieve for his people . . . and he will be successful. If I needed a cataract operation, I would come to Nepal and get Ruit to do it."

"I did a thing or two to help Ruit get going," Shore says, "but let's be clear: If Les Douglas hadn't been ambassador to Nepal, Tilganga would never have been founded."

Douglas arrived at a transformative time in Nepal's political history. Nepal was still a kingdom, and the royal family's power was firmly entrenched. But a nascent democracy movement had spread from rural areas to Nepal's cities and had forced concessions from King Birendra. These culminated in 1991's elections, which made Nepal a constitutional monarchy, with the king as the head of state and a prime minister as the head of government.

Prime Minister G. P. Koirala had made his reputation as a leader of the labor movement, organizing workers in the jute mills of his hometown, Biratnagar, and he came to office promising to press for further democratic reforms. "What that meant, practically, was that Nepal's political system was in chaos when I arrived," Douglas says. "A lot of the politicians and bureaucrats I met with seemed to have no idea how to help the Nepalese people, and they were puzzled about who was actually in control of the country."

Douglas saw Ruit as someone who could get something done. "Before Ruit left the Nepal Eye Hospital, I went to watch him operate, and I came away impressed not just with his skill as a surgeon but by what an extraordinary human being he was. Ruit taught me not only a lot about Nepal, about the inefficiencies and corruption of the bureaucracy; he taught me how to live a meaningful life. And he explained very clearly that his vision was to develop a world-standard medical facility which was owned and run by the Nepalese."

During his twenty-eight-year diplomatic career, Douglas had become disenchanted with most development programs. He had seen too many aid efforts pander to what the donor countries wanted to do, rather than what the local people needed. "That wasn't the case with Ruit," Douglas says. "He knew exactly what he wanted to do, and he had no problem telling me not only what he needed but what I should do to make myself useful."

The first priority was finding a piece of land on which to locate the facility. "We were a pretty formidable little team," Douglas says. "Rex was the administrator, zipping from meeting to meeting on his motorcycle. And as a diplomat, I used my influence to press the decision makers. That left Ruit free to focus on the big picture."

Douglas met regularly with Prime Minister Koirala and pressured the government to donate a suitable piece of land. "It was quite funny, actually," Douglas says. "We went to the city surveyor's office, pulled out maps of available land, and the prime minister said, 'Pick whatever you want and I'll make sure you get it.'" Unfortunately, the most recent survey maps available were from the 1940s. Every time Douglas contacted Koirala to request a particular piece of undeveloped real estate, he'd receive a phone call weeks later from a functionary who'd explain that the site he'd selected was already built up or reserved for a relative of the royal family.

Finally, after months of runaround, Ruit and Douglas found a piece of land so modest that they couldn't imagine any royal wanting to claim it. The land was on the eastern fringe of Kathmandu, near the airport, and across the Bagmati River from the cremation platforms of Pashupatinath. Occasionally, it was used to park buses that carried pilgrims to Pashupatinath from India. The rest of the time it served as the neighborhood dump. But the land belonged to a trust headed by Queen Aishwarya, which had no intention of donating property near the country's most sacred Hindu site to a group led by a casteless Bhotia from the frontier of the kingdom.

Embarrassed by his repeated inability to deliver, and determined to send a message to the royal family about a shift in the country's power structure, the prime minister insisted that the land be handed over. And, grudgingly, it was.

Ruit visited the site regularly, after excavation was under way. To the casual observer, it may have looked like little more than a dusty lot, strewn with mounds of rotting trash, scented with the smoke of burning flesh drifting across the Bagmati. But to Ruit it was a foundation sturdy enough to support a dream. He noticed a narrow, trash-choked stream, trickling through the lot toward the Bagmati from the slum in the hills above. He asked an old man hobbling by for its name and learned that the local people called it Tilganga, the "Stream of Sesame Seeds."

"In Nepal," Ruit says, "hospitals and other institutions tend to have great big grand names—King this or Queen that—and achieve very little. I thought it was correct that we start with a very modest name like Tilganga and prove our worth with achievements. Besides, even the smallest, dirtiest stream eventually finds its way to a river and runs its course through the country."

Ruit rented a small office with NEPA funds and selected a team of board members for Tilganga formidable enough to break through Kathmandu's daunting bureaucracy. He recruited Hari Bamsha Acharya, Nepal's most famous comedian, for help publicizing their efforts; Shambu Tamang, the first non-Sherpa Nepalese to summit Everest, for his ability to organize expedition-type medical outreaches; Jagdish Ghimire, the local director of OXFAM, for his experience running an NGO; Suhrid Ghimire and Rabindra Shrestha, two successful entrepreneurs, for advice on managing a growing business; Sushil Pant, a powerful lawyer, to help steer Tilganga through Nepal's corrupt legal system; and the industrialist Diwakar Golchha, so Tilganga would have access to his peers, Nepal's wealthiest potential donors.

Prime Minister Koirala laid Tilganga's first foundation stone himself. With only $40,000 in hand from NEPA and the Australian government, little more than enough to lay a foundation, Ruit ordered architects to draw up plans for a fully outfitted three-story facility, built around the courtyard he pictured as Tilganga's heart. The plans included a modern surgical center, a clinic, and a separate building for the Fred Hollows Intraocular Lens Laboratory, since a steady supply of inexpensive artificial lenses was the key to all the doors Ruit hoped to kick open. Ruit told the contractors he had funds to pay for the entire project, when, in fact, he had almost nothing. "I saw that there was a great light in front of me, so I knew I must keep my mind straight and move toward it," Ruit says. "I just felt the money would fall into place."

And with the good fortune that has defined so much of his life, it did. Ruit was devastated to learn that his friend and supporter the Third Jamgon Kongtrul had been killed in a car crash on the plains of India. But his disciple Tenzeng Dorjee, the director of the Jamgon Kongtrul's newly created trust, stepped forward as if the departed Rinpoche had read Ruit's mind, and pledged funds to construct Tilganga's operating theater. Additional money to keep the construction moving was donated by a Kathmandu temple trust, local businesspeople, and even a beer company. But whenever the cash on hand dipped dangerously low, Les Douglas scrounged up more from the Australian Agency for International Development.

Meanwhile, "Ruit was busy operating and Les was busy ambassadoring," Shore remembers. Even though he had no experience with construction, Shore found himself de facto foreman. Fortunately, his former porter Prakash had quit carrying loads, moved to Kathmandu, and started a contractor business. "My Sherpa brother was the only person in the trade I could trust," he says, "and I hired him." Together, they traveled to consult with Douglas. "I remember Les pointed at the brick walls of the Aussie embassy and said, 'Build it solid, like this,'" Shore says. "So we did."

Word of Ruit's project provoked jealousy among his superiors at the Nepal Eye Hospital. They wanted the lens laboratory built as an extension of the NEH and used their connections to promote it over Tilganga; they petitioned Prime Minister Koirala to stop the construction of Tilganga's lens lab, but Koirala refused. "They even tried to have me thrown out of the country and get the government to gum up renewing my visa," Shore says.

Prakash's crew completed the lens laboratory and the surgical center before turning their efforts toward raising the rest of Tilganga. The automated lathes, presses, and polishing tools required to produce the lenses were paid for by the recently founded Fred Hollows Foundation in Australia and installed by technicians sent from Sydney. Ruit recruited a brilliant local engineer named Rabindra Shrestha—no relation to the Tilganga board member of the same name—and hired him to supervise the lab's entirely Nepali staff.

Ambassador Douglas asked the Australian government to extend his appointment from three years to however long it took to open Tilganga. Douglas allayed Ruit's eagerness to begin operating out of his own facility by suggesting a diversion he knew Ruit couldn't resist.

Mustang, in north-central Nepal, was one of the nation's least developed and most inaccessible areas. Because of the ongoing conflict with the Chinese forces across its northern border, Mustang was militarily sensitive and restricted to outsiders. Douglas used his leverage with the newly democratic government to wrangle permission for Ruit to lead the first ophthalmic team into the region. Known within Nepal as Little Tibet, for its large population of Tibetan refugees and traditional Buddhist culture, Mustang loomed in Douglas's imagination as a sort of Shangri-La, preserved by its isolation from the modern world. For Ruit, a population near the border with Tibet with no access to medical care was a powerful magnet.

The team flew in prop planes to the district headquarters in Jomsom, where a train of twenty packhorses waited to take them into the mountains. Nabin Rai, along with five nurses and technicians Ruit had recruited to staff Tilganga when the construction was complete, accompanied them. And squeezed into one of Royal Nepal Airlines' undersized seats, with his feet propped up on a burlap sack of rice they'd brought to feed themselves and their patients, sat Michael Amendolia, his photographer's vest crammed with camera gear.

The presence of a foreign ambassador can open only so many doors. The evening the members of the expedition gathered in Jomsom's only guesthouse before their departure, Douglas asked Ruit, who'd invited Amendolia, how he'd arranged to get permission for a foreign photographer to enter a sensitive military region. "Oh," Ruit said, grinning conspiratorially, "I didn't worry so much about that." They decided to deplete some of their precious stock of scotch to smooth over any difficulties and invited the district commissioner to their room to share a glass or three. "When I judged he was ripe enough, I poured him another drink," Ruit says, "and asked him if he could help with our little problem."

"You've never seen a man sober up so fast," Douglas says. "You could see the fellow's career flashing before his eyes. He told us he couldn't help us, but at least he said he wouldn't report us, and we'd be on our own with the border guards."

"Bugger it," Ruit said, pouring each of them a splash after the commissioner had gone. "Something will work out."

"At that moment," Douglas says, "I remember thinking Ruit had never seemed more like our dear unflappable friend Fred."

They left at first light into a sharp-toothed wind, covering their faces with cloth, traveling within a long plume of dust stirred up by their small Tibetan horses. Ruit advised Amendolia to remove his photographer's vest and hide his gear until they were well past Mustang's border guards. And the doctor, who had never cared for riding horses, sat uncomfortably on his mount, his face covered tightly by a cloth.

"We rode up a narrow trail, no more than two meters wide," Douglas says. "I tried to enjoy the mountain scenery, which is stunning in those parts, and not look down at the sheer drop, but I confess I had a hard time keeping my eyes off our horses' hooves, and watching how close they came to the edge."

The guard post was on a small plateau above a perilously steep portion of the trail. Anxiously, Amendolia rode toward the soldiers, who had automatic rifles slung casually over their shoulders. Ruit, bringing up the rear, was spurring his horse, coaxing it to climb, when suddenly it reared up on its hind legs and rolled over backward onto him.

"Fortunately, when the horse fell on me, I landed in a sort of bathtub shape carved out of the rock and his weight didn't crush me as it would have done on level ground," Ruit says. "But then I was rolling downside, ass over teakettle. I couldn't tell which way I was falling, and I remember praying I didn't go off the edge."

When horse and rider came to rest, after tumbling more than twenty yards straight down the spine of the trail, Ruit was bruised, badly shaken, and relieved to be alive. Despite the long fall, his rugged mountain pony seemed to have suffered nothing more than a few scratches, and he led the spooked animal back uphill by the reins to the post, where the border guards gaped at the man whose corpse they'd been preparing to recover. In the wind and dust and confusion, Amendolia slipped past the guards without being asked to produce the permit he didn't have. And the expedition, complete with its photographer, proceeded on its way to Upper Mustang.

"That tumble on the horse changed me," Ruit said. "A few feet one way or the other and I would have fallen to my death. I told myself, 'You have your family and your work. You can't take this sort of senseless chance anymore.'" From that day forward, Ruit preferred to trust his own feet on the most treacherous portions of his travels. He avoided Nepal's accident-prone small planes whenever it was possible to drive to his destination. And his companions and coworkers learned to settle back onto their saddles, or the seats of their SUV, as Ruit plodded slowly and deliberately along the edges of cliffside trails or crumbling roads on foot, refusing to trust his survival to the hands or hooves of others.

They rode up a fourteen-thousand-foot pass toward Charang, where they had arranged to operate in the village veterinary clinic. Mustang was so sparsely populated that advance screening teams had been able to gather only fifty-five patients who could benefit from cataract sur-gery. "Charang was probably the poorest place I'd ever been," Douglas says. "It was such an arid, desolate area that you couldn't believe it could support human life. And the people were like something out of prehistory. They wore clothes made from the hides of their goats; you could smell them coming from a mile away." The single piece of furni-ture they could find was a bench too rickety to serve as an operating table. There were only two scrawny trees standing within several hours of the village. Douglas convinced the villagers to let him cut one of them down, and they used its timber to brace the bench so it was stable enough to support patients.

"Ruit was really in his element," Douglas says. "He operated as quickly and confidently as if he was in a hospital back in Kathmandu. I'll never forget the next morning. One woman had been blind for about ten years, and had never laid eyes on three of her own children. When her bandages came off and she saw them, we all just sat there on the ground and cried, me, Ruit, the woman, and her children. It was just so emotional."

Michael Amendolia proved worthy of the risks Ruit had taken to bring him along. He burned through roll after roll of black-and-white film, capturing indelible images of the harshly beautiful landscape, as well as the patients' elation. In the most famous photograph ever taken of Ruit at work, Amendolia caught a seventy-eight-year-old shepherd named Pemasumta at precisely the moment the doctor removed his eye patch. "I'm not only seeing the sun, I feel I *am* the sun!" Pema-sumta said as Amendolia's shutter clicked, raising his hands and press-ing them together to bless the man who had returned light to his life. Ruit is grinning so exuberantly, so soulfully in the photo, you'd think it was the first time he'd ever cured a blind patient.

"Michael captured the essence of Ruit right there," Douglas says. "I'll tell you a story about Ruit you don't have to believe, but it's true: Ruit is like a godfather to our son Zac and visits us whenever he's in Australia. Well, Zac was stricken with encephalitis before one of Ruit's visits, and even though Sanduk was late for a conference, he insisted on stopping by the hospital to check in on our boy. By then, Zac was in a coma, and my wife and I were sick with worry. Ruit sat next to Zac, took his hand in his, and at precisely that moment, Zac came out of his coma and sat up. I can't explain it, but if you spend enough time around Ruit, it doesn't seem so strange. In all my years as a diplomat, meeting prime ministers, presidents, and kings, he's the pinnacle. The greatest, most inspirational human being I've ever had the privilege to know."

Their last morning before turning for home, the members of the team were served their morning tea along with the news that an elderly monk had died in the night. They were invited to witness his sky burial. In an alpine region of permafrost, interment in the frozen earth is not a practical option. And wood is far too rare a commodity to consume for a funeral pyre. So the funereal tradition known as *jhator*, or sky burial, persists in high-altitude Tibetan communities. The literal meaning of *jhator* is "giving alms to the birds." And in a Buddhist worldview, where a corpse is an empty vessel and the soul has moved on toward rebirth, it's considered fitting that human flesh nourish other living beings.

Charang's living monks carried the body to the crest of the nearest hill. Two men serving as *rogyapas*—the word translates literally as "body breakers"—slit the monk's stomach open and summoned the vultures that had already begun to circle the hilltop by imitating their eerie cries. When the birds had consumed most of the monk's flesh, the *rogyapas* crushed his bones and mixed them with *tsampa* to spur the vultures on. And when only a skull remained, the men shattered it with a mortar and pestle and mixed the bone and brain matter together with *tsampa* and yak butter. They set the offering on a stone, and a lone black vulture circled the funeral party, beating its heavy wings. It was larger than the other birds, and they fled when it touched down to eat. The funeral party retreated stealthily; if the last remnants of the monk were not consumed, their hosts explained, his reincarnation could not be assured.

As the members of the medical team mounted their horses and rode through the narrow lane at the center of Charang, villagers crowded around Ruit's horse, touching his legs and straining to reach high enough to pat his arms as he passed. Douglas recognized several patients who had been blind days earlier, running confidently alongside Ruit and reaching out to touch him.

"Why are they doing that?" Douglas asked a young monk who was accompanying the pack train on the trip back down to Jomsom.

"Because they believe he is a god," the monk said. "Can you blame them? They've seen him perform miracles."

June 7, 1994, was one of the most memorable days in Sanduk Ruit's life. The facility he'd been struggling to bring to his country for years, an eye hospital capable of providing uncompromising care, was about to throw its doors open to any Nepali who needed its services. King Birendra and Prime Minister Koirala joined Ambassador Douglas to cut the ribbon officially opening the Tilganga Eye Centre. It was a landmark moment not only in his life but in the nation's history; it was the first time, Ruit says, that Nepal's royal and political leaders had ever appeared together in public.

The king, the prime minister, and the ambassador stood in the sturdy brick building's courtyard, surrounded by a cheering crowd. Amid the lush greenery Douglas had picked out himself, overseen by a larger-than-life portrait of the departed Fred Hollows peering wryly over his trademark half-glasses, Tilganga's first patients were led toward benches where a different sort of pilgrim would now gather on the site of the former festival parking lot.

The laboratory that bore Hollows's name, run by Rabindra Shrestha's team of Nepalese technicians in sterile, blue-hooded suits, struggled at first, but after retooling its assembly line, it began turning out hundreds of first-world-quality intraocular lenses a day, at a cost of $4 apiece. Ruit had overcome the prejudice of Kathmandu's elite, attempted sabotage by his former superiors at the Nepal Eye Hospital, and doubts that such a facility could be built in a developing country. Rex Shore remembers standing off to the side of the ceremony, away from the VIPs, as flowered garlands were exchanged and news photographers snapped pictures, biting his lip to restrain the emotions that threatened to spill out. Against all odds, it had happened. The vision had materialized in brick and mortar. The combined efforts of a dead man, a former ambulance driver, and an ambassador had helped a Nepalese doctor realize his dream.

CHAPTER 13

The Most Eyes on Earth

*If you don't know the kind of person I am and I don't know the kind of
person you are a pattern that others made may prevail in the world
and following the wrong god home we may miss our star. . . . I call it
cruel and maybe the root of all cruelty to know what occurs but not
recognize the fact. And so I appeal to a voice, to something shadowy,
a remote important region in all who talk· though we could fool each
other, we should consider—lest the parade of our mutual life gets lost in
the dark. For it is important that people be awake, or a breaking line
may discourage them back to sleep; the signals we give—yes or no,
or maybe—should be clear: the darkness around us is deep.*
—William Stafford, "A Ritual to Read to Each Other"

Tabin ran through Thamel, past shops selling counterfeit mountaineering gear manufactured in China, past galleries displaying
psychedelic *thangkas* of grinning or scowling gods, past T-shirt shops
pitching their yins and their yangs to hippies, past metalsmiths, hammering sets of singing bowls. He jogged at an easy pace, noting how
comfortable his body felt in the clear air and mile-high altitude.

Running past one of the neighborhood's innumerable bakeries, he
caught and held the lovely eyes of a woman setting out a tray of sweet
pastries. They were rimmed with black *kajal*, and a red tikka jewel
sparkled at the center of her forehead. He was considering stopping
and trying to strike up a conversation when the spell was broken by an
auto-rickshaw carrying a swaying load of bamboo building materials;
it passed between them with its engine belching blue smoke, and he
ran on.

It may be possible that the Nepalese have the world's most striking eyes; it is also likely that Nepal contains the most eyes, per capita, of any country on earth. There are the third eyes, or tikkas, that peer out from so many Hindu foreheads. There are the eyes framed by the carved wooden windows of Kathmandu, surveilling all that passes below them in the capital's crowded streets. There are the eyes that stare out from the headlamps of transport vehicles, painted there by drivers hoping for the foresight to avoid a collision. There are the all-seeing eyes of the Buddha, gazing mindfully from the flat surfaces of stupas, *mani* stones, and monasteries where they've been painted. And there are the commercial versions of these eyes, embroidered on the T-shirts, sweaters, and handbags marketed to tourists, who yearn to preserve a fragment of the visions they've experienced, to capture and carry them home.

Tabin picked up his pace, turning down a narrow alley that led to the Bishnumati River, running past the stalls of butcher shops, where the skinned and charred heads of goats and sheep rested on blood-slick counters and seemed to regard him with their blank, blanched eyes as he sped past.

Could Tabin be blamed for seeing eyes everywhere he turned? In Kathmandu, it was hardly possible to avoid them. But his life was now centered on diagnosing and repairing eyes, in a way it had been focused only once before—on mountains.

Hugh Taylor had sent him from the Royal Victorian hospital in Melbourne to Kathmandu, where his training would be put to the test. Taylor had developed great affection for Tabin after supervising his corneal fellowship; he had come to appreciate how useful Tabin's manic energy could be when properly directed. "Geoff may be untamable, but as a physician, he's first-rate," Taylor says. "He was certainly one of the best fellows I ever worked with. Geoff was hyperactive, superactive, but totally focused on learning. He asked endless questions. And every morning, when we began rounds at the Royal Vic, Geoff insisted that we climb the eight flights of stairs from the lobby to our patients. It's a practice we continue to this day."

Tabin ran across a bridge over the reeking Bishnumati, continued up past steeply terraced rice paddies, swerved to avoid a snarling dog with a skin condition, and reached the steps of the Swayambhunath Temple complex. Like the eight flights of stairs at the Royal Victorian hospital, this run was his routine each morning in Kathmandu. Through the Fred Hollows Foundation, where he served on the organization's board, Taylor had arranged for Tabin to work with Ruit. "I didn't know much about Dr. Ruit other than hearing he had a reputation as a maverick," Tabin says. "But I figured, I'll be back in Nepal. I'll be near the mountains if things don't work out. How bad can it be?"

Tabin ran between twin Buddhas guarding the stairs to the hilltop temple, quickening his pace. A homeless girl of five or six slept peacefully on the outstretched palm of the left-side statue. Beggars lined both sides of the staircase, their heads lowered and hands raised. Even if he wanted to put a few rupees into those hands, Tabin carried no cash in his jogging shorts. He was here to help people like them, he reminded himself as he sprinted up Swayambhunath's 365 steps. He'd help them not with money but with specialized skills he'd acquired from Hugh Taylor.

He paused at the top and leaned against a giant golden *vajra*, the thunderbolt that eradicates ignorance, to catch his breath. Buddha's eyes were painted on all four sides of Swayambhunath's central stupa, watching over, it was said, all the people of Nepal, regardless of religion. Tabin straightened up to take in the view. The dense, jumbled center of the city looked less frenzied from this height, surrounded by green parks and paddies. He scanned the brown ridgelines of the midhills, and beyond them he saw the unforgettable outline of the Himalaya. How satisfying, how familiar it felt to be back at the site of his greatest accomplishments, to return to his second home.

"I was blown away by Tilganga," Tabin says. "There's no other way to put it." Despite the heat and dust outside its gates, and the patients who crowded its corridors, he says, "The place was spotlessly clean—no garbage, no dirt, no dust. It reminded me of an American or Australian hospital, not a third-world facility."

He put on scrubs, entered Tilganga's operating theater, and stood in front of Ruit's table, waiting to announce his arrival. He'd prepared a short speech about how excited he was to be back in Nepal and how much he looked forward to working alongside someone Hugh Taylor had described as one of the world's standard-bearers for their profession. But if Ruit noticed Tabin's presence, he gave no sign. He finished his case and bandaged his patient's eyes with brisk, efficient movements. He looked up from his stainless steel operating table only after technicians had led the man away and slotted an emaciated blind woman into place. The doctor's dark, intense eyes gazed out, levelly, between his sky-blue mask and surgical cap. He fixed those eyes on Tabin and acknowledged him with a grunt before turning to his next patient.

Though the greeting was less welcoming than Tabin hoped, he'd been swept aside by the egos of eminent surgeons at Harvard and Brown and the Royal Victorian hospital, and the terrier in him had managed to win most of them over, eventually. Tabin ascribed Ruit's coolness to his total concentration on his patients and felt sure that when they were able to spend time together socially, the distant technician, the hard-closed case that Ruit seemed to be in the operating room, would warm to him.

But in their first days together, Ruit never offered Tabin that opportunity. After mutely observing as Dr. Ruit and Dr. Reeta Gurung performed one flawless cataract surgery after another in a matter of minutes, Tabin was finally given a turn at the operating table. During his hour-long struggle to remove one of the largest cataracts he'd ever encountered from an elderly woman's eye, he felt someone breathing by his side, and looked up to see Ruit observing his work through the microscope's second eyepiece. "Gently, gently," Ruit said, "not so much thrashing about."

Tabin felt off-balance and confused. "I'd never operated on a cataract as challenging as the one Ruit watched me try to remove at Tilganga. And I struggled with the microscope, a mediocre seven-thousand-dollar machine, not the crystal-clear seventy-five-thousand-dollar model I was used to." But he told himself he'd come this far; he'd win Ruit's confidence.

If Tabin thought his credentials from Yale, Oxford, Harvard, Brown, and Melbourne would dazzle a surgeon from the medical backwater of Nepal—one who hailed from a village without a school—he was mistaken. "Truly, when I first met Geoff, I wasn't impressed," Ruit says. "He was so hyperactive he made everyone nervous. And his surgical technique was still pretty lousy. Lots of foreign doctors came round in those days. Most wanted to do little bit of work and have a nice mountain vacation in Nepal. I chalked him up as just another one of those jokers."

When Nabin Rai announced plans for an upcoming cataract camp in Jiri, Tabin jumped at the opportunity to join the team. Jiri, the trailhead on his trek to Everest, was a place where he'd departed for one of his life's high points, and he looked forward to the chance to bond with Ruit on the long drive into the hills.

Ruit sent Tabin ahead, in a rented jeep with a junior ophthalmic assistant, to screen patients and decide which of them were suitable for surgery. Jiri was where Tabin had tugged on skintight spandex tights during the monsoon and begun his fruitless battle to keep leeches from establishing intimate contact. After enduring the bumpy ten-hour ride, he sprang out to stretch his legs on the muddy grounds of the school where the Tilganga crew planned to operate and was struck by the difference between the lighthearted, irreverent tone of mountaineers setting out on a long trek and the grim facts he was faced with on a medical mission. "There were more than a thousand people packing the school grounds, waiting for us," Tabin says. "There was no time to eat, drink, or even pee. It was straight to the examination table." Tabin had only a flashlight and an ophthalmoscope, a relatively crude magnifying device. But for many of the patients, his naked eye was enough to assess the damage. As the patients pressed forward, often accompanied by several anxious family members, Tabin could feel their hopes crowding around him. He had the wrenching task of telling too many of them that there was no chance they'd regain their sight.

On his first day, Tabin saw more pathology than he'd ever encountered in America or Australia; nearly every eye condition known to science was present, and many of the diseases had reached their terminal stages, something he'd never seen in the West, where most eye ailments were treated early. He found people blind from the effects of tuberculosis and leprosy, people who'd suffered severe untreated trauma months earlier, children with tumors that engulfed their eyes—death sentences, sure to travel up their optic nerves to their brains. "Telling their families that nothing could be done for them," Tabin says, "was one of the saddest things I've ever had to do in my life."

Tabin worked twelve hours that day, sifting the human ore for patients whose sight could be saved. He found 248 of these patients, these people.

That evening Ruit and his senior staff arrived in the white Land Cruiser that Gabi Hollows had pressured Toyota to provide Tilganga at cost. There would be no more riding the roof of VW buses for Ruit. He now had a reliable off-road vehicle in which to travel the high roads of the Himalaya, and a former ambulance driver at the wheel who had fitted the rugged Land Cruiser with frilly lace headrest-covers and christened the vehicle Hilda, after a powerful Scandinavian Valkyrie.

When Hilda rolled into the schoolyard, Tabin felt the center of gravity shift. Ruit's reputation was well established in the mid-hills, and Tilganga had run ads on the local radio station and handed out flyers announcing that the doctor was coming. Families of patients clustered around Hilda, straining for a look at the man on whom so many of their hopes rested. Ruit climbed out and strode through the crowd to the examination room, requesting, in Nepali, the count of patients screened for surgery. He listened with his head cocked and nodded.

"Busy day tomorrow," he said to Tabin. "Better get some rest."

Then he climbed a hill to the room he'd been given in the school headmaster's house. "Ruit's house had electricity and running water," Tabin says. "I stayed in the student barracks, with the junior staff, and was given a bunk next to two doctors from Tibet that Ruit had convinced the Chinese government to let him train."

The previous year, after delicate negotiations with Chinese authorities, Ruit had been one of the first foreigners allowed to practice eye surgery in Tibet. He'd demonstrated his surgical technique in Lhasa City Hospital, and the results had so impressed the officials that they'd agreed to send their two most promising eye surgeons to learn alongside Ruit in Nepal.

Dr. Olo and Dr. Kesang were eager students, but both had only two years of health sciences education after high school, followed by a single year of specialty training in treating eye diseases. Dr. Kesang had one additional specialty. An enormous man, he snored with more vigor than anyone Tabin had ever heard. When the doctors joined Ruit in the mess tent for breakfast the next morning, Tabin drank cup after cup of strong black tea, willing himself to wake fully up.

But when it was his turn to sit at one of the two microscopes the team had placed side by side in the schoolhouse Tilganga's staff had worked overnight to sterilize, his adrenaline more than made up for his lack of sleep. If operating at Tilganga had been a struggle, trying to remove the outsized cataracts of patients in a dimly lit schoolhouse, while balancing on an uncomfortable wooden stool, was more like torture for Tabin.

"I kept looking over at Ruit, bent to his work, turning out a perfect surgery every seven minutes, and for one of the first times in my life I began to doubt my own abilities," Tabin says. He averaged forty-five minutes to complete each surgery and often had to call Ruit over and ask for help with the most complicated cases. Ruit finished the surgeries quickly and silently, while Tabin waited for words of encouragement that never came.

Tabin was amazed, as so many before him had been, by Ruit's hands. "It was incredible," Tabin says. "Every movement was graceful. It was like watching Michael Jordan steal a basketball and sprint down the court for an effortless breakaway dunk." Tabin was also impressed by the elegant choreography of Ruit's staff. "The moment we were done, a technician would cap and tape the eye, briskly help the patient off the table, and slot the next one into place. There was no time or motion wasted." The first night, they worked until well after dark. And when they scrubbed out and walked together toward the mess table for dinner, Ruit had completed sixty surgeries to Tabin's seven. As his adrenaline drained away, exhaustion had set in, and Tabin couldn't recall any time in his life—in sport or in medicine—when he'd felt so thoroughly overmatched.

He expected a simple meal, then another attempt at sleep. But Tabin was surprised to see that Ruit's cooks had prepared a seven-course feast of vegetable and mutton curries, rice, and turnip salad, accompanied by freshly baked chapattis. "Like a wise general, Ruit knew he was pushing his troops hard and he had to keep them in top fighting condition," Tabin says. He had resigned himself to the fact that Ruit would remain gruff and distant during their time together and decided that if friendship wasn't possible, he would at least learn as much as he could from the finest surgeon he had ever seen.

As Ruit washed down his second helping of mutton curry with a mug of Nepalese rum, Tabin noted the doctor's transformation: Ruit shed his tense, tightly wound demeanor, and something appeared on his face that Tabin had rarely seen in the weeks they'd worked together: a smile. Twelve hours of surgery seemed not to have tired him at all. He filled Tabin's mug with a generous splash of rum and asked who among the twenty seated under the first spray of stars was willing to commemorate a successful day's work with a song. Singing was one of the few talents Tabin didn't possess. But Dr. Olo had trained in classical Tibetan opera.

Olo stood at the end of the long table, downed his mug of rum for courage, and opened his mouth. It was as if three separate people were singing at once. His voice was simultaneously sweet, guttural, and hypnotically rhythmic. Accompanied by brightening stars, he sang a ballad of conquest and betrayal, and the drinkers showed their appreciation by banging the plank table. When Olo was done, he passed the baton to Sonam, who sang Nepalese pop tunes with his achingly sweet voice. When the rum ran out, they switched to whiskey. And when the whiskey was finished, they drank *raksi*, the home-distilled rice liquor their hosts had provided.

Near midnight, after most of the staff had stumbled off to bed, three doctors remained at the table, contemplating a problem. Kesang had passed out and lay by their feet, snoring. Ruit and Olo tried to raise him to a sitting position, but he weighed nearly two hundred pounds. They couldn't move him. It was five hundred yards down a steep trail to the student barracks. "We'll have to leave him here," Ruit said. "He's Tibetan—it won't be the first time he'll have slept rough."

"Mind if I try?" Tabin said. He squatted, gathered himself, and heaved Dr. Kesang up and over his shoulder. "I'll put him in his bed." Tabin stepped carefully down the dark trail, carrying Kesang's dead weight as easily as he had hauled heavy packs of food, fuel, and rope during the years mountains had been his main ambition. He looked back over his shoulder at Ruit. "See you at breakfast?" Ruit didn't reply. It was too dark to tell exactly what registered on the doctor's face, but Tabin was fairly sure he saw a healthy dose of astonishment— and at least a grudging glimmer of approval.

CHAPTER 14

Three Shirts a Day

Fill your bowl to the brim and it will spill.
Keep sharpening your knife and it will blunt.
Chase after money and your heart will never unclench.
Care about other people's approval and you will be their prisoner.
Do your work, then step back. The only path to serenity.

—Lao-tzu

"Thirteen–two." Tabin heard the score, but he still couldn't believe it. The loss of the first set he had chalked up to a fluke. Ruit must play badminton regularly, Tabin thought; the soldiers at the gym on the police base near Swayambhunath Temple had all nodded to him and swung the gates open without suspicion, even though it was still dark when they'd arrived. But that didn't explain the agony of this thrashing. He was still holding a racquet, after all. Swinging a racquet was something Tabin was so good at, he'd come prepared to muff a few shots and build camaraderie with Ruit. Now he was fighting for his life.

Ruit's eyes revealed nothing as he served with a quick flick of his wrist. Tabin lunged to his left and, with sheer athleticism alone, managed to get the face of his racquet on the shuttle just before it touched down in the farthest corner of the court. He lofted up a desperate, defensive shot. Ruit didn't move his feet a millimeter. With the same blinding whip crack, he fired a smash that nicked the baseline to Tabin's right.

"Fourteen–two."

Tabin heard giggles from the policemen who'd stopped their exercise to watch. As he'd been losing the first two sets, there had at least been the distraction of a group of young men in the blue camouflage fatigues of Nepal's police, grunting as they did their early-morning calisthenics. But they had cut their workout short to take seats on the sidelines of the court and enjoy the spectacle of the unathletic-looking Dr. Ruit showing a fit and cocky foreigner how relentlessly badminton could be played.

"Game point," Ruit said mildly, holding up the white shuttle for Tabin to see. If Tabin trusted his eyes, the last thirty minutes made no sense. Ruit stood on the opposite side of the court, his great, square head topping his equally broad body. He looked no more mobile than a boulder, and by the logic of someone who'd played tennis at Tabin's level, he should have been a pushover. Yet Tabin couldn't make him budge. Instead, Ruit controlled the center of the court with lightning flicks from his racquet, running Tabin from side to side until he was soaked with sweat. Tabin couldn't recover quickly enough to hit a shot capable of moving Ruit more than a foot or two in any direction.

Ruit wound up to serve, and Tabin anticipated a long drive deep to his left. He sidestepped neatly and prepared his backhand. But the shuttle floated lazily, clearing the net by no more than an inch, and died there, dropping like a bird shot from the sky. Tabin looked at the little white object lying on the court fifteen feet in front of him and heard the laughter of the policemen echo throughout the gym. He hadn't even taken a step in the right direction.

"Match," Ruit said.

Tabin handed his borrowed racquet back to Ruit and gulped from a water bottle. "That was incredible," he said, patting the back of Ruit's clean white polo shirt, noting with annoyance that he hadn't broken a sweat. "How long have you been playing?"

"Oh, some years," Ruit said, and Tabin was sure he detected restrained laughter just beneath the surface of the expressionless reply.

If Tabin could get Ruit on a tennis court, he knew, the outcome would be radically different, but somehow that knowledge wasn't satisfying. He wasn't on his own ground. It was badminton, not tennis. Nepal, not America. Finicky, rather than first-rate microscopes. And massive, calcified cataracts, rather than the manageable variety he'd trained on in Australia. Still, Tabin wanted to succeed on this ground, on this man's terms.

After the eye camp at Jiri, Tabin had returned to Melbourne for six months and completed his fellowship with Hugh Taylor. Then he'd flown home to Chicago to visit his family and tell them what he'd seen Ruit's hands perform. Tabin had acquired many mentors—at altitude as well as in operating rooms—but no one had ever challenged him the way Ruit had. Tabin burned to go back to Tilganga, felt that if he could only penetrate the guarded surface of this infuriatingly masterful man, his vague lifelong ambition to help others could finally be realized.

Tabin hoped he'd made a positive enough impression at Jiri to convince Ruit to accept him as an apprentice. Carrying Dr. Kesang to bed might have opened Ruit's eyes to Tabin's usefulness on rugged trips to mountain communities, but it was his performance at the microscope that Tabin felt would be the deciding factor. He had sat beside Ruit during four twelve-hour days of surgery at Jiri, and he had worked as hard at improving his technique as he ever had at anything. By the fourth day, he'd shaved a few minutes off each operation and had interrupted Ruit less frequently to ask for help.

He called Ruit from Chicago and pleaded his case, talking about how much he wanted to learn and how hard he was willing to work. The silence on the other end of the line was so pronounced that Tabin feared he'd been disconnected. Finally, he heard the doctor exhale. "Come along then," Ruit said. "We'll see if you can be of some use."

Tabin stuffed as much as he could fit into two large expedition bags and returned to Nepal with only his savings and two credit cards whose credit he was prepared to exhaust, determined to do whatever it took to earn Ruit's trust.

After his humbling on the badminton court, Tabin shared a ride to work with Ruit in Hilda. The Land Cruiser crept through the dense morning traffic, as motorcyclists with special steel roll cages welded around their engines to protect riders from frequent impacts sped past only inches on either side, ignoring lanes of traffic, slowing all large vehicles to a crawl.

There was plenty of time to talk in the stagnant stream of traffic, so Tabin asked how he could be most helpful. "There's lots of work to be done," Ruit said. "And I have an idea how we might make use of your . . . energy. But you need more training. You should work with Dr. Reeta. She's a wonderful surgeon. And much kindlier than me."

Ruit was conflicted about the hyperactive creature at his side, even now tapping his feet impatiently at the stalled traffic. "Geoff *had* shown me some iron at Jiri," Ruit says. "But I still had doubts. I needed to know he was there—hundred percent—for the patients."

Rex Shore, who'd by then become Tilganga's official driver, as well as its unofficial liaison with Kathmandu's diplomatic community, knew how hard it could be for outsiders to penetrate Ruit's protective shell. "Let's be honest," he says. "Ruit can be a cranky bugger. I always tell him he's damned lucky he's got a lady like Nanda in his life, to smooth over his difficulties in Kathmandu society. And he's equally lucky to have Dr. Reeta on staff. Sanduk can be so damned impatient, always rushing forward, feeling his work is too important to be polite to people. Getting Ruit to go to a meeting or put in the kind of fifteen-minute appearances with officials that make this country go round takes a lot of arm-twisting, I can tell you. But Dr. Reeta is all patience and no ego. She holds the whole operation together."

Reeta Gurung grew up in the Annapurna range, west of Kathmandu. In 1993, she wrote to Ruit from England, where she'd completed her ophthalmic training, and explained that she understood exactly how radical a leap he'd made by operating in remote villages. She wrote that she'd also been born where resources were scarce, and she said she believed in his mission. When they met in Kathmandu, Ruit took to her immediately. With her Mongolian features and her matchless work ethic, she was, Ruit felt, a member of the same breed he belonged to: the underestimated.

Reeta's family came from Ghandruk, one of the last settlements before the base camp of Annapurna II. Ghandruk, like Olangchungola, had no school, so her family sent Reeta and her sister to boarding school in Kathmandu. Reeta's father was a soldier employed by the Indian Army. The Gurung were renowned warriors and hired on with India as professional soldiers. As a teenager, Reeta was studying in Kathmandu when her father was killed in an exchange of artillery along the India-Pakistan border, where running battles for the disputed region of Kashmir were common. Reeta's mother was widowed at the age of thirty, with a small pension from the army and three children to raise. After her husband's death, she leased property the family owned in Nepal's flatlands to growers who gave her a small portion of profits from crops, and she borrowed money to pay for her daughters' education.

"Why do you want to learn about me?" Reeta said, in the British-inflected English she'd acquired during her medical study abroad, waving away my notebook when I asked about her childhood. "My story is nothing special. If you want to write about a really impressive woman, write about my mother. I can't emphasize how difficult it is to be a single woman in Nepal, even now. My mother was very courageous and fought for our futures like a wild animal. She let nothing stand in her way. My sister is a doctor too, a gynecologist who works much harder than me. Whatever we've achieved is because of our mother."

Sitting beside Reeta in Tilganga's operating theater, Tabin watched her easily remove the kind of massive cataracts that had given him so much trouble since arriving in Nepal. Her hands lacked the balletic grace of Ruit's every surgical movement, but they were rock steady, each gesture fast and efficient.

Since training with Hollows, Ruit had been tirelessly making small improvements to his technique. Hollows had taught, for example, that after inserting an artificial lens, one should seal the wound with a single line of sutures and leave the stitches exposed to the air. One of Ruit's many innovations was to tuck the sutures under a flap of tissue; because of this, his wounds healed faster and were less likely to leave the eye misshapen. Ruit had also taught himself, year after year, to carve progressively smaller tunnels in his patients' eyes, scarcely wider than the cloudy cataracts that needed to come out.

Fashioning such a minute escape hatch for a patient's diseased lens was difficult to master. "Imagine using tiny, sharp tools, trying to coax a marble through a drinking straw without damaging the straw," Tabin says. When Reeta asked Tabin to change places with her and operate on the next patient, he did his best to impress her. But the first incision with the point of his blade brought a grunt of disapproval. "Try not to jab at the patient like you're killing a pig," Reeta said. "Let your hand widen the wound gently."

Tabin pictured the way fencers held their foils as they sized up opponents—swaying gently side to side—and attempted to send that image to receptors in the fine muscles of his fingers, so that they enlarged the opening one delicate cut at a time.

"Much better, Dr. Geoff," Reeta said. "If you keep this up, you'll hardly blind anybody!"

After two weeks of training alongside Reeta, Tabin felt he'd reached a new level of proficiency. Ruit absented himself, trancelike, in each of his cases. But Reeta was encouraging, coaxing Tabin's callused climbers' hands to wield the cutting tools ever more gently. The enormous cataracts he addressed each morning through Tilganga's microscopes had begun to feel not like outsized challenges to his dexterity but a normal, manageable condition he was able to cure. With so few doctors trained in Ruit's technique and such an enormous backlog of blind patients in Nepal, Tabin hoped Ruit would soon consider him capable of traveling to eye clinics in the country's mountains and, with the lessons he was learning at Tilganga, helping to teach more of the nation's ophthalmologists modern skills. He hinted to Ruit how much he'd like to work someplace like Phaplu, where the fuse had been lit that had led him to a career in ophthalmology.

As the days passed in the crowded capital, Tabin tried to fill his hours away from Tilganga with entertainment. Into the duffel bags he'd brought from Chicago, he'd stuffed tennis racquets, expedition-grade outerwear, and a full rack of climbing gear. Tabin found a tennis partner, Krishna Ghale, who coached the national tennis team and worked as the resident pro at the American embassy's tennis facility. They were perfectly matched, and Tabin looked forward to a long rivalry on the courts of Kathmandu. He planned to move from his guesthouse in Thamel to a spare room in the home of his summit partner Nima Tashi, whose extended family lived in a large house near the Pashupatinath compound, an easy walk to work at Tilganga.

Thanks to Tabin, Nima Tashi's ankles had healed well enough for him to rise to the top of his profession, as a climbing *sirdar,* the chief Sherpa on high-altitude expeditions. When he wasn't working in the Khumbu, Nima Tashi and Tabin discussed mountains they might tackle together if Ruit posted Tabin to work at a higher altitude.

"I'm sending you to Biratnagar," Ruit told Tabin while they were both scrubbing out after surgery one day. "Let's see if you can be of use there."

Biratnagar? Tabin thought, scanning his mental map of the country. Wasn't that way down in the south, where it was broiling hot . . . and boringly flat? Tabin leaned against the hospital's cool tile walls, trying to absorb what Ruit had said.

"I wanted to settle the question that troubled me. I didn't know if Geoff was a climber or a doctor," Ruit says, with the startling giggle that often slips out when something especially delights him. "So I decided to test him by sending him as far from the mountains as I could."

Biratnagar sits at sea level near the country's border with India, on the flat portion of the Gangetic Plain known in Nepal as the Terai. When Tabin stepped out of the propeller plane that bumped to a stop on the Biratnagar airport's single runway, he was hit by such a comically oppressive blast of heat and humidity that he laughed out loud. "After walking a few minutes from the plane to the terminal, my shirt was completely soaked through with sweat," Tabin says. "The thermometer on the terminal wall read one hundred and four degrees. And the humidity must have been one hundred percent."

The northern horizon was completely obscured by a shimmering screen of heat haze. To the south, a sere, scorched-looking agricultural landscape extended to the Indian border. Before dispatching him to the airport, Ruit had made Tabin's mission clear: The Golchhas, one of Nepal's wealthiest families, who'd made their fortune from jute mills

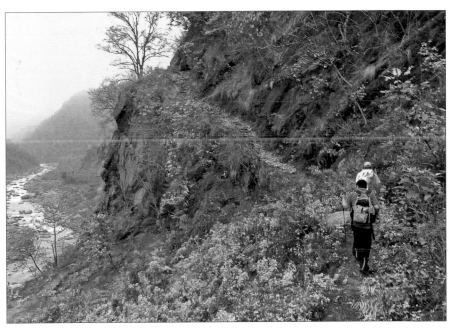

Sanduk Ruit and Geoffrey Tabin on the third day of the trek to Sinwa.
David Oliver Relin, 2010

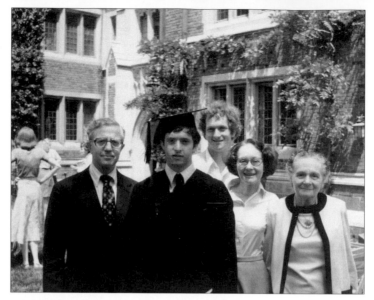

The Tabin family at Geoff's 1978 Yale graduation.
From the left: Julius, Geoff, Cliff, Johanna, and Geoff's
maternal grandmother, Sara Krout. *Geoff Tabin, 1978*

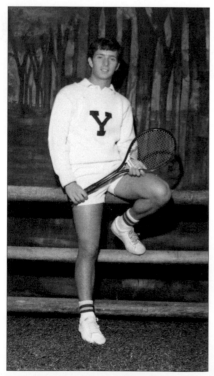

Tabin captained the Yale tennis team
his junior and senior years.
Geoff Tabin, circa 1977

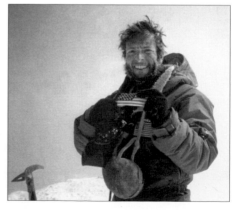

Tabin on the summit of
Mount Everest, October 2, 1988.
Geoff Tabin, 1988

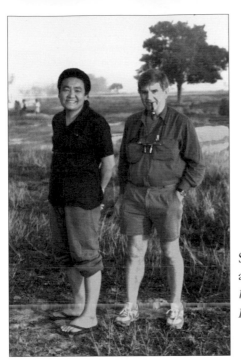

Sanduk Ruit with his friend
and supporter Fred Hollows.
*Rex Shore, courtesy of the Fred Hollows
Foundation, 1990*

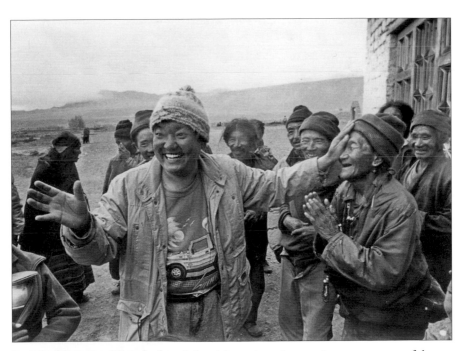

Ruit in Mustang, Nepal, elated that his patients' surgeries were successful.
Michael Amendolia, 1992

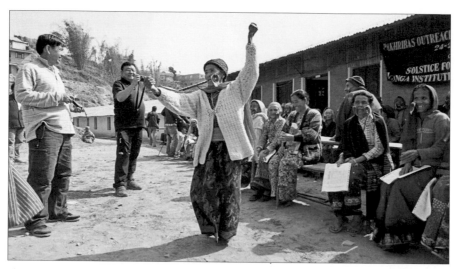

With Khem Gurung, left, and Ruit looking on in Pakhribas, Devi Rai jumps to her feet and begins to dance after her sight is restored.
David Oliver Relin, 2010

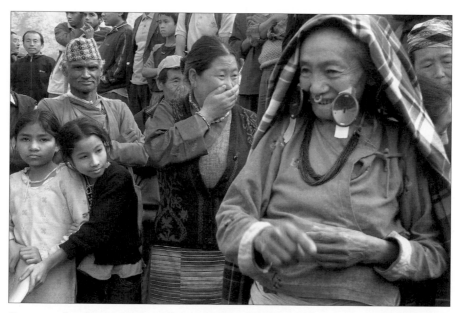

Scene at the Sinwa camp as formerly blind patients begin to walk unassisted.
David Oliver Relin, 2010

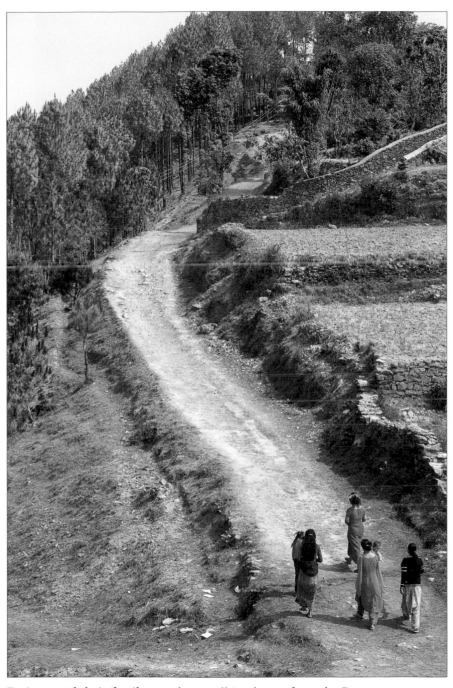

Patients and their family members walking home from the Rasuwa camp.
David Oliver Relin, 2008

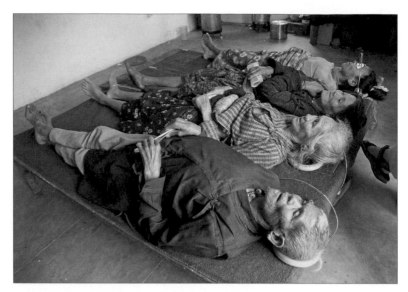

Patients being prepared for cataract surgery at Rasuwa.
David Oliver Relin, 2008

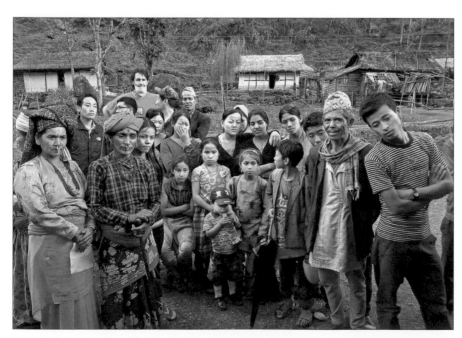

At Sinwa, watching surgery on a monitor outside the makeshift operating
theater. *David Oliver Relin, 2010*

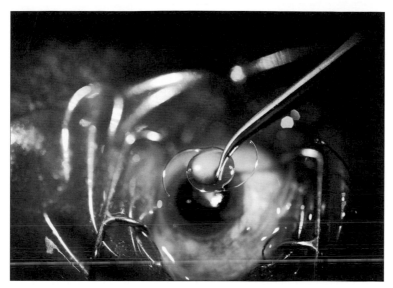

An intraocular lens, about to be inserted in a cataract patient's eye.
Ace Kvale/TandemStock.com, 2009

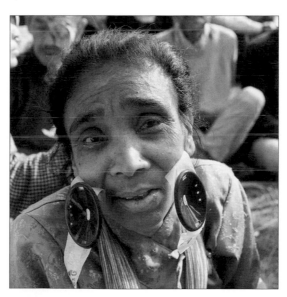

Patali Nepali seeing for the first time after
having her bandages removed. *David Oliver
Relin, 2008*

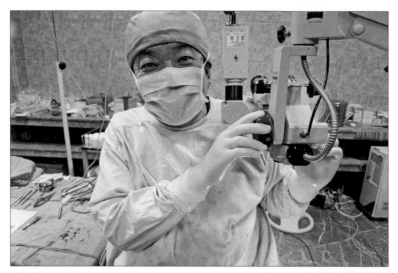

Ruit pausing between patients in the shiny new operating theater
of the HCP-supported Hetauda Community Eye Hospital.
David Oliver Relin, 2008

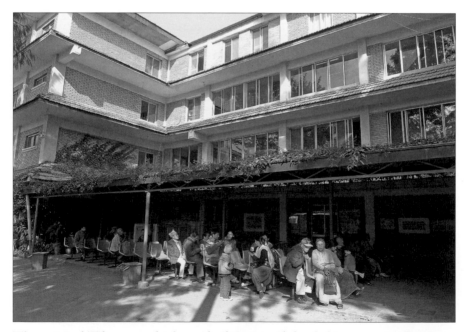

The original Tilganga, which was built in a modular fashion so extra floors
could be added as needed. *David Oliver Relin, 2008*

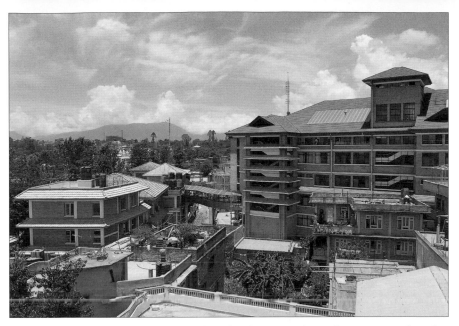

The new Tilganga Institute of Ophthalmology, on the right, connected to the original Tilganga, on the left. *Himalayan Cataract Project, 2009*

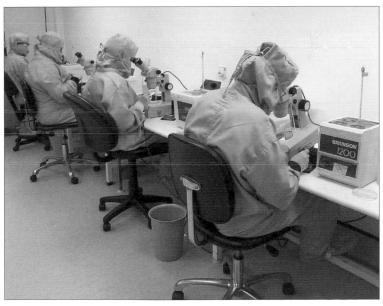

Technicians at the Fred Hollows Intraocular Lens Laboratory, manufacturing lenses to exacting standards.
David Oliver Relin, 2008

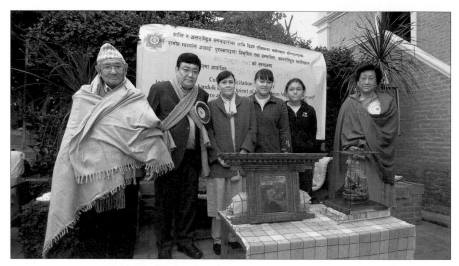

The ceremony honoring Dr. Ruit's career, at a restored palace in Patan. From the left: Ruit's father, Sonam; Ruit; his wife, Nanda; his daughters, Serabla and Satenla; and an official of the Nepal Ophthalmic Society. Ruit's son, Sagar, was away at college. *David Oliver Relin, 2008*

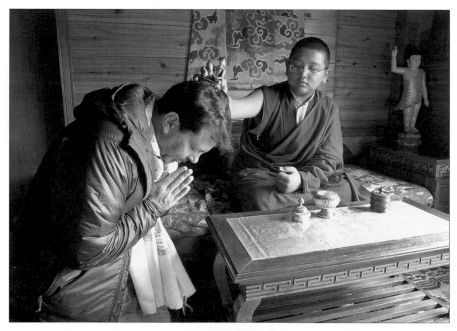

Relin receiving a blessing from the Fourth Jamgon Kongtrul at his monastery in Lava, India. *David Oliver Relin, 2009*

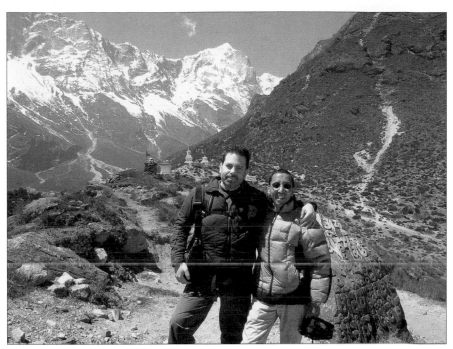

Relin and Apa Sherpa visit Apa's home village of Thame.
David Oliver Relin, 2008

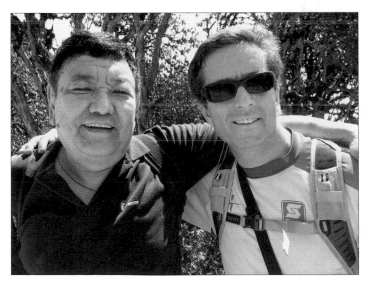

Ruit and Tabin, trekking on the trail toward the Sinwa
surgical camp. *David Oliver Relin, 2010*

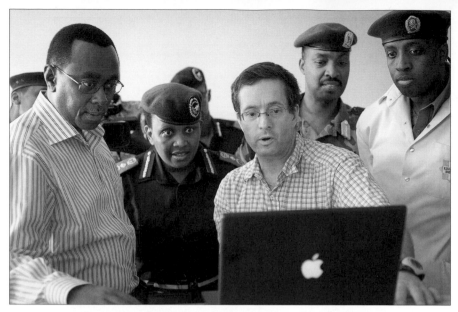

Tabin, center, and John Nkurikiye, right, showing a video of cataract surgery to Rwandan officials, including Prime Minister Bernard Makuza, on the left.
Ace Kvale, 2009

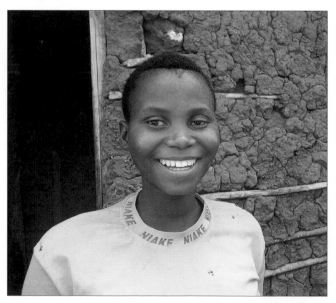

Eminante Uzamukunda returning home after her successful cataract surgery at the Nyamata hospital.
David Oliver Relin, 2009

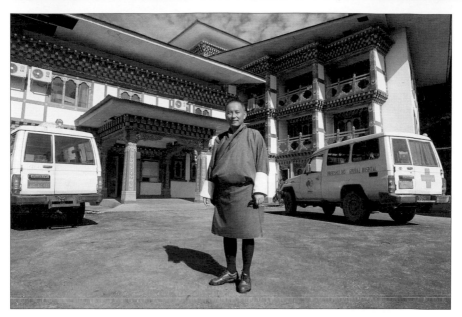

Dr. Kunzang Getshen, wearing the traditional Bhutanese *gho*, at the Phuentsholing General Hospital, in the town his father helped to build.
David Oliver Relin, 2009

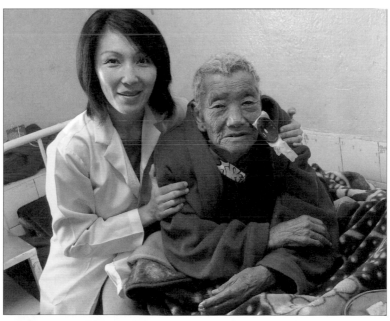

Dr. Dechen Wangmo, after operating on her aunt at Bhutan's National Referral Hospital in the capital, Thimphu.
David Oliver Relin, 2009

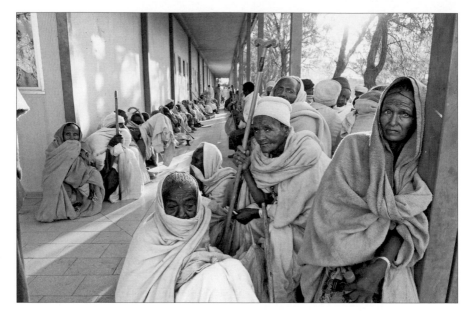

Patients and family members gathered at the Quiha Zonal Hospital, Ethiopia. *David Oliver Relin, 2009*

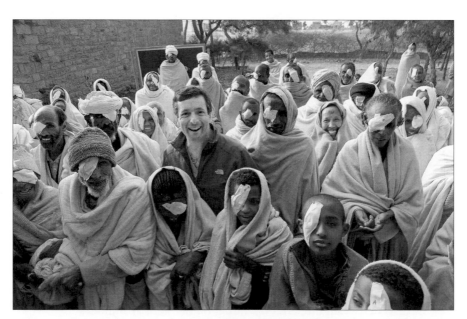

Tabin, surrounded by some of the cataract patients who were operated on at Quiha Zonal Hospital the previous day. *David Oliver Relin, 2009*

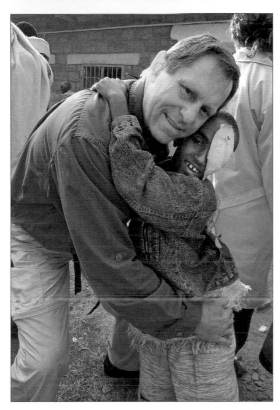

Ten-year-old Temesgen
thanks Dr. Alan Crandall
for restoring his sight at
the Quiha Zonal Hospital.
David Oliver Relin, 2009

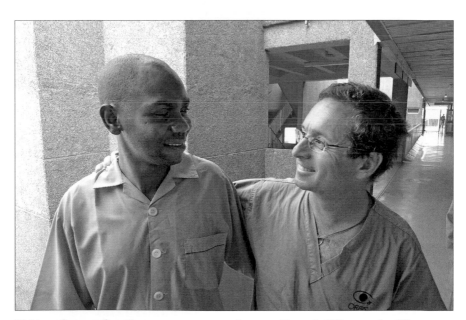

Tabin, after performing a cornea transplant on Francis Kiiza, at the King
Faisal Hospital, in Kigali, Rwanda. *David Oliver Relin, 2009*

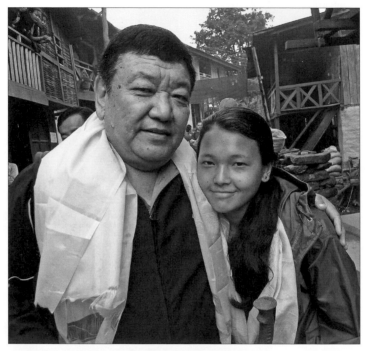

Ruit and his daughter Satenla—draped with *kata*s from grateful patients—setting out on the trek to Olangchungola, Ruit's home village. *David Oliver Relin, 2010*

and steel foundries, had recently built a modern eye hospital in Birat-nagar. It was staffed by two senior ophthalmologists, but Ruit had been receiving disappointing reports about the quality of their surgeries. Tabin's task was to help raise the hospital's standards.

On his ride from the airport to Golchha House in a chauffeured black sedan, Tabin felt as if he'd entered another country. Off the main highway, the streets were rutted tracks. Motorized vehicles were rare. And bicycle-rickshaw drivers with weathered, sun-darkened faces lounged under the awnings of their pedal-powered carts on every cor-ner, immobile as lizards, following the limousine with their eyes only, as if turning their heads took too much effort in the heat.

The Golchhas provided Tabin with a private suite in one wing of the sprawling white marble mansion they'd built in a walled compound at the center of Biratnagar. A staff of ninety cooks, cleaners, chauffeurs, and gardeners attended to the Golchha family, as well as the livestock, orchards, vegetable beds, and meticulously pruned ornamental gardens that surrounded their home.

Tabin was assigned his own valet, Sunil, an older, stooped gentle-man with unfortunate teeth who hovered constantly at the periphery of Tabin's vision and insisted on carrying the doctor's ophthalmoscope and day pack on Tabin's walk from the compound, past the Tip Top Tailor Shop, the Sweetie Pie pastry store, and the Lord Buddha Nurs-ing College, to the Golchha Eye Hospital, a mere two blocks north, at a busy intersection on Goshwara Road. "I felt pretty silly with Sunil walking behind me with my bags," Tabin says. "But the Golchhas were unbelievably generous. It took me weeks to convince them I didn't need a chauffeur to drive the two blocks. But I never persuaded them that I didn't need a servant waiting on me twenty-four hours a day."

Tabin's reception by the senior staff of Golchha Hospital was con-siderably chillier. "The doctors weren't *openly* hostile the first day I arrived at work," he says, "but they were cooler than most Nepalese, and it was obvious they were offended by the idea of a young Western doctor telling men who'd been in ophthalmology for decades what to do."

The elder of the two surgeons, the balding, round-faced Dr. I. C.

Biswas, pointed out to Tabin that he had practiced in Biratnagar for more than twenty-five years and had previously served as president of the local medical association. "Young man, I've seen every eye condition that exists," he told Tabin, asserting his status in a country consumed by caste and rank. "Furthermore, I haven't needed to consult a medical text in more than twenty years!"

"That last comment really alarmed me," Tabin says. "Because I knew how radically eye surgery had improved in the last few decades."

Dr. Joshi, a decade younger, thinner and lighter-skinned, seemed equally aloof. The doctors suggested that since Tabin spoke very little Nepali, he wouldn't be of much use dealing with the examination and diagnosis of the patients. So they suggested that he shoulder the heaviest surgical load during the months he remained in Biratnagar.

"As I got to know him, I realized Dr. Biswas was in fact a lovely guy, a dedicated doctor and a pillar of the community. But his name was a real misnomer. He may have been known as I.C.," Tabin says, laughing, "but very few of his patients could." Both Biswas and Joshi still clung, stubbornly, to outdated intracapsular cataract surgery. "Dr. Biswas boasted that his eyes were still so excellent he could operate perfectly well without a microscope," Tabin says. "So I watched Dr. Biswas and Dr. Joshi slice patients' eyes nearly in half, forcibly wrestle out the lens with forceps, and sew the eyes shut with sutures as large as those used for general surgery in America. After the surgery, patients needed a week to recover in the hospital's filthy wardrooms. And when their eyes healed they were discharged with the kind of thick Coke-bottle glasses that, at best, horribly distorted peripheral vision, if they didn't break when they returned to lives of hard labor in their rural villages. It was considered a good result at Golchha Hospital if postoperative patients could avoid walking directly into objects in their path."

Since its construction, the hospital had completed only a few hundred cataract surgeries a year, in a region where it was the only facility serving nearly a million and a half people. "I thought the staff was doing a pretty miserable job of serving their patients," Tabin says, "and the more I watched them work, the more I struggled to keep my criticism diplomatic."

One morning an eight-year-old girl arrived after suffering extreme trauma to her eye. She and her father had walked for three days from their village to buy basic necessities in the big city. While strolling the streets of Biratnagar, the girl had been playing with a stick, spinning and tossing it, when the sharp end stabbed her in the eye, lacerating her cornea.

With Dr. Joshi translating, Tabin examined the girl. Her wound was so deep that her iris, the colored tissue that contracts and expands to control the flow of light through the pupil, was prolapsed, bulging outside of her eyeball. The girl was in great pain, and Tabin struggled to calm himself and think clearly. He asked Dr. Joshi to explain the situation to the girl's father: Her iris needed to be coaxed back within her eye and the wound sealed to prevent infection; if nothing was done, she would lose her eye, and it was possible that an infection could travel to her brain along her optic nerve and kill her. Surgery was the only option, and Tabin instructed Dr. Joshi to prepare the operating room while he ran back to Golchha House, to consult his textbooks on the exact dose of general anesthesia a girl her age and weight would require.

Tabin returned twenty minutes later, drenched with sweat and trailed by Sunil, carrying his medical bag and a spare, freshly laundered shirt. Dr. Joshi sat in an examination room, drinking a cup of tea. The girl and her father were nowhere in sight.

"Where are they?" Tabin asked, panting from his run in the midday heat.

"They are gone," Dr. Joshi said.

"What do you mean, gone?"

"They have returned to their village," Dr. Joshi said, calmly sipping his tea.

"Didn't . . . didn't you explain the girl could die if we don't operate?" Tabin said, his voice rising to a shrill, accusing complaint.

"Yes," the doctor replied. "I told them. But her father decided it was best not to wait for surgery. He said he needed to return to his village."

Tabin's long-simmering disapproval finally boiled over into scalding criticism. He was appalled by the low standards and wasted resources in a region where a million and a half people needed better care. And he told everyone, from the administrators and surgeons to the technicians and janitors, how he felt about the hospital, how unclean and inefficient it was, despite being stocked with modern equipment. Diplomacy had never been Tabin's strength. He spoke bluntly to the staff at Golchha Hospital, aiming his harshest criticism at Drs. Biswas and Joshi, whom he accused, point-blank, of failing their patients.

The next morning, as he was about to sit down to the lavish breakfast of mango, pineapple, and papaya salad, spicy *masala dosas*, and feather-light puffs of puri the Golchhas' chefs knew he particularly liked, he was summoned by Sunil to the hallway for a phone call.

"What the devil are you doing down there?" Ruit's voice bellowed, clearly, from Kathmandu. "I've heard how disrespectfully you've been speaking to the staff! What are you thinking? They haven't had the advantages you've had in life, or your training. Your duty is not to beat them down. Your responsibility is to lift them up! Are you capable of that? Because if you're not, you should pack your bags and leave for America today."

While Tabin fumbled for the right response, he heard Ruit slam down his desk phone. Then the line went dead. When Sunil ushered him back to the breakfast room and heaped the usual delicacies on his plate, Tabin could only stare at his food.

"Ruit can be rough," Tabin says. "In the years I've worked with him, he's said a lot of harsh things. But I've never been reamed out like that, before or since, by someone I respected so much. The worst thing about what Sanduk said to me was that I knew he was right. I'd been sent to Biratnagar to lift the staff of the hospital up. I didn't know if I was able to do that, but I decided to start trying. And I figured the best chance I had was by doing what Ruit did so well—leading by example."

For the next two months, Tabin dedicated himself to improving his own skills. "I worked methodically on the small-incision extracapsular surgery Ruit taught me," he says, "making sure to go slowly enough that the patients would end up with excellent vision. I averaged only ten surgeries a day, but the good results began to add up." Each afternoon, Tabin returned to Golchha House for lunch, where he'd find a freshly laundered shirt laid out on his bed by Sunil. And when he came home at the end of a long shift he'd spent hunched over the microscope, he'd shower before dinner and change into his third shirt of the day, which was always neatly pressed and awaiting his return, a gift he wasn't sure he deserved.

Siddhartha Gautama, known by the name he chose, the Buddha, or "the enlightened one," was born in Lumbini, far to the west of the hills where Tabin ran to clear his mind. As the story goes, Siddhartha, born into great wealth and privilege, grew disenchanted with his comfortable life when he witnessed the poverty and suffering of ordinary Nepalese beyond the gates of his family's walled compound. Meditating on the inequity and misery that defined the lives of much of humanity, he abandoned his wife and children, took a seat under a pipal tree, and resolved not to leave until he discovered a way to release himself—and, by extension, all of humanity—from the endless cycle of birth, death, rebirth, and suffering.

Tabin may not have achieved enlightenment running past the sorts of trees where the Buddha once sat, but he did have time to refine his priorities. None, he realized, ranked higher than alleviating suffering. When he returned to Golchha Hospital, he not only focused on curing his patients but labored to repair his relations with Dr. Biswas, Dr. Joshi, and the entire staff. All it took was respect and, perhaps most crucially, compassion.

After two months, so many of the formerly blind had walked out of Golchha Hospital the day after Tabin operated on them with excellent vision that word had spread, and new patients began arriving every day, asking for the foreign surgeon. Seeing irrefutable proof that Tabin's results were superior to their own, Dr. Biswas and Dr. Joshi finally took an interest in learning Ruit's technique and began scrubbing in to watch Tabin work.

"Both Dr. Biswas and Dr. Joshi had done phenomenal numbers of operations in their careers," Tabin says. "And they both had excellent, steady surgical hands. Once they adjusted to the novelty of working under a microscope, and learned how to construct small wounds and implant IOLs, they quickly began achieving excellent results."

As the flow of people seeking treatment at Golchha Hospital increased, Tabin helped to raise the skill level of the hospital's general staff as well. He had noticed that two young technicians, Mukesh and Bhupendra, were extremely bright and capable but weren't being asked to do much more than serve as orderlies. Tabin challenged them to work to the limit of their abilities, as Ruit demanded of all of his employees. He taught them how to recognize and care for most minor eye problems, how to prescribe glasses, and, most critically, how to properly anesthetize patients' eyes for surgery. Tabin noticed how quickly they thrived with their added responsibility, how they began to take pride in the hospital, how committed they were to keeping it orderly and clean. "I finished surgery each day ecstatic that we were finally managing to create the atmosphere of excellence that our patients deserved," Tabin says.

After work, he returned to Golchha House not tired but rejuvenated by the progress he knew he was making. The extended Golchha family had a dozen young children, and Tabin would greet them all by name with a barrage of high fives, then entertain them in the evening with sleight-of-hand tricks, making red sponge balls disappear between his fingers and pulling them out of the mouths and ears of the astonished Golchha children.

"We've had many foreign doctors stay in our home over the years, and help with the hospital," Madame Rajluxmi Golchha told me one morning, years later, while I was visiting the family compound with Tabin. "But I've never seen a person as dedicated as Dr. Geoff. Maybe 'dedicated' isn't the precise word," she said. "I mean 'fanatical.'"

Since establishing the eye hospital, Madame Golchha hadn't withdrawn to a life of ease within the gilded walls of her palace. She has been hard at work providing another service for the citizens of Biratnagar: building a school for children with special needs. When I asked why she didn't just stay at home and enjoy the pleasures of Golchha House, she simply pointed at Tabin. "I blame *him*," she said. "Geoff is literally the most inspiring person I've ever met. He was always running to the hospital night or day if the patients needed something. How could I sit inside these walls when he set such an example? You know, the children and I had a special name for him." Madame Golchha laughed as she retrieved it. "We called him Dr. High Five!"

On one of his last evenings in Biratnagar, Dr. High Five left the hospital after a satisfying day of surgery just as the leading edge of a tropical storm swept into town. His familiar two-block walk took on the flavor of an adventure as he squelched through ankle-deep mud and leaned into the liquid wind. Sunil tried to cover him with an umbrella, but it was blown inside out. Children celebrated escaping the heat by jumping and splashing in puddles.

Tabin gave up any hope of remaining dry and turned his face up into the commotion, welcoming the change in weather. He didn't know what plans Ruit had for him, or where he was bound next, but he felt his time in Biratnagar had been an unequivocal success; he was now firmly on the path he'd been trying to follow ever since the day he'd seen the Dutch doctors working minor miracles. Tabin hadn't known the question Ruit had asked about his American apprentice's dedication to doctoring, but he had answered it for himself. He was now there—hundred percent—for his patients. Geoff Tabin had spent years seeking a kind of clarity in the earth's high places. As the rain fogged his glasses in the flatlands of Nepal and he tried to find his way through muddy crowds toward the gate of Golchha House, Tabin felt he'd never had a clearer vision of his future.

CHAPTER 15

The Wave Is Water

Do not accept any of my words on faith, believing them just because
I said them. Be like an analyst buying gold, who cuts, burns, and
critically examines his product for authenticity. Only accept what
passes the test by proving useful and beneficial in your life.
—Siddhartha Gautama, the Buddha

R uit wiped the window with the meat of his palm and squinted into
the rain. He couldn't see a thing. Somewhere out there, hidden by
impenetrable clouds, were Cho Oyu, Makalu, Lhotse, and Everest,
four of the ice giants of the Himalaya. Only the rumble of the plane's
jet engines hinted at the speed they were traveling past the peaks.

They were flying north, through angry gray storm clouds, soaring
over the sort of steep high passes and smoke-blackened villages his father and his caravans would have trudged through, on month-long
treks to trade goods in Lhasa. But they were due to reach Tibet's capital in a mere two hours. It wasn't the sort of travel Ruit could appreciate. There was no time to study the land as it rose, scouring away all
but the hardiest plants and people, no opportunity to ponder the collision of the Indian Plate and the Tibetan Plateau that had thrust these
mountains five miles into the atmosphere. In this thrumming aluminum tube, with windows that looked, to Ruit, as scarred and scratched
as traumatized corneas, he couldn't even say if they had crossed into
Chinese airspace or whether they were still flying over his own country. During his childhood, not knowing which side of the border he
was on might have meant the difference between life and death. How
odd it felt that they could simply soar past it.

In the aisle seat beside Ruit, Geoff Tabin twitched with nervous energy, gulping his handful of roasted peanuts all at once, while Ruit tucked the package into his rucksack, where it might come in handy while they waited out a landslide blocking one of Tibet's rural roads. Tabin wanted to talk, but Ruit had too much on his mind to make polite conversation and kept his face pressed to the window. After Fred's death, the Hollows Foundation had grown into a large and prominent Australian institution since the massive funeral they'd arranged and promoted in the Australian media with the slogan "Don't bring flowers. Bring a fiver." Ruit hoped that might mean a reliable source of funding for Tilganga, but he concluded the Fred Hollows Foundation was more interested in mining Tilganga's success for publicity than in funding it. Still worse, the FHF had written to Australia's latest ambassador in Kathmandu, Brendan Doran, warning him that the foundation planned to work with doctors countrywide, and not to become exclusively involved with Ruit.

Sarah Elliott, who worked as the Nepal program manager for the Fred Hollows Foundation at the time, remembers being stunned by the discourtesy of her organization toward the man she so admired. "Ruit was never content to sit on his accomplishments," she says. "He was always worrying about sustaining what he'd built, and those plans depended on our support. I did my best and tried to calm him down, without much success. Ruit felt like we'd betrayed and abandoned him, and I couldn't blame him because I felt the same way."

Ruit, as always, took inventory. Tilganga was nearly in a position to sustain itself. He had structured patient services on a cost-recovery model: middle-class and wealthy Nepalese paid for their surgeries on a sliding scale, which enabled Tilganga to offer free care to as many poor as were able to make it through the hospital's doors. But keeping the best staff meant being able to offer competitive salaries. The outreach and expansion he had in mind would take more substantial funds than they could raise in Nepal. Ruit knew he needed a foreign partner, but the future with the Hollows people was looking bleak.

Despite the positive reports he'd received from the staff at Golchha Hospital about Tabin's dedication, the inexperienced American doctor beside him, now polishing off his carton of mango juice like a greedy child, might have had all the ambition in the world, but ambition without fund-raising experience couldn't pay for the sort of expansion Ruit had in mind. He had invited Tabin to the eye camps in Tibet both as a reward for a job well done in Biratnagar and to gauge his commitment firsthand.

Just before the air turbulence struck, Ruit was considering just how poor his own Buddhist practice had become. He knew he should be grateful that Tilganga had reached the capacity of patients he'd designed the hospital to treat each day and was running smoothly, but he seemed incapable of living in the moment, except when he was at his microscope. Otherwise, his mind was always sprinting ten years ahead, toward the plans he was forming to expand quality eye care across the Himalaya. Ruit recognized a strain of that impatience in Tabin and appreciated that he, too, dared to leap toward the unknowable, striving toward something larger than the comfortable life of conventional doctoring.

The turbulence grasped them like the great hand of one of the scowling gods of his childhood that had so scared and fascinated him in the charged gloom of his village monastery. It shook the plane so violently he was sure the wings would snap free of the fuselage, and kept shaking it as they passed over the crest of the Himalaya, bouncing off the jet stream while the winds buffeted the solid metal aircraft like an illustration of the mutability of matter. While the flight attendants rushed to strap themselves into their jump seats and tried, unconvincingly, not to let any fear show on their smooth, doll-like faces, Ruit was living very much in the moment.

He reached out and grabbed Tabin's hand.

"Ever since I'd met him, patients had always told me how gentle Dr. Ruit's hands were." Tabin says. "But not then they weren't. He had me in a death grip, and I was shocked by his strength. I was afraid he was going to break my fingers."

The turbulence continued without relief. "I didn't like it much either," Tabin says, "but I'd flown a lot more than Sanduk, so I just started talking, trying to calm him down—anything that came into my head, really, how I'd been through worse in little tents on big, windy mountains, how much I'd enjoyed the breakfasts at Golchha House, but none of that seemed to help." So Tabin turned to a subject sure to engage Ruit and asked what his plans were for Tilganga, what he could do in the future if they could arrange funding and support from American sources.

Once he'd confirmed that the wing was still attached to the fuselage, Ruit pried his eyes away from the window to look at Tabin. He discussed the importance of not settling for taking shelter within a shiny new facility but expanding efforts to reach patients across the crests and folds and crenellations of the Himalaya, so the Kamisya Tamangs of the world wouldn't have to waste away for years in isolation, waiting to be released from darkness. He confided that he could no longer depend on the Hollows Foundation and he needed to find a new source of foreign capital.

Tabin talked about an idea that had been fermenting since he'd gotten to Biratnagar: creating a formal connection between Tilganga and American medical schools, so ophthalmic fellows could train in Kathmandu, where they were sure to find more challenging caseloads than at American hospitals, and Tilganga could benefit from the funding and prestige associated with bettering the skills of America's up-and-coming ophthalmologists. Tabin was a graduate of some of the world's most famous universities, he told Ruit, but he'd learned more about surgery in the months since he'd met Ruit than those institutions had been able to teach him in years. Other Western doctors, he said, should have the same opportunity.

They flew on, threshing out the details of how this sort of partnership might work. It was not lost on either of them that Tabin, technically, was unemployed. So finding a job at a university would be his first task after he returned to America. He would need to land at an institution that supported international health initiatives and permitted frequent foreign travel. It would take some searching, Tabin said, but he was sure it could be done. And though the turbulence tapered off soon after they crossed the highest point of the range and reached Tibet, Tabin noticed, as they approached the stony, sunbaked plain

surrounding Lhasa, descending along their glide path through mercifully smooth air, that Ruit was still holding, though no longer crushing,
his hand.

Since his last trip to Tibet, Lhasa had become another sort of city,
Tabin thought. They rolled into town on a freshly paved, four-lane
highway from Lhasa Gonggar Airport. During his first two visits as a
climber, Tibetans in traditional dress had dominated the population.
The Potala, where a succession of Dalai Lamas had lived among the
palace's thousand rooms and served as their people's spiritual guides,
still hovered over the heart of the town like a man-made mountain.

When Tabin had come to take his second crack at the Kangshung
Face, in 1983, heavily armed Chinese soldiers had stood guard outside
the stronghold of Tibetan Buddhism, barring entry. But by 1995 the
Potala and many of Tibet's religious monuments had become tourist
attractions, besieged by armies of camera-toting Han, the ethnic group
that made up more than 90 percent of China's population. As their bus
neared their hotel, Tabin noticed that the majority of faces they passed
in the street belonged to ethnic Chinese in Western clothes. And the
historical center of Lhasa, with its low, wooden traditional homes, sea-
soned by centuries of wood smoke, was surrounded by a modern Chinese city, which encircled the Tibetan quarter like a stockade.

What Beijing hadn't been able to do by force—crush the heart of a
Buddhist rebel movement that resented China's occupation—they
were trying to achieve by dilution, by making Tibetans a minority in
their own land. During the last decade, tens of thousands of Han Chinese had accepted Beijing's offer of cash incentives and relocated their
families to Tibet.

Tabin's sense of discomfort only increased when he and Ruit arrived for their first day of work at Lhasa City Hospital. Drs. Olo and
Kesang had continued their studies since Jiri, and they hoped to hone
their skills further alongside Ruit and Tabin. But many of the hospital's
senior staff were Han Chinese, and Tabin was appalled by the generally low medical standards. "Lhasa City Hospital, despite the grandeur

of Lhasa relative to Kathmandu, was a backward and unsanitary place compared to Tilganga," Tabin says. "And seeing how bad it was, I had even more admiration for what Ruit had been able to build."

Tabin says he witnessed a devastating breach of medical ethics his first day at the hospital, when he saw poorly trained Chinese surgeons attempt to perform an appendectomy on a teenage boy. They were unable to locate his appendix and ruptured several blood vessels trying to reach it, Tabin says. He watched the boy's abdomen fill up with pus and blood as each probe and thrust of their scalpels made the situation worse. "I was kicking myself," Tabin says, "because if I'd jumped in right away, I could have performed a reasonable appendectomy. But by the time they'd made a mess of his bowels, repairing the damage was beyond my abilities." Tabin watched the doctors give up and sew their doomed patient's incisions shut. "Later, I learned they told the boy's parents that they'd found incurable cancer and informed them that he was likely to die."

Tabin wanted to pursue the matter and report the doctors to the authorities, but Ruit restrained him forcefully. "You can't do everything at once, Geoff," he told Tabin, something he would repeat to the man who would become his partner so often over the years that it would become a kind of mantra. "We have to choose our battles strategically."

Ruit and Tabin operated side by side, as Drs. Olo and Kasang observed. Ruit was still much faster, completing four surgeries to every one of his, but Tabin hoped the progress he'd made in Biratnagar was apparent. He looked over at Ruit's table each time he finished a case, hoping for a sign of approval or encouragement, but none came. Ruit appeared oblivious to his surroundings.

After four hours, Tabin stood up and prepared to scrub out for a bathroom break.

"Where are you going?" Ruit inquired the second Tabin pushed back his stool.

"Out to take a pee, back in a flash," Tabin said, but something in Ruit's tone of voice as he'd asked the question kept him rooted to the spot instead.

"You know, Geoff," Ruit said gravely, "you really must learn to control yourself better."

Tabin, gritting his teeth, sat back down. While working on patients, the sensation was bearable, but after he taped the eye of each completed case shut and swiveled on his stool, tapping his feet, waiting for the next Tibetan to be led to his table, the pressure was intolerable. After two more hours, Tabin could take it no longer. He pushed back his screeching stool, scrubbed out, and jogged toward the hospital's mercifully vacant squat toilet. He could hear Ruit's high-pitched giggle all the way down the hall. "I don't know how he does it," Tabin says. "I've seen him operate sixteen hours without a break. If the *Guinness Book* had a category for bladder control, Ruit would hold the world record."

That evening, Tabin and Ruit sat on the balcony of their hotel, continuing their conversation about collaborating after Tabin returned to America, as the sun sparked fiery reflections in the tiers of windows that climbed the Potala toward the darkening sky. "This morning your post-op patients looked really first-rate," Ruit said, pouring each of them a tumbler of whiskey. "Your surgery is coming, Geoff, don't you think?"

"I'm trying," Tabin said.

"You're trying *hard*," Ruit said. "Now we have to get our Tibetan friends up to snuff."

Tabin liked the sound of that "we."

Their final morning in Lhasa, the last batch of postoperative patients assembled on benches in the hospital's courtyard. Tabin and Ruit bent to examine each of them. Ruit used a cheap plastic flashlight and Tabin studied their handiwork with a climber's headlamp, but they both saw the same results: All 155 of the eyes Ruit and Tabin had operated on appeared clear and without complications. Olo and Kesang's clumsier surgeries had mildly traumatized some of their patients' eyes, but the redness and swelling would disappear in a few days, and both Tibetan doctors had progressed to the point that they were now capable of operating on their own. All in all, a cause for celebration. Ruit threw his arm over Tabin's shoulder as they walked toward the hired bus that would take them toward the surgical camp they planned to conduct in Medrokongga, three hours from Lhasa. "Well," he said, "we've managed to light two more candles, isn't it, Geoff?"

North of Lhasa, the paved highway disintegrated into a gravel road, then a rutted track, as it left the plains and climbed along the Tsangpo River Gorge. The river coiled back on itself as they rolled along the wall of the canyon it cut, into the mountains that towered over Medrokongga. They were able to see the route they would have to travel, miles ahead, where the road doubled back in their direction, following the river, clinging to the face of the gorge. And they could clearly make out the series of pale scars that blighted the hillside, where the road had been washed out by landslide or flood and local workers had buttressed it against the sheer slope with stones.

At thirteen thousand feet, the site where they planned to operate in Medrokongga County looked more like a nomad encampment than a permanent settlement, Tabin thought. Hundreds of families had settled on the stony grounds of a dilapidated clinic, warming their hands over yak dung fires or stirring *tsampa* in blackened pots. At the sight of the medical staff disembarking from the bus, the hundreds who could see stood as one, cupped their hands together in blessing, and bowed. Tabin could feel the longing and hope rising from them as palpably as the smoke from their cooking fires.

Ruit was touched to see that even in these modern times, when foreign influence obliterated so much tradition, many of the families greeted them in the venerable Tibetan way, sticking out their tongues respectfully. He had chosen to come here because preliminary screening had indicated that this community had the highest percentage of blindness he'd ever encountered. Among Medrokongga's eight hundred residents, nearly two hundred were suffering from severe cataracts.

The optimistically named Medrokongga County Hospital was, in fact, a one-story bunker with peeling paint that had once been white. The hopes of the crowd outside the door weighed on Tabin as he inspected the place where he was expected to cure them. "There was no heat and no power," Tabin says, "and somehow it felt even colder inside. The place was ripe with the stench of excrement and stale urine. Welcoming committees of flies greeted us in each of the three rooms. I was only relatively sure we could make this place sterile enough for surgery."

He stepped back out into the early-afternoon chill and saw that the sun had already sunk behind the canyon's western wall. Tabin stared at the crowd, mentally adding up the hours it would take to cure such a quantity of blindness. Beyond them, on the trail that descended from the upper settlement, more blind patients in rags rolled toward them on flat carts with wooden wheels, pulled by rusty tractors.

When he looked away from the smoke and filth and torn clothing and turned to his colleague, Tabin was stirred by the expression on Ruit's face. Ruit stood on the hospital's stoop, looking over the encampment, beaming like he'd never been happier in his life.

"Don't you see how perfect this is, Geoff?" Ruit said, pointing toward the swelling crowd, elated to accept the absolute fact of their suffering, and the power he had to make it cease. "This is where the people need us!"

Buddhist scholars preach the importance of learning to distinguish between relative truth, *samvrti-satya*, and absolute truth, *paramartha-satya*. To understand relative truth, the Vietnamese Buddhist monk and teacher Thich Nhat Hanh explains in *The Heart of the Buddha's Teaching*, study the movement of water. Watch how a wave moves, absorb the temporary beauty of its unique shape as it swells, crests, and collapses. To comprehend absolute truth, he teaches, look deeper, and remember that, whatever form it takes, the wave has always been, and will always be, water. "It would be sad," Thich Nhat Hanh says, "if the wave did not know that it is water," if it thought, *"when I arrive at the shore, I will return to nonbeing."*

Growing up privileged in a Western world that offered him limitless opportunities, Tabin had flowed like a shape-shifting wave through the ocean of relativity that is modern American life. He could be a tennis player, a bungee jumper, a magician, and a mountaineer. He could commit to medicine. Or he could try to be all these things at once.

Since the day Tabin had made eye contact with Ruit over an operating table at Tilganga, he had learned more crucial lessons more quickly than he had imagined possible. Confronting suffering at Tilganga and Jiri and Biratnagar, he had learned to lessen it, as Reeta had taught him, by wielding a blade like a fencer's foil. He had learned that the best way to lift others up was by example. And he had learned about the bone-deep satisfaction that comes from working to the limit of your abilities. But standing beside Ruit on the steps of the Medrokongga County Hospital, and staring at these people, his patients, he got a glimpse of a deeper, more absolute truth. He hadn't come to this windswept settlement to find his path, further his training, or win Ruit's favor. He was not only a wave; he was water, at one with this ocean of humanity who looked toward him and Ruit with such hope. He was here because he was needed. And now he needed to get to work.

Over the next three days, Ruit and Tabin operated in the dank room where the staff had scrubbed and disinfected every surface before nailing plastic tarps straight into the concrete ceiling and over all four walls. When their generator ran out of fuel, which was often, they continued working while technicians held flashlights over their patients. After the quarts of sweet tea Tabin drank at breakfast, trying to stay hydrated and warm, he still had to schedule his surgeries around the clarion call of his bladder. Ruit no longer made mention of his absences, other than allowing himself a brief smirk of pride.

"I had learned something important about Geoff," Ruit says. "He was a persistent cat. Like me. He kept climbing over whatever obstacles I threw in his path. And I saw that he was relentless in the best way. You don't often find people with such stamina. What we were doing was hard—no one had ever tried to cure people in this place—but I never heard him complain. There aren't many like that, who are willing to stand by you hundred and one percent."

Each morning, after warming their fingers around scalding mugs of tea, the doctors examined the previous day's patients before scrubbing in. Tabin had been alarmed, at first, when one of these patients had been placed on his operating table. She was covered with so many cuts and bruises that Tabin worried she was the victim of domestic violence. When he asked about her injuries through an interpreter, sixty-three-year-old Sonam Detchen told him she was a widow. Without living sons, she explained, she had no one to help her, so she often bumped into farming implements, cut herself while trying to cook, or fell into ditches.

The morning after Tabin repaired her eyes, seconds after he re-moved her white gauze patches, Detchen burst into tears of relief that streamed past the bruises on her broad, sunburned face. "You don't get many moments in your life when you're absolutely positive you're doing exactly what you were put on earth to do," Tabin says. "That was one of them."

Tabin watched Detchen squint, then stare at the serrated tips of the eastern ridgeline that cut into the pure blue sky with the precision of a freshly sharpened saw blade. "There is a new sky for my eye! I'm free from the hell of darkness!" she shouted, hauling herself to her feet. The day before, Detchen hadn't been able to see the shadow of a hand waving an inch in front of her face. "Now," she told Tabin proudly, "I can see well enough to take care of myself."

Their last night in Medrokongga, after nearly two hundred patients had received the same gift as Detchen, the village elders and the medi-cal team gathered inside the community center, a big structure built in a disheartening style, with walls of unpainted concrete blocks. But the large single room at the interior of the building was purely Tibetan. Around a metal firebox that warmed the air a few degrees, low benches were arranged against the wall, and covered with handwoven rugs.

After dinner, their hosts lunged around the room, topping up their cups every time they took a few sips with more sweet Chinese liquor. While Tabin tried to calculate how much he'd drunk, a musical com-petition broke out. It started innocently enough, with the Nepalese, led by Sonam, singing their traditional songs. Both groups danced to the rhythm Nabin banged on his bench in accompaniment, since he had no *madal* at hand. The Tibetans responded with selections from their own classical operas, which unfolded leisurely enough for Tabin and Ruit to remain upright, swaying on their feet, despite the alcohol and the altitude.

A local boy of no more than nineteen upped the ante when he unveiled a boom box, slid in a cassette he'd produced from the pocket of his torn dress shirt, and pushed Play. Michael Jackson's "Thriller" thumped out of the overstressed speakers. This whip-thin boy, with bowl-cut hair, brick-red cheeks, and castaway clothing, transformed himself into a credible King of Pop. Mirroring moves he'd perfected studying Jackson's video of "Billie Jean," he spun in place, spread his legs, and flipped up the collar of his shirt. The elders took their seats and the Tilganga team tried to keep pace, but dancing so fast in air so thin sent them panting toward their benches.

"Nabin," Ruit said, "don't give in so easily."

Gamely, Nabin stood back up, kept pace with the boy for a few more steps, and was even feeling cocky enough to attempt a spin before the altitude asserted itself. He gasped for air and collapsed back into his seat.

"Sonam!" Ruit ordered, playing his ace. "Get out there and kick his ass!"

Sonam, slim and fit, always at the head of every trek up the steepest trails in Nepal's mid-hills, fared no better above thirteen thousand feet. He faced off against the boy, and their two pairs of thin legs flailed together in time, at first, but the Tibetan danced faster and faster, swinging his arms wide and raising himself to balance on his toes, posing to hold his arm above his head, brandishing Jackson's imaginary fedora. After two minutes, Sonam's chest heaved and he slunk back to his seat, defeated.

"Bugger this," Ruit said. "I'll beat him myself!"

"You should know that Ruit never dances," Tabin says, laughing at the memory. "And he wasn't exactly light on his feet. By then he already had a potbelly beginning to poke over the edge of his belt. But Sanduk stood up and tried to match the boy step for step, grimacing with the effort of upholding Nepal's honor." Ruit lasted longer than anyone else, perhaps three minutes, until the song ended. But when the next song began, the boy went for broke. He started moonwalking, gliding backward and turning, gliding backward and turning, describing a square around Ruit, who staggered in place like a gut-shot bear. Then the boy took pity on the Nepalese doctor. He grasped Ruit in his arms and spun him gently around the room until the song ended, and Ruit hugged him with relief. The audience broke into wild, alcohol-fueled applause.

Much later, when the others had tottered off toward their beds, Ruit and Tabin sat together, near the smoldering coals. "You know, Geoff," Ruit said, "these really are the most deserving people in the world, don't you think?"

"I do," Tabin said. "Not only the people here, but everywhere in the Himalaya."

"So let's do something about it, everywhere in the Himalaya," Ruit said.

And by the barely warm stove, under blankets that smelled of yak dung and hay, they shook hands and made a vow. They would work together to wipe out all preventable blindness in the Himalaya. They would train and equip doctors not only in Nepal and Tibet, and they wouldn't rest until every surgeon across the entire range was trained to implant artificial lenses under a microscope. Tabin looked down at his hand, crushed once again by Ruit's startlingly strong grip. This time, they were not up in the air but on absolutely solid ground, and he didn't mind the pain at all.

CHAPTER 16

Rock Meets Bone

It is the spotless precious clear crystal.
It is the glow of the lamp of self-luminous mind.
When you intensify devotion in your heart,
Rock meets bone in insight.
—His Eminence the Third Jamgon Kongtrul, *Cloudless Sky*

The brand-new BMW hugged the curves so well on the seven-thousand-foot descent from the monastery above the Indian town of Lava toward the airport at Siliguri that its driver gained more confidence with every mile. The sporty sedan the Jamgon Kongtrul's brother bought for him promised to make the frequent travel that was required of the Rinpoche, to oversee his charitable projects, faster and far more comfortable.

The Rinpoche rode up front, admiring flashes of cloudless sky through gaps in the leaf-dark forest canopy. The driver pushed the powerful sedan hard, after they'd finished the hazardous descent, and the flat road stretched temptingly straight.

Tenzeng Dorjee, one of the Third Jamgon Kongtrul's closest disciples, remembers the events of that day well. He can't say the precise speed they were traveling, because he was sitting in the backseat with another monk, but he knows they were moving fast. Suddenly, he saw several pigeons dart in front of the car. "As you know," Dorjee says, "in our tradition, every life is significant." The driver did his best, swerving to avoid the birds, but he lost control and they pitched toward the forest and slammed into the rock-hard trunk of a large tree. "The Rinpoche's earthly mind was dissolved into *parinirvana*. My companions also were killed. I alone lived," Dorjee says, "and was left to consider why such a sadly tragic thing had taken place."

The Jamgon Kongtrul and the Karmapa are leaders of the Kagyu, one of the four major sects of Tibetan Buddhism. The Kagyu is also known to some as "the Whispering School," since it places great stock in the oral transmission of Buddhist wisdom from scholarly leaders to their disciples. Replacing a leader as charismatic as the Third Jamgon Kongtrul was no simple matter. His absence left a Rinpoche-shaped hole in the hearts of those who had come to respect him, like Sanduk Ruit. "Too many of our monks are content to sit in comfortable monasteries, meditating," Ruit says. "The Third Jamgon Kongtrul traveled throughout Asia, and even to Europe and America, telling people it wasn't enough just to chant *Om mani padme om*. He taught that true compassion means rolling up your sleeves and making people's lives better."

Though he was only thirty-nine at the time of the crash in April 1992, the Rinpoche left a lifetime's worth of inspiration for his disciples. He built a medical clinic at the gate of his monastery in Lava, where local people could come for free treatment. He bought land and set aside funds to build Pullahari, a retreat center for both Asian and Western scholars in the hills outside Kathmandu. He founded a combination orphanage and old-age home on a shared site in the former British hill station of Kalimpong, in northeast India. And, though his Rinpoche didn't live to see Ruit conduct surgery near his monastery in northern India, Dorjee sold the wrecked BMW and used the proceeds to fund Ruit's first camp in the region, where the doctor and two local trainees operated on more than seven hundred patients over the course of ten days.

The search for the Fourth Jamgon Kongtrul lasted more than three years. Even as a boy, the Seventeenth Karmapa, the head of the oldest lineage in Tibetan Buddhism, was noted by his disciples for his uncanny ability to predict reincarnations of Rinpoches like the Jamgon Kongtrul. When he was twelve, the Karmapa summoned Tenzeng Dorjee and told him he'd been having visions indicating the spot where the Fourth Jamgon Kongtrul could be found. He wrote a prediction letter, detailing images that had come to him in dreams: He had seen a great black mountain near the Tsurphu Monastery in southern Tibet; he'd seen the smiling face of the Third Jamgon Kongtrul materialize within a rainbow just south of the monastery, by a turbulent river, and at that exact spot, he'd watched the Rinpoche's face dissolve into spectral colors; and he had been granted a glimpse of a two-story home, populated by eight people, with the door facing east, where the young boy could be found. "Be attentive to these signs," the Karmapa wrote, "and to the presence of rainbows, and you'll find the Rinpoche."

Tenzeng Dorjee led a search party to Tibet. They combed the villages south of the Tsurphu Monastery, looking for a house matching the Karmapa's description. They found it in the village of Sehmed Shang, with a door facing east toward rapids that surged over boulders in the Tsangpo River. The boy, eight months old at the time, was the youngest of a family of eight. He was plump, with outsized ears. "When I entered the home," Dorjee says, "the boy, who was bound to his mother's back, smiled at me like a long-lost friend, like the Third Jamgon Kongtrul."

Dorjee returned to the Karmapa and informed him of his discovery. The Karmapa rummaged in a wooden trunk until he found what he wanted. According to Dorjee, the Karmapa placed a replica of the home he had just visited in Sehmed Shang on the carpet before him, which the Karmapa had crafted from his vision out of a children's set of Lego building blocks. "Is this the residence of the Fourth Jamgon Kongtrul?" he asked.

"It is, Rinpoche!" Dorjee replied, his eyes flooding with tears.

They whisked the boy out of Tibet and into India. At the seat of the Tibetan government in exile, in McLeod Ganj, India, the Dalai Lama wrote a formal letter of recognition, hung a scarlet cord around the boy's neck, and performed the traditional hair-cutting ceremony to welcome the reincarnation of the Rinpoche, whom he named Tenzin Osel Choying Gyatso. The Dalai Lama agreed to supervise the Fourth Jamgon Kongtrul's Buddhist education, and sent tutors with the Jamgon Kongtrul's entourage when they departed to take up permanent residence at Lava.

Stopping at the partially built Pullahari, on his way through Nepal back to the home of his previous earthly incarnation, the Fourth Jamgon Kongtrul was greeted by a crowd of thousands of monks, lamas, and devotees of the Kagyu faith who had come from around the world, straining for a glimpse of the spiritual leader they believed had been returned to them.

Ruit and Tabin rode in Hilda, driving up the same road the Third Jamgon Kongtrul had descended on the last day of his life. They crossed the British-built Coronation Bridge over the slow-moving Teesta River, where, even at this early hour, gangs of thin, sun-darkened workers heaved large rocks from the shallows to shore, for others to break into manageable bits with sledgehammers. The air became noticeably cooler as they climbed, and Hilda's engine roared, hauling them up the steep grade, tilting around tight curves cut from dense vegetation, as vines slapped at the windshield and monkeys, sitting inert in the middle of the road, stood and ambled insouciantly into the foliage at the last possible second.

Since Ruit and Tabin had made their pact in Medrokongga, more than a year ago, Tabin had taken up residence at a lower altitude, in New England. When he'd returned to America, only one academic position in ophthalmology with the specialization in corneal surgery he sought had been posted. The process had been extremely competitive, but Tabin had prevailed—in part because of the experience he'd gained working alongside Ruit. After the University of Vermont offered him the job, Tabin negotiated unconventional terms of employment. He says he turned down $150,000 and five weeks of vacation to press for less money and more time away, agreeing instead on a salary of $105,000 and three months a year in which he would be free to work overseas. If he didn't have at least three months a year to devote to international work, Tabin felt, he wouldn't be able to dedicate himself to his partnership with Ruit.

They settled on the name Ruit had suggested for their charity, the Himalayan Cataract Project, though Tabin's ambition was to equip both Tilganga and their new organization with specialists trained to treat every type of preventable blindness. Tabin would eventually file paperwork making the HCP a 501(c)(3) nonprofit organization, capable of accepting tax-deductible donations, but for the time being, they were an NGO in name only; the few donations Tabin had been able to collect were small contributions from friends and relatives.

After this trip, he told Ruit, he'd devote himself more vigorously to the process of charming cash out of colleagues and acquaintances. "One positive thing about my checkered academic history," Tabin says, "is that I knew high-earning graduates from every institute of higher education I'd bounced between. And I planned to target them all."

As Hilda crested the ravine, the landscape softened and spread its wings, soaring past the sculpted hillocks of tea plantations, toward the wide, ice-encrusted summit to the west that moved both the mountaineer in Tabin and the Walung in Ruit. Kangchenjunga billowed like a sail set to capture the breath of the rising sun. They had been discussing the number of surgeries they could expect to perform when they reached Kalimpong, and the challenge of training the local doctors, but the sight of Ruit's mountain silenced them both.

Tabin sensed that this wasn't simply a trip they were taking together to cure another group of blind patients. They could drive in almost any direction from Kathmandu and the level of need would be nearly the same. When Ruit had suggested that they work so close to the region where he'd been raised, a door had slid open slightly. Tabin felt he was being invited to peer through the crack, to look a bit more deeply at the forces that had made his partner a person he was still only starting to understand.

This view of Kangchenjunga was nearly the same Ruit had seen as a schoolboy in Darjeeling. Kalimpong, another former British hill station gone gracefully to seed, was separated by only a few miles of tea plantations—folded back on themselves like bolts of green velvet—from the site where his formal education had begun. Ruit hadn't been back to Olangchungola since his trip as a young doctor, accompanying the border survey team, and he wondered if circumstances would ever permit him to return. But being able to work so close to Kangchen-junga was nevertheless a kind of homecoming.

The Jamgon Kongtrul the Third Memorial Home sprawled across a hilltop at the edge of town. The low, latticed Victorian bungalows of the original compound had been connected by garden walkways and trellises of tropical plants to concrete dormitories for the orphans and elderly, who regarded the residence not as a dead Rinpoche's experi-ment in social engineering so much as simply home. Thirty-odd chil-dren gathered on the stairs leading from the drive to the upper compound, shyly cocking their heads and scrutinizing Tabin as he leapt out of the vehicle in running shoes, trekking pants, and an un-zipped orange fleece jacket that exposed his bare chest. Tenzeng Dor-jee bowed and placed a white silk *kata* around Ruit's neck as he climbed out of the Land Cruiser. Tabin, too, lowered his head to receive the lama's blessing.

Ruit raised his eyes and saw how healthy and well cared for the chil-dren looked. They had come from villages like his own—last places—where everything, especially opportunity, was scarce. He saw his younger self in them, recalled the boy who had been frightened, at first, by the store-bought clothes and sophistication of students raised in towns and cities. These children, too, would have suffered in their journeys down from the moon. He stared at them and felt so much tenderness he could hardly speak.

Tabin was also touched by the children. He performed nightly magic shows for them. And when he made his set of sponge balls ap-pear and vanish at will, or seemed to swallow a lit cigarette without suffering any apparent injury, he was greeted with gales of laughter and wild applause, until he slipped in the set of plastic vampire teeth he'd hidden in his pocket, growled, and the laughter turned to delighted screams.

Ruit was pleased to see how comfortable Tabin was with the chil-dren. "When I saw Geoff entertaining them with magic and scaring them with a set of artificial dentures," Ruit says, "I wondered why he didn't have any children of his own. He was nearly forty years old at the time, so I advised him to think about starting a family before it was too late." Ruit wasn't the only one. Tabin's mother had gradually resigned herself to the dangers he faced as a climber—he'd cheerfully ignored her protests for decades—but she'd never stopped hoping he'd settle down or hinting how much she longed for him to have children. For his thirty-fifth birthday, Johanna Tabin had gone so far as to send her son a package containing two sets of baby clothing, one pink, one blue, and a note that read, "Just in case."

"I've always related well to kids," Tabin says. "Maybe that's why I tend to spend more time socially with climbers than with doctors, who tend to be pretty serious. Climbers retain that sick, twisted, immature sense of humor, like children who've never grown up. I always figured I'd have children someday, but that day hadn't come and I was beginning to feel a little concerned that the twisting path I'd taken in life meant it might never happen for me."

"Fourteen–seven, Geoff, isn't it?"

"If you say so," Tabin said, hands on his knees, laboring to draw a full breath.

This pre-breakfast match was played, mercifully, without spectators, except for the wall of stuffed and mounted animal heads the British had hung when this had been a colonial social club. Tabin was still losing badly, but he knew that his badminton, like his surgical technique, was steadily improving. He'd moved Ruit around the court enough this time that a small patch of sweat darkened the center of his sky-blue polo shirt.

Like most of the colonial relics in the hill stations, the club building sagged somewhat, under the weight of moisture, overgrown vegetation, and time. Its stuffy rooms were hung with fading framed black-and-white group portraits of British officers in tennis whites, but the clay courts outside had reverted to mud, and the furnishings stank of mold.

"Have you thought about what I told to you, about finding a suitable woman?"

"I'm trying not to think about anything right now," Tabin said, "except beating you at this ridiculous game."

"Never!" Ruit said, giggling happily as he served a final ace for match point. As they zipped their racquets back into their cases and set out toward a day of surgeries, a silent gallery of dusty glass eyes—of musk deer, ibex, mountain goats, and Marco Polo sheep—looked on, without apparent judgment.

During most of his days in Kalimpong, Tabin was too busy to ruminate about his romantic life. At Tenzeng Dorjee's invitation, they were holding one of the few cataract camps the area had ever seen. Tea plantation workers, exposed to the sun all day, had extraordinarily high rates of cataract disease. So did the Lepcha people, who lived in the forest between the hill stations and worked as woodcutters and stone breakers, providing basic heating and building materials for the more affluent residents of Darjeeling and Kalimpong. Nuns of Mother Teresa's Missionaries of Charity, wearing the traditional white saris bordered with blue, scoured the valleys between the hill towns ahead of Ruit and Tabin's arrival, urging Lepcha families to bring their blind up to Kalimpong.

Thinlay Ngodup, a lay Buddhist with a scraggly goatee, windblown hair, and a wild cackling laugh, whom Dorjee had chosen to direct the Jamgon Kongtrul the Third Memorial Home, says finding patients for the dozens of eye camps the HCP has since held in Kalimpong has rarely been a problem. "For years, we could throw out a net from our perch on top of this hill and catch two or three hundred blind people," he told me.

Ruit and Tabin operated for a week in a school where the orphans ordinarily studied; formerly a storehouse for Tibetan trade goods owned by the Third Jamgon Kongtrul's father, it was a half-hour walk uphill from the memorial home. Dorjee, well aware of the thousands more in the surrounding hills who needed surgery, suggested to Ruit over dinner one evening that the Jamgon Kongtrul's trust fund the construction of an eye hospital in Kalimpong, based on the Tilganga model. "My Rinpoche may not have lived to see it," Ruit says. "Still, I was happy that those, like Dorjee, charged with grasping the baton and continuing what he started were committed to carrying out his vision."

Ngodup, full of tireless good humor, seemed to be everywhere at once, helping to screen patients, feed and shelter their families, or translate. Tabin could see why he'd been chosen to run a facility with such wide-ranging responsibilities. One morning Tabin operated on a Lepcha man with a single cataract. His healthy eye had enabled him to keep his job, breaking rocks on the road to Siliguri. His wife had worked hammering them into smaller stones alongside him, until she'd lost her sight completely. Tabin was sure the surgery he'd performed on both of them the previous day had gone well and that the couple could expect good results. But when their bandages came off, they began behaving strangely. Though Tabin couldn't understand their language, they appeared to be arguing, and the woman, wearing a freshly laundered crimson sari, poked her husband in the chest and twisted the fabric of his faded dress shirt. It had been scrubbed and washed against river rocks so many times that its original color was a mystery, and all that remained was a faint paisley pattern.

Tabin called Ngodup over. "What are they saying?" he asked. "Is there a problem with their eyes?"

Ngodup squatted in front of the couple and cocked his head to listen for a moment, before laughing. "The wife is very angry at the husband," he explained to Tabin. "She says to him, 'The last time I saw you, three years ago, you were wearing that same ugly shirt. Are we so poor that you can't afford another? Or have you stopped taking pride in your appearance altogether?'"

More than six hundred patients had gathered at Kalimpong, taxing the small surgical team of Tabin, Ruit, and two local doctors who'd done only a few hundred microsurgeries between them. Ruit put the pedal down and drove through an enormous caseload each day, leaving Tabin in charge of training the two surgeons, who had come from Sikkim, twenty miles to the northwest.

Sikkim had spent much of its history fending off foreign powers with designs on the strategic thumb-shaped land straddling the mountains between India and Tibet. In the late 1930s, eager to avoid being absorbed by British India, the *chogyal*, or king, of Sikkim signed an alliance with Nazi Germany. Nazi dignitaries visited on the verge of World War II and were greeted with all the ceremony that the small nation could muster. Banners decorated with the traditional Buddhist pinwheel signifying good luck—the *svastika*, as it's known in Sanskrit—were displayed in honor of the regime that had appropriated it as a state symbol, and for years thereafter Sikkimese children were christened with unlikely Teutonic names. Following India's independence, Sikkim was gradually absorbed by its neighbor to the south, first becoming an Indian protectorate, shielded from China's military by India's armed forces. Finally, in 1975, the Sikkimese, frightened by repeated border skirmishes with the Chinese and worried that they might suffer the same fate as Tibet, voted to officially become the twenty-second state of India.

Which is how Tabin came to be training not only a Sikkimese surgeon named B. P. Dhakal but an ophthalmologist with the unforgettable name of Hitler Pradhan. "At first I got a big kick out of the idea that a Jew was teaching Hitler how to heal the blind of Sikkim," Tabin says. "But training them was tough. B.P. had excellent academic credentials, but he was too cocky for someone who had hardly performed any surgery. B.P. would charge ahead, make mistakes, then come to me very obsequiously and ask for help. Hitler was an experienced surgeon, but he had rather heavy, clumsy hands. He would just bumble on and giggle when he wasn't able to do some of the more delicate work."

Tabin took over cases when Dhakal or Pradhan ran into trouble. He tried not to bother Ruit, but he often had to ask for his partner's help. Tabin sensed the goodwill and trust he'd been accumulating with Ruit starting to slip away, and with each interruption, his felt Ruit's annoyance rise from a simmer to a boil.

"What are you here for?" Ruit barked at Tabin, sliding off his stool to repair the damage after Dhakal's blade had plunged too deep, rupturing a patient's iris. "You have to be better, Geoff, you know?"

"I tried to let the criticism slide," Tabin says. "I'd had much more insulting things said to me by big-shot surgeons during my training in the States. But Ruit's disapproval was really hard to take. He had a way of making everyone around him feel like they were failing if they weren't always getting better." Tabin experienced uncharacteristic doubts about whether he and Ruit had aimed too high. The goal they'd set for the HCP—"to eradicate preventable blindness across the entire Himalaya and beyond"—was so overwhelming that at moments like this, Tabin felt the weight of the communities they'd yet to cure pressing down so hard he could barely breathe. He had to be better, Tabin told himself, not only at the operating table but by working to turn the HCP into an organization capable of keeping such an ambitious promise.

Back amid the noise and bustle of Kathmandu, which seemed busier and dirtier every time Tabin returned to town, he pushed himself to the point of exhaustion at Tilganga. He operated when Ruit or Reeta were in the clinic, examining and diagnosing patients. He contacted Hugh Taylor and helped arrange a retinal fellowship in Melbourne for Govinda Paudyal, Tilganga's most talented young surgeon. And he spoke with Reeta about the HCP funding a fellowship so she could work with him in Vermont, where she could hone her skills as a corneal specialist.

During the evenings, he roamed the pubs and cafés of Thamel, the place where he had been happiest during his climbing days, hoping for temporary refuge from Ruit's scrutiny. At the Rum Doodle bar—where, on a block of wood bolted to the wall, his signature was inscribed alongside those of such luminaries as Sir Edmund Hillary and Tenzing Norgay—he met a barefoot young Australian backpacker on her first trip to Asia. "I don't remember her name," Tabin says, "but I know that she'd shaved her head, and for some reason being bald made her unusually attractive to me."

Tabin had a card the restaurant had issued him, as it did to all who summited Everest, entitling him to free meals for life. But the management of the Rum Doodle wisely made these climbers, notorious for their bottomless ability to consume alcohol, pay for their own drinks. Tabin bought himself and the woman a beer, and then another, and another, telling tales about his climbing days and the way his life had swerved and become more serious, maybe too serious for him to maintain, since he'd met Ruit.

He woke up in her shabby guesthouse room the next morning, his head throbbing. By the light streaming through the room's tie-dyed curtains, he watched the woman while she slept, taking in details he hadn't paid much attention to the night before. Her arms were heavily covered in tribal tattoos. Metal studs pierced her eyebrows and upper lip. When she woke up, she reminded him that he'd promised to show her Tilganga. So after the Asian backpackers' staple breakfast of banana pancakes, he brought her to the hospital.

Tabin walked the woman, still barefoot, to Ruit's table so she could observe him at surgery. Ruit's face was covered by a mask, but when he looked up and took the measure of Tabin's companion, his raised eyebrows told Tabin all he needed to know.

"This was really too much," Ruit remembers. "I mean, this person was a completely unsuitable presence. She had metals sticking out all over her face! And Geoff hadn't thought twice before bringing this barefoot, tattooed girl to a place so respectable as Tilganga. I had some doubts about Geoff's judgment before, but after seeing her, those doubts doubled."

A week later, when the bald backpacker left for Australia, Tabin had dinner at the Ruits' cramped apartment over Archie's Photo Shop. It was the evening before his own flight was due to depart for America, and before heading home, Tabin hoped to patch up the offense he'd obviously caused his partner. Nanda had done what she could with the modest space, covering the linoleum floor with a Tibetan carpet and hanging lace curtains over the narrow windows. There was no dining table and no kitchen, so she cooked upstairs in Sonam and Kasang's apartment, and they ate the mutton curry and rice she brought downstairs seated on cushioned benches, holding the plates in their laps. The Ruit family had grown, despite the close quarters, and now, in addition to seven-year-old Sagar, they had two daughters, Serabla, five, and Satenla, two.

Most of the meal passed in silence, with Tabin aware of the tension he'd caused, but unsure of how to defuse it, and Ruit trying not to raise the subject. Tabin admired the cozy domestic scene, compared it with the squalid guesthouse where he'd spent the last week, and wondered whether the advice his mother and Ruit felt free to give about his personal life mightn't have some merit. With a faint twinge of jealousy, he watched the natural way Ruit and Nanda sat side by side, a hand or hip in constant contact, always finding an excuse to brush against each other. After dinner, the Ruits' pretty, dark-haired daughters climbed down from the benches to lounge on the carpet against their father's legs.

"I tried to keep my mouth shut," Ruit says. "And I made it through dinner, but knew I couldn't last much longer."

He'd formed a partnership with Tabin, and beyond their professional ties, he enjoyed the American's company. But Ruit still wondered if he could depend on him, if this man only a few years younger than himself was so immature that he was willing to risk everything they were trying to build for a pointless affair. "I mean," Ruit explains, "taking up with a woman like her, he could get diseases. He could be disgraced. He could fall down very fast and very far. I'd come to care about Geoff, and I felt it was my duty to tell him so."

"Really, Geoff," Ruit said, after Scrabla and Satenla had gone to bed, unable to contain himself any longer, "don't you think it might be time for you to grow up?"

Tabin opened his mouth to speak, but words wouldn't come. He settled for pressing his lips together and firmly nodding, once. The most infuriating thing about his partner, Tabin thought as he thanked Nanda for dinner, zipped up his fleece jacket, and patted his passport, was how often, and how indisputably, he was right.

CHAPTER 17

Sir Is Willing

When waking a tiger, use a long stick.
—Mao Tse-tung

The war came to Kathmandu on February 13, 1996. The Maoists fired the first shots of their revolution, launching small, coordinated attacks across the countryside at police posts, landlords' homes, and banks that extended loans to farmers at extortionate rates. They hurled Molotov cocktails at a Pepsi-Cola plant on the outskirts of Kathmandu, which they'd chosen as a symbol of capitalist oppression. The explosions left scorch marks on the exterior of the factory and burned a few outbuildings, but it failed to cut the supply of Pepsi products to the capital.

Most of the other attacks were also symbolic, targeting the institutions that oppressed Nepal's poor while carefully limiting human casualties. Prachanda, one of the movement's most charismatic leaders, told the press that the rebels limited their assaults on the capital because they didn't want to kill innocent people or scare the country's intellectuals away from revolution in one stroke. It's equally plausible that they avoided attacking Kathmandu because a poorly equipped peasant fighting force was reluctant, at first, to challenge a harder target, since the city was surrounded by military garrisons.

Ruit sympathized with the Maoists' cause. But he worried that if the violence grew from symbolic attacks to a bloody campaign, the ambitious expansion he and Tabin had set in motion would become infinitely more challenging.

The uprising was rooted in the desperate poverty of Nepal's rural population, and its power base rose from Rolpa, one of the most economically depressed districts in the country. Just before the first wave of attacks, the rebels had issued a declaration of forty demands, including the establishment of a democratic secular republic, the elimination of caste- and gender-based discrimination, and free education and health care for all Nepalese. "Nepal had been a feudal system for so long," Ruit says. "Countries in the region, like India, made tremendous advances in democracy and public welfare. But in Nepal, despite decades of protests, nothing changed. Certainly not the inequity between the elites and the rural people. And the anger had really been building. The country had reached the burning point."

The rebels called themselves "Maoists," which Ruit considered misguided, since the former Chinese leader had never been popular in Nepal. And history was increasingly judging Mao's legacy by the brutal excesses of his Cultural Revolution, when professionals were forcibly removed from cities to work in agrarian collectives and brigades of armed children were encouraged to denounce and even kill the parents, teachers, and other adults they judged to be enemies of the revolution.

Despite their unfortunate name, Ruit shared many of the goals of Nepal's new guerrilla army, and he certainly agreed with their grievances. "Out of that list of forty demands, I agreed with about thirty-eight of them," Ruit says. "Everything except extremism and violence. Most of their demands were about improving people's lives."

Even after downgrading the power of the monarchy in the early 1990s and taking tentative steps toward democracy, Nepal remained one of the world's poorest countries. Despite a healthy tourist industry and the capacity to produce abundant hydropower, the nation had a crumbling infrastructure and frequent power outages. Wealth accumulated through foreign investment pooled in the accounts of corrupt police, politicians, and the Kathmandu elite, rarely trickling down to communities in the countryside, where 81 percent of Nepal's population labored in subsistence agriculture and most lived, as Ruit was acutely aware, as impoverished peasants.

After dark, one chilly evening late in the winter of 1996, when the children were tucked under heavy quilts, asleep in their unheated apartment, the People's War approached Sanduk and Nanda Ruit via a ringing phone. Sanduk put down his newspaper and answered it. The voice was female and sounded very young. The Maoists used idealist young women to communicate in Kathmandu during the early years of the war. They often wore their hair in the twin braids common among college intellectuals in Kathmandu that year, a style suggested by the posters depicting fearless female soldiers—rifle in one hand, the clenched fist of the other held high—that the Maoists had pasted all over town. That was how Ruit pictured the woman—a girl really, he judged—on the other end of the line.

"I'm sorry to disturb you so late, Doctor *dai*, but there has been a blast."

"A *blast*?" Ruit said, seeing Nanda draw aside the curtain that separated the sleeping area and lean into the living room. He nodded toward her, assuring her that all was well, even though the news had shocked him, and she withdrew, sliding the curtain closed.

"A *bomb* blast," the girl said, choosing her words carefully. "A . . . *comrade* of ours . . . has been injured in the eyes. A commander. If sir is willing, we'd like to bring the commander to hospital."

"Sir is willing," Ruit said. "I'm a doctor, not a politician. An eye is an eye."

Ruit imagined that he could see her face flood with relief.

"How shall we manage it?" she asked.

"Tomorrow, we see the last patients by two-thirty," Ruit said. "Bring your commander by after that. I'll make sure everything is in readiness."

He made the first incision gently, widening the wound bit by bit with his blade, as he'd done so many times before, every movement delicate but brisk. Once he'd captured it with a cannula, the slightly opaque cataract slid easily out through the tunnel of tissue he'd constructed. After all of the challenging cataract operations he'd performed, this case was simple and stress-free.

Tabin inserted the intraocular lens smoothly and centered it in his patient's eye. He snuck a glance at his new supervisor, an ophthalmologist whose wavy, flame-colored hair escaped her surgical cap, wisp by wisp. Tabin pushed his stool away from the operating table, and his supervisor leaned in to look through the microscope's eyepiece, inspecting his work. "Lens is lined up well," she said. "The eye is clear and clean. I'd say it looks perfect, Dr. Tabin."

"Geoff," he said.

"Jean didn't remember me at first, but we'd met years before," Tabin says. "It was at a conference of the New England Ophthalmological Society in Boston, when I was a senior resident at Brown. I saw this hot redhead sitting alone during a lecture and introduced myself. As I recall, her first words to me weren't really that romantic. I think she said, 'Stop bothering me.' "

Tabin hadn't known it at the time, but her husband, Eugenio DeMarchis, an Italian anesthesiologist, had been killed a few years earlier, when the car he was driving home after he'd been called in for emergency, middle-of-the-night surgery at St. Vincent's Hospital on Staten Island, swerved into oncoming traffic and hit a truck head-on. He wasn't wearing a seat belt and survived the blunt impact of the steering wheel on his chest only long enough for an ambulance to rush him to the hospital before he died.

Widowed, with three daughters aged two, five, and seven, and a growing fear that she wasn't strong enough to raise them alone, Dr. Jean DeMarchis was in no mood to be romanced the day Tabin flirted with her at the conference. "I was trying to pay attention to the lecture and was having a hard enough time keeping my mind on my work when this guy started hitting on me," Jean says. "He looked young enough to be a medical student. You know how Geoff kind of hops when he gets excited? He was doing that, and I just wanted this hyper, hopping guy to leave me alone."

In Burlington, Dr. DeMarchis had been assigned to proctor her department's newest employee, which meant she was required to observe Tabin performing surgery. "When I saw Geoff's climber's hands, I thought, 'No way is this guy going to be any good.' But he was a terrific surgeon. His hands were a lot more delicate than they looked."

One evening soon after Tabin was hired, the chairman of the oph-thalmology department held a party in Tabin's honor, at his home on the shore of Lake Champlain, formally welcoming Geoff to the University of Vermont. Tabin sought out his redheaded supervisor. He took a draw from his beer and studied her. By the dusky lake, with lanterns lighting her wavy red hair, she looked, he thought, lovely. She didn't seem to remember their encounter in Boston. He considered reminding her, but he'd bought a small house only a block away from hers in Burlington, and he didn't want to give Jean the impression that he was stalking her.

"I thought he was exciting," Jean says. "He was telling stories about climbing and Nepal. You could definitely say he made an impression on me."

They often saw each other socially after that, and Jean got to know and like Tabin's Australian girlfriend, Samantha, who lived with him for much of his first year in Vermont. Jean was in a relationship herself, but she felt it might not have a future. "The man I was dating told me he wanted to wait to get serious until the kids were older," Jean says. "He said that would be healthier for them. I took that to mean he didn't want to commit, and eventually we split up."

In the spring of 1996, Jean attended an ophthalmology conference in Boston, where she found herself seated next to Dr. Mike Wiedman, Tabin's mentor at Harvard who had encouraged him to climb Everest. "Observing that I was from Burlington, he mentioned that I must know Geoff Tabin and that I should get to know him better, as he was such an amazing man," Jean says. "His stories about Geoff fascinated me."

Samantha moved back to Australia to continue her studies, and Jean found her thoughts turning, increasingly, to Tabin. She was training to run the Boston Marathon, and each time she ran by his house, she was tempted to stop. One evening she saw him standing in his kitchen window and knocked on Tabin's door. She left with an invitation to run with him. After one of their runs he invited her over for dinner.

During the meal, Tabin told carefully selected stories about climbing and his work with Ruit in remote Himalayan villages. "I remember at some point Geoff placed a statue of a fertility goddess he'd picked up during his travels on the table as we talked. I found him fascinating and brilliant and goofy and adorable," Jean says. "I'd never met anyone like him." That night, after she'd walked home, Jean tossed in bed, replaying highlights from their conversation. "I woke up at three A.M.," she says, "and I thought, 'This guy is the most incredible person I've ever met.' He was like a combination of Albert Einstein and Mr. Magoo."

"From the moment we started dating, I was crazy about Jean," Tabin says. "We had so much fun. And as I got to know her girls, I fell for them, too." Ali, Jean's crimson-haired, freckle-faced youngest, shared Tabin's sense of humor. She was eight, and she'd walk around Burlington with Tabin while he did errands. He'd pretend to be Himalayan and speak Nepali-sounding gobbledygook to the clerks at the supermarket or the ice cream shop, and Ali would translate his nonsense into plausible English. "She was really good at it," Tabin says, "and was able to keep a straight face until we walked back out into the street, where we'd both lose it."

But Tabin felt conflicted. He'd bought a two-bedroom house a few blocks from the campus that suited his bachelor's life perfectly. He'd installed a hot tub in one of the bedrooms and converted the attic into a climbing gym, which became a party center and focal point for Burlington's mountaineers. "Jean's place was hyperfemale and not my style at all," he says. "It was frilly and full of antiques and lace curtains. And I really loved my little house and the lifestyle I had there."

Still, Tabin adored Jean's daughters, so much that he found himself daydreaming about what it would be like to form a large family and add children of their own to the mix. They used birth control but joked about the "puppy" they might have if the potency Julius Tabin had passed on to his son found a way past the imperfect barriers they put in place. "That would be great," Tabin told Jean. "I've always wanted a puppy."

In October 1996, while Tabin was packing for his next trip to Kathmandu, his mother, a shrewd assessor of current events, phoned to ask whether it was safe for him to work in Nepal. He told her not to worry, but, in truth, he wasn't sure; he wondered how the Maoists' declaration of war would affect the HCP. The glimpse he got of the city, on the short ride from the airport to Tilganga, revealed little out of the ordinary. There were no crowds of rebel protesters, no unusually heavy military presence in the streets.

The next day, sitting together in Hilda's backseat, Ruit and Tabin inched out of town, beginning the long drive to an eye camp Nabin had organized in the Maoist-dominated district of Dhading. Nabin had gone ahead with Tilganga's advance team to convert a rural clinic into an operating theater capable of meeting Ruit's standards. "Without any complications," Ruit said, "we should catch Nabin by midafternoon and begin operating tomorrow morning."

"Complications," Tabin said, "meaning Maoists?"

As the traffic thinned out at the city's western edge and they sped toward the hills, Ruit briefed Tabin on what he thought the insurgency would mean for the HCP. He explained that the Maoists were extremely active in the countryside, where they had wide support among the rural people, but rarely made their presence felt in the capital. He told Tabin about the Maoist commander whose shrapnel-scarred eyes he'd repaired after hours at Tilganga. Since then, Ruit said, several high-level Maoists had come to him clandestinely for treatment, most often for ordinary complaints like cataracts or glaucoma, and less frequently for injuries inflicted by weapons. "From what I've seen, they're a fairly sensible lot," Ruit said. "If we run into trouble in rural areas, I think they'll look kindly on our work, once we tell them clearly who we are."

For someone who'd come to Kathmandu as an outsider, Tabin admired how thoroughly Ruit had been able to establish relationships with people of influence at every level of Nepalese society. "Basically," Tabin says, "he seemed to have the whole country wired; he had lines of communication open to everyone who mattered, and I felt like as long as I was under his wing, there was really nothing to worry about."

Two hours from Kathmandu, at a checkpost constructed of felled trees, Ruit and Tabin were stopped by teenage Maoist soldiers waving antique British rifles that looked too rusty to fire. They inspected Ruit and Tabin's papers, then demanded that the doctors make a donation to the Maoist cause before they'd be allowed to pass. Ruit stepped out of Hilda, inflated his chest, and brought his large, square head right up to the face of the boy who appeared to be in charge. "Listen clearly, *bhai*," he said, calling the anxious camouflage-clad teenager "younger brother" to emphasize his own standing. "My contribution to the Maoist cause is that I have stitched back together the eyes of your commanders when the bombs they were building exploded too soon. That, *bhai*, is the only contribution I'm willing to make. You won't rob a single rupee from me. We're here to help the poor, the people you say you're fighting for. Can you say the same?"

"Sorry, Doctor *dai*," the boy said, leaning his gun against a tree trunk like he was embarrassed by it. "You and the foreigner are free to pass."

Not every encounter was settled so easily. At other checkpoints, deeper into Maoist territory, they were often detained until a senior officer could be contacted to grant them the right to pass. During one of these mandated rest stops at a rebel checkpoint, they left Hilda idling by the roadblock and strolled for a few hundred yards back the way they'd come, passing Maoist symbols—raised red fists, hands breaking the chains that bound them—spray-painted on boulders. As they walked along the line of stilled vehicles waiting for permission to proceed, Tabin finally told Ruit about Jean: about her career, and her children, and both the doubts and enthusiasm she sparked in him.

"An ophthalmologist, isn't it?" Ruit said, his eyebrows raised in approval. "But three children by another fellow. That is rather a lot to take on, I agree. Still, you're not getting any younger. And she sounds like a woman of character. I'd advise you to proceed."

During other enforced delays, Ruit lectured on one of his favorite subjects: whether Maoists could really be trusted to combat rural poverty as aggressively as they were battling the country's elite institutions, and if they could provide the decent, democratic governance he felt his people so urgently deserved.

"The countryside is really burning, eh, Geoff?" Ruit said while they were waiting for permission to pass still another checkpoint, the barrels of the young and inexperienced soldiers' guns waving uncomfortably close; they were near Dhading, the heart of rebel country. "One of their commanders told me the Maoists already control eighty percent of the country. Everything but the cities. Our work here," Ruit said cheerfully, as if he almost relished the challenge, "is becoming a bit more complex, isn't it?"

Once they'd reached Dhading and settled into the all-consuming routine of surgery, their medical team operated as flawlessly as they always had before the Maoist revolt. But traveling less than a hundred miles to treat rural patients had proved far more difficult than Tabin had expected. How could the HCP reverse the tide of blindness across Nepal, not to mention the entire Himalaya, if they couldn't drive ten minutes without finding themselves at the mercy of teenage rebels?

When Tabin returned to comparatively uncomplicated Kathmandu in early November, he found a fax from Jean waiting for him at Tilganga. "Remember that puppy you wanted?" it read in her sloppy doctor's scrawl. "We're getting one."

On the succession of long flights home, Tabin felt a potent cocktail of confusion and exhilaration swirling inside him. Jean's fax made the obstacles the HCP faced seem either simpler or much more difficult, depending on the shifting currents of his emotions. During his flight to London, it seemed that having Jean by his side might make the insanely difficult task he'd set for himself easier. But hours later, on his last leg across the Atlantic, he stared at the endless, comfortless expanse of ocean and wondered whether being tethered to a family might make him question the risks working with Ruit required.

"I'd thought about a future with Jean and the girls, and it appealed to part of me immensely," Tabin says. "But when you're a bachelor for forty years, and you're used to your freedom, you don't necessarily picture a widow with three children as your romantic ideal. I had doubts about whether I was ready to take on all that responsibility."

Those doubts were obvious to Jean when Tabin returned. The man she'd fallen for, the risk-taking traveler, ready to dive into the unknown, was nowhere to be found. "I don't want to put pressure on you," she told him. "I'm going to have the baby. You can be a part of it if you want."

Tabin alternated between soaking in his hot tub and climbing in his attic, brooding about the choice he had to make. Whether he was in the water or hanging from holds, he knew that his decision would alter the way he assessed himself. Stepping off the railing of the Royal Gorge Bridge, tethered to survival by an elastic rope that hung nearly a thousand feet above the Arkansas River, hadn't felt half as frightening as the leap he was considering.

"It felt like my life had spiraled away from the possibility of having a family of my own," Tabin says. "So, on the one hand, I was thrilled about the idea of our child growing inside Jean, about seizing the chance I thought had passed me by. But there was also big-time fear; I was terrified about jumping from bachelorhood to the Brady Bunch overnight."

A few weeks after he'd arrived in Burlington, Tabin woke early, groggy from a night of fitful sleep, and phoned his parents. It was even earlier in Chicago. But he imagined, after all the years of waiting and hinting, that they wouldn't mind. "Do you still have Grandma Sara's diamond ring?" Tabin asked when he heard his mother's voice.

The shriek of delight from the central time zone stirred Tabin fully awake.

They held the wedding two months later, on January 4, 1997, so that Jean wouldn't be showing too obviously, and booked the posh Topnotch Resort at the Stowe ski area for the affair. Most of Tabin's tennis teammates from Yale attended the ceremony, along with his classmates from Harvard and Oxford and Brown, and his expedition mates from Everest's Kangshung Face. They had plenty of material to work with for their toasts, and they dredged up embarrassing anecdotes about Tabin's unharnessed days, trying to top one another at a roast they held for him the evening before the wedding, in a dive bar they'd rented for the night called, appropriately enough, the Matterhorn.

Paul Burke, Tabin's roommate at Yale, recounted an incident from their freshman year when his alumni father had taken the teenagers to Mory's Temple Bar, one of Yale's exclusive private clubs, and poured punch bowls of various liquors into the inexperienced drinkers. Burke had the crowd howling in appreciation as he related how Tabin, staggering around their dorm room and judging the distance to the bathroom too daunting, had opened their window and urinated from the second story of Wright Hall at precisely the moment Burke's formally dressed father, on the way to his car, was passing below.

But it was one last adventure as a bachelor that Tabin concocted just hours before the ceremony that nearly caused him to be late for his own wedding. Tabin could almost hear Ruit's disembodied words— "Remember, Geoff, you can't do everything at once"—as he drove away from the resort where the guests were gathering, into the Green Mountains. Along with two friends, the Alaskan climbing guide Carl Tobin and the Colorado-based mountaineer Neal Beidleman, Tabin attempted a first ascent of one of the toughest ice climbs in Vermont. "The frozen waterfall was a freestanding pillar the width of a tree trunk. If you hit it too hard, the whole thing could collapse and kill you," Tabin says. "But we took our time and worked our way up it, using our ice tools as delicately as kitten's claws." At the top, the three embraced and gave Tabin the honor of naming the demanding first ascent. He chose "Prenuptial Agreement."

Tabin made it back moments before the six o'clock ceremony was scheduled to begin, showered quickly, threw on his suit (a tasteful black, far from the mothballed, Oxford-era white tuxedo with the wide lapels), and arrived at the altar just as the string quartet started playing.

"I was still learning about the way Geoff worked," Jean says. "Thank God I didn't know he was out climbing just before the ceremony or I would have been a wreck."

Tabin had hired his favorite local musician, Big Joe Burrell, and his band played the electric Chicago-style blues Tabin considers the bedrock cultural contribution of his hometown. He and Jean were carried on swaying chairs by their guests, in the Jewish tradition, as Big Joe fought his way through "Hava Nagila." Then the newlyweds descended to the dance floor, where they were surrounded by a hundred friends, relatives, climbers, and coworkers, shaking their hips to the Chicago groove. Livia, Emilia, and Ali, Jean's—and now Geoff's—three daughters, joined their parents on the dance floor, along with another addition to the family, riding along to the rhythm beneath Jean's cream-colored wedding dress.

Tabin had stepped off the ledge and taken the leap. And this time, though he wasn't turning somersaults, tethered to a cord, swinging at the mercy of unpredictable winds between granite canyon walls, the sensation was no less exhilarating.

CHAPTER 18

Load Shedding

Though born in a dark age, I am very fortunate.
I may be unworthy, but my guru is good.
— The First Jamgon Kongtrul, instruction to his new disciples,
to be repeated aloud when facing obstacles

The twelve corneas traveled on dry ice, in a white Styrofoam box sealed with duct tape. The box, carried under Geoff Tabin's arm, was plastered with stickers, alerting authorities that it contained human tissue. Customs officials at Tribhuvan airport had delayed one of these deliveries before and had been unlucky enough to face a furious Ruit, warning them that their actions might prevent blind people from regaining their sight. In a culture where karma factors into so many decisions, no one wanted such a potent black mark ticked against them for eternity.

After a cursory glance at the bleary-eyed foreigner, they waved him around the line of people waiting to load their luggage onto scanners. In the arrivals area, Tilganga's new driver, La La, greeted Tabin with a slap on the back and plowed a path through the shouting touts, toward Hilda. In the passenger seat, with the box cradled in his arms, Tabin saw that Tilganga's vehicle had a large "H," for hospital, affixed to the windshield with blue painter's tape. "Everything okay, Dr. Geoff?" La La asked. "The trip was good?"

"Waaayell," Tabin said, "it was a bit long."

He'd been traveling for more than thirty hours since the corneas that had been FedExed to Vermont from eye banks across the country had arrived. He'd slept for a few hours on a padded bench in the Bangkok airport before boarding his flight to Kathmandu.

"Going to be little bit longer," La La said, laughing apologetically. "We're having *bandh.*"

"A what?"

"A *bandh*. I think you can call this thing 'strike' in English."

"Why's that?" Tabin said.

The driver answered with a shrug. The explanation was beyond his limited English. Even in Nepali, people could tie themselves in knots trying to talk about the Maoists and what motivated them. As Hilda pulled away from the airport, Tabin saw that the streets were thronged. The city always seemed to contain about twice as many people as it was equipped to support, but something was different this time. The stream of slow-moving traffic hit a human dam. Most of the protesters were young students, wearing red headbands painted with hammers and sickles.

Hundreds of them had surrounded a long black sedan a few vehicles ahead of them and were shaking their fists, chanting something over and over, and rocking it from side to side. It was dusk, and Tabin couldn't see the passengers through its tinted windows, though he could imagine their panic.

"What are they yelling?"

"They say, 'No corruption in the new Nepal,' something like that."

"Who's inside?"

"The rich person," La La said. "Maybe government man or family of king." He rolled down the window, waved over the nearest headbanded boy, and began speaking rapidly, pointing to the blue "H" on Hilda's windshield. Suddenly they were moving, the mob parting with unlikely organizational discipline, and Hilda was waved through the gauntlet. Protesters had blocked the main route from the airport into Kathmandu with a cross-country bus covered in red banners. It spit diesel smoke and backed up precisely enough to let them pass.

"What did you say?" Tabin asked.

"I told them we worked with Dr. Ruit," he said as they accelerated past Pashupatinath. "I say some poor people need to see and we carry them a box of brand-new eyes."

Twelve corneas meant, if they made no mistakes during surgery, that twelve people would have a second chance at sight, courtesy of American cadavers. The quality of donated corneas is measured by the number of functional cells remaining in the tissue when it's removed. Some of the corneas Tabin had procured from American eye banks had cell counts too low to be considered optimal and had missed the cut for use in U.S. hospitals. But in Kathmandu, where donated corneas were as rare as uncongested streets, viable but imperfect tissue was a treasure. Whenever possible, Tabin brought a batch to Ruit.

Fresh corneas degrade rapidly once they're harvested. The sterile solution they're packed in can preserve them for only five days. And each hour, more of the corneas' functional cells die. So they would operate into the night.

"Ready to work hard?" Ruit said, throwing an arm over Tabin's shoulder.

"Do I have any choice?"

"None," Ruit said merrily. "None at all."

Tabin downed two weak cups of instant coffee, then, considering the surgeries he had ahead of him, stirred up two more, hoping they would counteract his jet lag, and scrubbed in. Reeta allowed herself only one cup of black tea, so her hands would be steady.

In Tilganga's early years, Ruit had been the only surgeon qualified to transplant corneas. But Reeta, like Ruit, was relentless about learning the latest advances in her chosen specialty, and she'd quickly surpassed Ruit as a corneal surgeon. She'd returned from the fellowship in Vermont that Tabin had arranged for her so skilled that Ruit's surgical burden at Tilganga had been dramatically lessened, and he'd begun to leave the most difficult corneal cases in her able hands.

Ruit had been refining his skills, too. "It seemed like every time I returned to Nepal, Ruit had tweaked his cataract technique," Tabin says. "I'd gotten a lot faster, but he kept making so many innovations, it was impossible to keep up with him." Ruit had switched from the common practice of sitting by the top of the patients' head, and operating over their forehead, to sitting beside their temple and performing his surgeries from the side of the eye he was working on, which created less scar tissue and decreased postsurgical astigmatism. This way, he was able to have his staff bolt two operating tables together and prep one prone patient while he worked on the other, shaving valuable seconds off the time it took to slide his next patient into place. By the time Tabin arrived in 1996, Ruit had succeeded in carving unusually small tunnels in the side of his patients' eyes, no wider than the diseased cataracts that needed to come out. These wounds were so tiny that they allowed the eye to heal itself without needing to be sewn shut.

Ruit stayed long enough to make sure Reeta and Tabin had the supporting staff they needed; then, thanks to the blockade, he rode home through quiet streets to spend the rest of the evening with his family.

Tabin blew out his breath and bent to his work. The traumatized portion of his first patient's cornea, the clear tissue at the front of the eye, had to be excised in such a way that the shallow cavity he would cut into the surface would precisely match the disk of donor cornea he planned to cut, then sew into place there. His scrub nurse lifted the donated cornea out of the solution of sterile liquid that had been preserving it and placed the flap of clear healthy tissue, about the thickness of grape skin, onto the center of a punch, then slid the device onto a stainless steel tray in front of Tabin.

He made sure the cornea was properly lined up, then pressed down hard on the punch with the heel of his hand. Despite its appearance of fragility, corneal tissue is surprisingly tough, and a surgeon must use a fair amount of force to cut through it cleanly. He picked up the disk gently with tissue forceps and draped it over the hole he had prepared. The fit was perfect, and after rotating it a few degrees so that it was optimally aligned, he began suturing the graft in place.

After several careful stitches ensured that the transplant was firmly affixed, he snuck a glance at Reeta, who had finished her first case and started her next. When Tabin tied off his last suture, his patient's eye looked as good as new, except for a cat's cradle of fine black filament encircling the graft.

Tabin pushed his stool away from the operating table and asked

Reeta to confirm that he'd done as well as he believed he had. Holding her gloved hands carefully away from the microscope, she leaned in to look through the eyepiece, inspecting his work. "Tissue looks lined up well," she said. "Stitches are neat and tight. I'd say it looks perfect, Dr. Geoff."

Tabin was just beginning to stitch his next cornea into place when Tilganga's operating theater went dark. The dim emergency lights were just bright enough for him to avoid poking the healthy portion of his patient's eye with his suturing needle.

"Load shedding," Reeta said, in a calm, resigned voice that betrayed none of the stress she surely felt in the dark, with a patient's open wound waiting for her attention. "Nowadays it's become so common you can practically set your clock by these power cuts."

"Do you think the power will come back soon?" Tabin asked.

"That's rarely the case," Reeta said. "But our staff will be tinkering with the generator presently, and we should have lights then. That is, if the *bandh* hasn't blocked our petrol supply." They sat quietly in the dark, and in Reeta's serene company, Tabin permitted himself to relax. All he could hear, other than his breathing, was steam escaping from the propane-fueled autoclaves boiling their instruments in the adjoining room. Then the motorboat throb of the generator started up outside, and the light in Tabin's microscope flickered, then flared back on.

The next morning, Ruit arrived at work well rested. He found Reeta and Tabin slumped in the tea room next to his office on the second floor, sipping from chipped china mugs, working to wake themselves. They had been up the better part of the night and had completed eight transplants. Having snatched four hours of sleep, they planned to finish the rest shortly. Eight patients were settled in recovery rooms. And if their bodies accepted the foreign matter, and the corneas knit themselves into their patients' tissue and remained clear, all twelve would be given a second chance to see.

"You know," Ruit said, "this is ridiculous. We can manufacture all the artificial lenses we need. But we have to go to such great lengths to acquire these corneas, and there is an unlimited supply just the other side of the river. The question is, can we collect them?"

After completing his morning rounds, Ruit tried to cross the airport road where it spanned the Bagmati River. Growing impatient, he held out his arms, trying to slow the endless stream of traffic. He dodged a speeding Bajaj motorcycle, telling himself to take care, and sidestepped down the steep embankment to the Bagmati. He was on his way to speak to a cremator, not to become kindling for the man's fires.

The fuel that sent Nepal's most fortunate dead on their journey of transmutation was stacked higher than Ruit's head, in piles calculated to consume an average corpse. Ruit walked between the human-sized towers of hardwood for hundreds of yards, until he emerged from this forest of final transmission at the ornamental brick gates of the temple complex.

Hindus argue about the exact number of gods in their pantheon, since many appear in multiple guises. Some scholars poring over the ancient scriptures of the world's oldest religion, the Vedas, Upanishads, and Puranas, count as many as 330 million. Many Hindu sects consider them various manifestations of a single supreme being; others consider them separate deities. But all Hindus agree that Lord Shiva is a god among gods, the creator and the destroyer, an ultimate arbiter of life and death. Pashupati is one of Shiva's many names, and the temple built sixteen hundred years ago in his honor is the holiest Hindu site in Nepal. Hindus in the kingdom aspire to end their days by the banks of the Bagmati, believing that a cremation at Pashupatinath might lead them toward the gates of paradise, or at least to reincarnation in the most appealing form possible.

Ruit strode through the sprawling temple complex, admiring the statues of Shiva in his various guises: as Pashupati, lord and protector of animals, holding a deer in the palm of his hand; as Sadashiva, a fierce five-headed figure holding a trident and a snake; and as all-seeing Talagaon, an imposing anthropomorphic pillar covered with one thousand eyes and endowed with unblinking watchfulness, a god it was impossible to deceive. The task ahead of him was tricky, and the pitfalls for a Bhotia at Nepal's holiest Hindu site were numerous.

Ruit found Krishna Thapa, Pashupati's chief cremator, at Bhasmeshvar Ghat, stacking firewood around the corpse of an emaciated woman shrouded in homespun white cloth. Thapa, too, was dressed all in white—a short white dhoti and a long, flowing white shirt, appropriate for both the solemnity of the death rituals and the warm work his position required.

Ruit kept a respectful distance while the woman's family members clung to each other in their grief and Thapa placed rice on the funeral pyre, so her soul wouldn't face hunger as it traveled, and chanted prayers, speeding her to her next incarnation. He covered her with straw, to shield her from the final indignity of having her family watch the details of her disintegration, then poured clarified butter from a golden urn through the thin shroud covering her face, into her open mouth, until it overflowed and spilled down her cheeks. Thapa gave her son a lit candle and guided his hand to his mother, lighting the holiest human spot first, in the traditional manner, until flames leapt from her burning lips like last words.

When the fire spread to the straw, Thapa left the mourners in the hands of his assistants, who would be sure to tend the pyre until, ideally, only ashes and fragments of bone remained, ready to be swept into the river.

"May I speak with you for a moment?" Ruit said. Standing face-to-face with Thapa, he saw what a tiny man he was, barely larger than a boy, with delicate, birdlike bones. Ruit started to explain who he was and why he'd come, but his growing prominence in Kathmandu made an introduction unnecessary.

"I know who you are, Doctor," Thapa said. "We all know about the work you do on the other side. I've heard people say when you make their eyes, you tear out the eyeballs entirely and sew in new ones. Is that the case?"

"That's what I wanted to talk to you about," Ruit said. "We do no such thing. To cure the most common kind of blindness, cataract disease, we make a tiny cut and insert a small piece of plastic, no larger than your fingernail. To cure the next most prevalent sort, corneal disease, we take a small scraping from the eyes of the dead and use that to give sight back to the living. When you're free, why don't you come across the road and see for yourself?"

They agreed on a time the following morning, and Ruit left Thapa to his next task: joining his fellow shepherds of the dead in carrying the shrouded remains of a man so corpulent, it took four cremators to escort him to his point of departure. The supply of corneas at Pashupatinath was limitless, Ruit thought, as numerous as the cords of wood waiting to consume them. Walking along the trickling Bagmati toward Tilganga, Ruit saw packs of dogs rummaging in the shallows, fighting for unburned bits of flesh. "I can fight for scraps, too," he thought.

"We already had an eye bank at that time," Ruit says, "but we had very little tissue coming in. So the next day Shanka Twyna, the eye bank director, gave Krishna a very VIP tour. He put him in a sterile suit so he could see the lenses being cut and polished in our laboratory. I had him stand beside me during cataract surgery, and sometimes that can be a problem. I've had government ministers or big rugged mountaineers pass out cold the first time they see me make a tiny incision. But you can imagine Krishna wasn't shy about human flesh. He's Chhetri," Ruit explains, "the caste who're allowed to touch the dead. He'd been handling corpses since he was a boy. So he had no problem watching me work. Then I had him observe Reeta doing a corneal transplant. He was amazed that it took such a small flap of tissue to complete the surgery. Twyna and I walked him through the recovery rooms and let him watch blind patients weep with joy when their bandages were removed. It's a powerful thing, you know. It catches me up every time I see it, and I've seen it so many thousands of times. But Krishna was unusually touched. Maybe because in his work, he only saw people going one way, down, and he saw the possibility of helping bring others back up. After that, he was devoted to creating a partnership between Pashupati and Tilganga."

With one foot in the crematory door, Ruit launched a campaign to convince Kathmandu society to donate the corneas of their dead. "I'd made a study of our practices of dying," Ruit says. "At first I was convinced Buddhists would be the answer, because I knew I could convince them that the dead, who are no longer inhabited, should be of use. But Buddhists keep the bodies of their relatives at home until a day they consider auspicious for their cremation, and corneas have to be harvested quickly. So I shifted my focus to Hindus, because they cremate ASAP.

"We put up signboards at Pashupati, saying, IT'S NICE TO DONATE YOUR CORNEAS. WHEN YOU DIE YOU CAN GIVE TWO PEOPLE THE GIFT OF SIGHT, and such like that. And that year, I think it was 1998, we started filming commercials for television, telling people donation was the right thing to do. This upset some powerful people. The head royal Hindu priest summoned me and said, 'Young Doctor,' even though I was in my forties, 'don't you ever take any eyeballs!' But I don't mind a fight," Ruit says. "You have to get brushed a bit, you need a little resistance, before you can get stronger, you see? So I ignored his threats and pushed on. We had a really uphill battle. We had to break a big taboo in our culture that you don't defile the dead."

Ruit had assembled Tilganga's board of directors carefully, so that its members came from diverse castes and careers and had influence on many sectors of Nepalese society. The popular comedian Hari Bamsha Acharya was the board member Ruit selected to sway public opinion. Even before the rise of the Maoist revolution, his comedy had begun to cut increasingly close to the bone, skewering the corruption of the old regime. He filmed a public service spot mocking those who thought modern eye surgery meant yanking out eyeballs, and announcing that he planned to donate his corneas when he died.

But it was Krishna Thapa, unknown to most Nepalese until their final hours, who was most helpful obtaining corneas, in reliable quantities, for Tilganga. "Coming from his mouth as he counseled families about to say farewell to their loved ones, it meant more than anything we could do," Ruit says. "He told them they would be giving a gift not only to the blind but to their relatives, because of the merit the dead would acquire on their way to their next life."

In the early days of their collaboration, Krishna would call when he'd convinced a donor's family, and technicians would rush across the river and harvest the corneas right on the burning ghats. But the pace of donations picked up so dramatically that Tilganga acquired a small office in the Pashupatinath complex where the fifteen-minute procedure could be done under more sanitary conditions. They now had an on-site eye bank, staffed twenty-four hours a day, ready to collect tissue whenever their partner across the river called.

In 1998, the year they launched their campaign, the number of locally harvested corneas Tilganga received grew from a handful to 240. In 1999, it rose again, to 547, requiring Tilganga to train a second corneal surgeon. At a time when the word "sustainable" was not yet in fashion, Ruit had reached across his country's holiest river and set in motion a mutually beneficial exchange of resources with no end in sight.

Ruit had become so accustomed to swimming alone against his profession's mainstream that he struggled to let go of any responsibilities, though he knew it was necessary. The lineup of patients waiting on benches by Fred Hollows's portrait grew longer each morning, and Tabin, Rex, Reeta, and members of the board pressed Ruit to hire more staff.

For years, Ruit had kept his eyes on Nepal's most promising medical students, nurses, and technicians. He knew he should hire some of them, bring in others who could help to shoulder his load, but he'd run Tilganga on limited funds since its launch, and his frugality had become ingrained. He didn't know any other way to operate, other than trying to squeeze the work of two staffers out of each Tilganga employee. But with Tabin proving a dedicated fund-raiser, Ruit finally began to relent.

Khem Gurung was one the first significant new hires Ruit approved. Gurung's father had been a regional governor in the mid-hills, and when he came to Tilganga with a fresh degree as an ophthalmic technician in hand, Ruit asked him why he wanted the job. "I've seen too much corruption. I want to work someplace free from corruption." Gurung's resourcefulness and easygoing attitude would overcome many obstacles, Ruit judged. And his wiry fitness and willingness to trek to Nepal's most difficult terrain would free Nabin Rai, who was less enthusiastic about roughing it in rural areas, to concentrate his duties at Tilganga, where he could became the hospital's roaming troubleshooter and its resident public health advocate, plotting out where to build rural clinics and devising the most effective means of reaching the largest number of rural Nepalese.

For years, Ruit had rebuffed most of the potential employees his board had suggested. "I can't take just anyone," he'd tell them. "I'm growing my staff like a crop. Many of them are still in school." By the millennium, that crop was finally coming in. With some money still arriving each year from the Fred Hollows Foundation, and modest but reliable funding from the slow-growing HCP, Ruit was able to do something he'd never imagined possible: offer competitive salaries to the candidates he wanted most.

Tabin, too, was struggling to adapt to new circumstances. He and Jean bought a large white Victorian house in a neighborhood of old shade trees near the campus of the University of Vermont. Every time he walked up the drive after work, and saw the manicured lawn and the wraparound porch, he couldn't believe he was rooted someplace so solid; a few years earlier, he'd been living out of a duffel bag. But it was the strong, opinionated women who inhabited this home that made him realize how radically his life had changed.

Livia, the eldest of Jean's children, was a standout student applying to elite colleges. Emilia, the middle child, was an athlete; she joined Tabin in jogging early-morning laps around slumbering Burlington. Ali, Jean's youngest, had embraced climbing and was ready at a moment's notice to join her father on a sprint to New Hampshire's granite pitches. The first child they'd had together, two-year-old Sara, was currently a mobile force of chaos, scattering toys throughout the house and sweeping Tabin's academic papers off tables where he'd left them carefully stacked. Jean had become pregnant with another child, Daniel, after she and Geoff had agreed that Sara would be happier with someone closer to her own age in the home.

Hyperactivity has its advantages. Especially when you're trying to work full-time as a surgeon, give your growing family enough attention, and raise money to combat a global health crisis most people in wealthy countries have never heard about. Still, Tabin felt the tyranny of time; there weren't enough hours in the day for him to devote himself properly to his family, and his long absences added to the burden. At first, Jean and the girls accompanied Tabin on trips to eye camps in Nepal and Bhutan. "I loved the travel," Jean says, "and getting to see Geoff in action. But I underestimated the difficulty of having both teenagers and toddlers. The frequent absences from school created all kinds of problems. So I decided I needed to be there for my kids. That meant staying home and making sure their lives weren't always interrupted. Geoff wants to have everyone along with him all the time. This is sensitive stuff; Geoff and I really love each other, but it's put a lot of stress on our marriage."

John Frymoyer, the dean of the University of Vermont's College of Medicine and the CEO of its hospital, understood the pressure Tabin felt, and the multiple lives he was trying to lead, and allowed university staff to create HCP promotional materials and send out letters soliciting donations. Tabin organized fund-raisers, which, in typical Tabin fashion, he dubbed "fun-raisers," twisting the arms of famous climbing friends to give slide shows, trying to sweep up donors in the romance of the world's highest mountains and the needs of the people who lived among them. "It was a lot of work," Tabin says. "I had to keep records of every five-dollar check and write thank-you notes to every donor. But I don't want to overstate my role. It's not like Ruit wouldn't have survived without me."

As the balance of the HCP's bank account slowly grew, Tabin phoned Ruit nearly every day, discussing how they could make the most of the funds and planning their upcoming trips. Tabin was especially keen to raise the skill level of Tilganga's staff by training a full roster of subspecialists, doctors who were able to treat retinal disorders, care for glaucoma, and practice pediatric ophthalmology, so the hospital would be qualified to care for any eye condition. They also talked about purchasing excimer lasers, so Tilganga could recover at least part of the cost of providing free care to the poor by charging Kathmandu's upper class for high-tech procedures like Lasik surgery.

Ruit and Tabin discussed creating a network of community eye centers in Nepal, so they wouldn't have to depend solely on eye camps to reach rural areas, and so patients with urgent conditions wouldn't have to travel for days by bus to Kathmandu. Tabin wanted to recruit a corps of dedicated young doctors, drawn from both America and Asia, send them to Tilganga for training, and unleash them on the region's hot spots of preventable blindness.

After five years of operating beyond its capacity, Tilganga was beginning to show the strain. A hospital designed for twenty-five surgeries a day was doing double that, and the building didn't have room to train more than a few foreign doctors at a time. Tabin and Ruit began discussing an expansion of the facility onto a vacant plot of land, uphill from the hospital, that Tilganga owned. "That would take money," Tabin says. "Lots more money than we had."

In the meantime, Ruit and Tabin worked on ways to expand Tilganga's influence throughout the region. In the fall of 1999, they designed a seminar to teach Ruit's technique and invited Himalayan eye-care leaders to Kathmandu. At a dinner they held at the Yak and Yeti to welcome attendees, Tabin's name card was placed beside Ruit's, but he kept jumping up between bites of food, introducing himself to surgeons and health care officials around the long table, clapping them on the back and shaking their hands warmly in both of his.

"Over the years, Geoff has surprised me many times," Ruit says. "And that evening I saw something clearly I'd failed to properly appreciate. Geoff's personality drew people to him. I realized you could put him on an airplane, or at a fund-raising event, or at a table of doctors we were trying to convert, and in five minutes, he'd make friends with everyone, right, left, and center. I can't do that. I'm not so outreaching. And I was glad to have him as my partner. Behind all of his naughtiness, I realized, he really cared. He had a golden, compassionate heart."

One of the doctors who'd come to Kathmandu that day was precisely the sort of person who could help them expand their outreach. As the tiny kingdom of Bhutan's first trained ophthalmologist, Kunzang Getshen was largely responsible for the eye care of his entire country.

Getshen had short-cropped hair, graying at the temples, gracious manners, and an incongruous laugh that barked out of him when he was titillated by something Tabin said, which was often. But he was dead serious about improving eye care in his isolated kingdom, and once Tabin identified the flame that burned in him, the terrier was all teeth.

Getshen told Tabin about the challenges facing him in Bhutan. He had recruited an Indian ophthalmologist to work with him and had begun training a second local eye surgeon, but he had virtually no funding or infrastructure. In a country where health care is free but doctors are few, Getshen was forced to send his most serious cases to surgeons in India.

"I'd love to visit you in Bhutan," Tabin said. "I've studied your rates of blindness, and together we could really bring them down."

"I'd be delighted to have you as my guest," Getshen said, in erudite English that he seemed to construct, a paragraph at a time, before he spoke. "But every major development in my country must be approved by the royal government. And His Majesty wants to concentrate on removing primary obstacles for my people, such as providing basic medical services and building roads and schools."

"I'd argue curing blindness is about the most primary thing you can do to improve people's lives," Tabin said.

"Of course I agree," Getshen said. "I've prepared an eye-care plan for my country. Perhaps you could take a look at it and give me your suggestions? As the chief ophthalmologist for seven hundred thousand Bhutanese, I have less time for such things than I'd like."

By the time he was home in Vermont, Tabin had read Getchen's plan and completed a proposal of his own for an HCP-led initiative in Bhutan. He contrasted Bhutan's rising rates of blindness with Nepal's, which had been steadily falling in the years since Ruit had moved home from medical school in India. He compared the modest cost of cataract surgery with the income lost to a country's economy when blind people, and the caregivers they require to have a decent quality of life, are banished from gainful employment. And he detailed how Bhutan's eye-care system could be transformed, providing he could find the funds. He sent the document to Getshen, hoping it would help pry open the door for the HCP to work in Bhutan.

With one of the lightning bolts of luck that have struck Tabin almost too many times to be believed, he received a call from an old friend and fellow Marshall Scholar at Oxford, Mark Haynes Daniell. Daniell had been hired by Mitt Romney to work at Boston's Bain & Company and had done well enough to eventually leave and launch his own investment firm in Singapore.

Daniell, who'd been contributing modestly to the HCP's general fund for a few years, told Tabin he'd been following the HCP's work with admiration. "But I don't want to give indiscriminately anymore," Daniell told Tabin. "I've benefited from some investments, and I'd like to make a targeted donation that could begin to turn back blindness in a single country. Can you think of any place where, say, five hundred thousand dollars could really make a difference?" Tabin knew that Daniell had long been fascinated by the small mountain kingdom and its protected Buddhist culture." "I believe you're familiar," Tabin said, "with a country called Bhutan?"

In a place often called the "world's last Shangri-La," Jigme Singye Wangchuck, the fourth Dragon King of Bhutan, relished the role of gatekeeper. K4, as he is affectionately known to his people, was less than a year older than Tabin, and as close to universally beloved as any head of state could be. He refused to throw the doors of his mountain kingdom open to the corrupting influences of the West, setting a slow, cautious course toward modernization. He denied visas to backpackers and limited tourism to high-paying group travel, mandated that his citizens wear traditional clothing to work, and banned television. He, too, had been educated in Britain, where he'd learned about the excesses of capitalism and the pervasiveness of poverty, even in so-called wealthy nations. In London he had swum briefly in the waters of the modern material world, before deciding to protect his people from it for as long as he could.

The king had attracted media attention when he'd announced, in 1972, shortly after ascending to the throne following his father's sudden death, that Bhutan would swim against the tide of simply accumulating wealth. He'd declared that "gross national happiness" was more important than gross national product, igniting a firestorm of both admiration and derision among foreign academics, who'd debated whether he could shelter his people from the realities of the twentieth century. Now the government of this monarch who'd worked so hard to keep foreigners out of his pristine mountain kingdom had invited the HCP in.

With Daniell's money, Tabin was able to launch the HCP's first major expansion beyond Nepal and Tibet. Where he and Getshen wanted to begin was by giving teachers and basic health care workers throughout the country simple training, so they could identify those who might benefit from eye surgery. Simultaneously, Tabin and Getshen would select a group of the nation's most promising medical students and send them to Tilganga for training. It would be a complex process, Tabin told Getshen, but in a country with such good governance, and a population of only 700,000, they could effect change quickly.

"The idea that Geoff would take a hands-on role was very important," Daniell says of his decision to donate the money. "This ensured the funds were well spent and the operating procedures and equipment well suited to the objectives of both an international eye-care standard and the country's stage of development."

In the winter of 2000, at the Queen Mother's invitation, Daniell traveled to Bhutan and pledged $100,000 a year for each of the next five years to transform eye care in the country. Afterward, Tabin flew in, met with the minister of health to discuss implementing the plan he'd honed with Getshen, and signed a five-year memorandum of agreement with the royal government, giving HCP staffers freedom to work in every far-flung community of the mountain kingdom.

Five years to turn a nation's entire eye-care system around. It wasn't a lot of time, but Tabin felt sure they could do it. Since the day five years earlier when Tabin had taken Ruit's hand and pledged to form the HCP, he'd relied exclusively on Ruit's judgment about who they would work with in Asia. Now Tabin had helped open a new front in the battle against blindness and had forged a partnership with one of the world's most reclusive monarchies. It had been a long time coming, but he was finally learning to shoulder his own load.

CHAPTER 19

Burn the Old House Down

*Even the bravest warrior with the sharpest eye who finds himself in a
dense forest on a moonless night is unable to see and may soon be lost.
The world, so rich in bright promises of happiness, is in truth, Oh King,
such a forest. By night it becomes black. Love becomes brutal
selfishness, wisdom becomes calculation. Prosperity becomes rabid greed,
and justice, a means of oppression. This kingdom will rise and fall
a thousand times. Even your own wisdom and power will wax and wane.
There is no moment at which great exertion is not required.*
—The Warrior Song of King Gesar, an epic oral legend
about the royal leader, believed to be a reincarnation of Guru Rinpoche,
who unified the warring principalities of the Himalaya

"How are you doing, Doc?" the king asked. "Is everyone in the
family well?"

"Very well, Your Majesty," Ruit said. "Now let's have a look at
those uncooperative eyes of yours." King Birendra Bir Bikram Shah
Dev slid his chair toward Ruit's slit lamp and removed his glasses. He
was familiar with the process after years of regular visits to Tilganga so
that Ruit could monitor the pressure in his eyes, which might lead to
glaucoma.

"The king always spoke to me in English," Ruit says. "He was a
thoughtful fellow who didn't want to be stiff with me. He knew that if
we spoke Nepali, I'd have to use lot of formal words, archaic language
specially for royalty, so I'd be groveling to him like serf to master."

"How does it look?" the king asked, leaning back in his chair.

"You probably won't go blind today or tomorrow," Ruit teased.

"But we need to keep an eye on your pressure. I'll need to see you in another three months."

"Okay, Doc, you're the boss," the king said, and he changed the subject to a topic he found more interesting, a topic everyone in Nepal was discussing: the Maoists. Birendra asked Ruit if he'd met any of their leaders. Ruit admitted that he'd had a look at a few of their eyes in the line of duty, adding that the leaders he'd encountered had seemed reasonable enough. Not as radical, certainly, as the students in the street.

"I advised the king that, in my opinion, the Maoists had a silly name but a valid point of view. The poverty in the countryside *was* unacceptable," Ruit says. "I told him I'd operated in some of the angriest districts, and cautioned him about the fires the government could start by cracking down too hard."

By the spring of 2001, Tilganga had become widely recognized as one of the kingdom's finest hospitals, ophthalmic or otherwise. By then, Ruit had prescribed glasses and performed cataract surgery for several members of the royal family. And after he'd replaced the Queen Mother's aging cataracts with crystal-clear locally produced IOLs, her daughter, Queen Aishwarya, had become one of his strongest advocates. Ruit was frequently invited to dinner at the palace. "During these visits, I became friendly with Prince Dipendra," Ruit says. "He was a good drinker, and we shared a fondness for a few pegs of scotch whiskey."

Dipendra, the twenty-nine-year-old heir to Nepal's throne, was even less formal than his father. He was a popular figure in Kathmandu, where he was known as "Dippy" for the carefree way he carried himself in public. "Dipendra was a modern fellow, educated in Britain," Ruit says. "He always had the latest-model computer, and one day, when I walked into the palace, he was talking on the first mobile phone I'd ever seen. He also had a reputation as something of a playboy who collected mistresses. But I never saw that side, or he never let me."

During Ruit's visits to the palace, he and Dipendra often discussed the Maoist uprising. The prince knew that the country's leadership would have to come to some accommodation with the Maoists, Ruit says, and he hoped to absorb them into the political system, rather than face them on the field of battle. During their drinking sessions, in the cozy billiard room behind the pink modernist palace's austere public spaces, the prince sought out Ruit's opinion as if he were speaking to an architect of social change rather than simply an eye doctor, and perhaps, if Ruit had his way, he was. "I wanted Tilganga to show other Nepalese, including the royals, that we can care for our own people," Ruit explains. "To be a model for what we can build when we don't let our efforts get buggered up by corruption."

Ruit believed that, by example, he could influence Nepal's monarchy to alleviate the poverty it presided over. But his hopes came crashing down on June 1, 2001. According to eyewitnesses interviewed by the official commission charged with making sense of that evening's events, the crown prince had a violent argument with his parents during a large family gathering over his desire to marry his girlfriend, an elegant aristocrat named Devyani Rana, rather than the wife they had chosen for him. During the argument, servants heard Queen Aishwarya threaten to disinherit her son if he refused to accept the marriage she'd arranged for him.

Servants saw the prince drink a tumbler or two of Famous Grouse whiskey and, at his request, brought him a pack of cigarettes laced with hashish. Multiple witnesses confirm that his voice was slurred and he was swaying, unable to remain upright, before four guests, including his brother, Prince Nirajan, helped him across the palace's inner gardens, over a footbridge, and to his room, where they left him.

Telephone records indicate that he made two brief calls to Devyani Rana that evening. Whatever the prince said worried his girlfriend enough for her to call his aides and ask them to check on him. Shortly before 9:00 P.M. one of these aides walked to the prince's room and saw him emerge from his bedchamber wearing black military boots, a camouflage army jacket and trousers, black leather gloves, and a camouflage vest with bulging pockets.

"Shall the emergency bag be brought, sire?" the startled aide asked.

"It's not necessary now," the prince replied.

Dipendra began firing the moment he entered the billiard room, strafing the ceiling with an MP5K automatic submachine gun. He strode toward his father, who was standing by a billiard table, and shot the king in the chest. Then he began firing indiscriminately. His brother-in-law, Gorakh, survived his wounds, but the prince killed his uncles, Dhirendra and Khagda, before throwing the spent weapon aside and hunting down the rest of his family with an M16 rifle.

The bodies of his sister, Princess Shruti; his aunt Shanti; and a cousin, Princess Jayanti, were all found just outside the billiard room. His brother, Prince Nirajan, was located by palace officials, unconscious and bleeding, by a hedge in the garden. He was rushed to the army hospital, where doctors pronounced him dead on arrival.

The body of the prince's final victim, his mother, Queen Aishwarya, lay crumpled on the staircase that led to his room. She'd been shot in the head so many times, at such close range, that she could be identified only by her clothing.

Security forces rushing into the palace found Dipendra sprawled on his back, with a head wound but still breathing, on a small bridge spanning a pond near his residence. They fished a nine-millimeter Glock pistol believed to belong to him out of the shallow water.

For three days, Dipendra lingered in a coma at Kathmandu's army hospital, where, according to Nepalese law, he was formally crowned as the nation's king while lying unconscious in his hospital bed. His reign lasted only the three days it took him to die.

As all of Nepal struggled to make sense of the massacre, Gyanendra, King Birendra's younger brother, who'd been away in the city of Pokhara during the killings, became the country's new king.

Despite the Maoist conflagration that had been burning steadily in rural Nepal for five years, the world still mainly associated the country with cheerful, ruddy-faced Sherpas and mountain tourism. The massacre, the most high-profile wholesale slaughter of a royal family since the slaying of the Romanovs after the Russian revolution, splashed Nepal onto front pages around the world. Foreign journalists unfamiliar with the intricacies of the kingdom's politics packed the daily flights from Delhi and Bangkok, and as Nepal's dazed public took to the streets in mourning, conspiracy theories were lobbed at them like grenades: The Maoists were responsible. They had long called for abolishing the monarchy; now their fighters had wiped out most of the royal family in a single storm of bullets. Prime Minister Koirala was really behind the murders. He had eliminated the royals so he could speed the nation's transformation to a republic, or to distract protestors calling for him to step down after his latest corruption scandal. King Gyanendra was guilty; he was a power-mad monarch who'd orchestrated the killings of his rivals, so that he could wear the crown he would have been denied by Dipendra. Indian or Chinese operatives were the culprits; they had infiltrated the palace and killed the king, so they could take advantage of the ensuing chaos and seize territory from their weakened neighbor.

Riots broke out across Nepal as the news spread. Two people were killed and nineteen others injured as mobs sought scapegoats for the violence they couldn't believe their beloved Dippy had perpetrated. "Like everyone else at that time, I was in shock," Ruit says. "I'd seen the prince only a few days earlier. And it just didn't seem possible that the free-and-easy friend I'd known could snap in such a way. But love can do surprising things to any human mind. And people I trust, people at the palace, told me what really happened."

The queen had had a long-standing feud with the family of the prince's girlfriend, Ruit explains, whom she considered lesser nobility, not fit to produce a bride for her son. But on the day of the massacre, the prince's grandmother had called Dipendra with good news; she'd told him that she'd convinced his mother to accept his marriage to Devyani. Just before dinner, where the prince was planning to announce the engagement to the entire family, the Queen Mother had approached the prince and given him devastating information: Queen Aishwarya had changed her mind.

To this day, many Nepalese don't believe that Prince Dipendra was responsible for the massacre. But Ruit does. "He started drinking and taking drugs," Ruit says. "His mind went dark, and that was that. The foreign press rushed in and stirred up all these conspiracies. All that was nonsense. What caused the killings was love. Blind love. I'm certain of it."

On June 2, Ruit shaved his head in mourning for his king and, like everyone else in Nepal with access to a television, watched the funeral. Twelve pallbearers wearing white vests and dhotis carried the flower-strewn body of King Birendra on a funeral stretcher. Queen Aishwarya was carried behind her husband, with a mask over her mutilated face, and both were accompanied by a palace guard of Gurkha soldiers in khaki dress uniforms. The procession traveled six miles, from the army hospital, through the streets of the capital, thronged with hundreds of thousands of mourners, to the burning ghats on the banks of the Bagmati.

Sitting beside Nanda and his parents, and surrounded by his anxious children, Ruit watched as the king's pallbearers circled his funeral pyre at Pashupatinath three times. The pyre had been built at an exclusive spot upstream, reserved for royalty, Nepal's caste system intact even in death. And when he saw his friend Krishna Thapa dutifully standing by the king as the sacred flames leapt out of the dead monarch's mouth, Ruit wept.

Nepal, despite its poverty, took pride in the fact that it had never been conquered. Several unusually shrewd kings had ruled during the Shah dynasty's two centuries in power. "King Mahendra, the assassinated king's father, was one of those," Ruit says. "He was a really sharp cookie who ruled with a hardened fist. He unified our country of so many tribes, castes, traditions, and languages into a modern nation and beat back foreigners who tried to tear us apart. His son Birendra was a weaker sort who at least had the wisdom to start our experiment with democracy and call for a constitution. But the new King Gyanendra was weaker still. I feared he would be easy for others to manipulate, and unfortunately I was right. Up to that point I felt, slowly but surely, we were making progress in Nepal. Taking baby steps toward true democracy. Now I was sickly with worry for the future of my country."

When the newly crowned King Gyanendra came to Tilganga to have his eyes checked, Ruit attempted to offer more than medical advice. He hoped to reprise his role as someone familiar with conditions in rural areas, an unofficial adviser who could convey to the monarchy the validity of many of the Maoists' grievances and the necessity of initiating peace talks. Ruit ordered a platter of tea and biscuits for the king and tried to discuss the crisis spreading through the countryside. But after Ruit examined his eyes, Gyanendra didn't stay long enough to touch his tea. He cut their conversation short in Nepali with a formality the former king had never shown.

The Maoist leader Baburam Bhattarai slipped into Tilganga two months after Gyanendra's visit to ask Ruit a favor. "He knew I'd been friendly with the former king," Ruit says, "and I'd treated so many Maoists by then that they trusted me. He asked if I could open a pipe to the palace."

Ruit told Bhattarai he'd try, but he advised him that he should consider changing his movement's name and turning it into a political party. "Everyone knows you're strong," Ruit said. "But they're not going to negotiate with you if they think you're crazy." Bhattarai said it was too late for that; the movement's most radical elements would turn on the leadership if they labeled what they were fighting for anything short of a revolution.

"That cat," Ruit says, "had crawled from the bag."

Ruit's worst fears were confirmed; with Gyanendra on the throne, his country's crisis was bound to escalate. After ordering a curfew to crush the rioting, the new king addressed the nation and denounced the Maoists. "He had a tremendous public mandate to move the country forward and bring the Maoists on board," Ruit says. "But he buggered everything up from the start. He was trying to be tough like his grandfather, but times had changed and the situation required more subtlety."

Three months later, on September 11, 2001, planes struck prominent American landmarks. Nepal, formerly a strategic backwater, a pleasure posting for American diplomats with a taste for trekking, was suddenly elevated, in coded diplomatic cables, to a "new front in the War on Terror." In the rush to take the fight to all their perceived enemies, the Bush administration formally declared Nepal's Maoists a terrorist organization. And that change in status triggered an olive-drab avalanche of American "advisers," automatic weapons, and ammunition, which swept across the runway of Tribhuvan airport.

"I'm trying to keep a clear mind and calm my voice while I'm telling you this," Ruit said when I pressed him to talk, at length, about his country's crisis. "But you're an *American.*" The edge in his voice when he said that word revealed the strain it took for him to remain polite while discussing my country's foreign policy. "You've done so much harm jumping into situations you don't understand. The Maoists were not a terrorist group. They were not leading a terrorist uprising but a social uprising. Their target, primarily, was *poverty.* In the early years of their revolt, they carried sticks. But your Bush and his British friends flooded Nepal with modern weapons. Then the Maoists began attacking police posts and army barracks to seize them up. And where did that leave us? Standing knee-deep in the shit you stirred up."

On September 11, 2001, Tabin, Ruit, and his friend Him Gurung, the deputy inspector general of Nepal's police force, were dining at the Jolly Gurkha restaurant on Tridevi Marg. Gurung's mobile phone began ringing, and he took call after call as they ate. The news nearly, but not quite, quashed Tabin's appetite. "First he told us that two planes had crashed into the World Trade Center," Tabin remembers. "Then he took another call and explained that the Pentagon had been hit. My mind was spinning, and I told him that was impossible."

"Why is that?" Gurung said. "Do you think Nepal is the only country that can have a crisis? Now it appears your United States is also at war."

Tabin finished the surgeries he had scheduled and flew home to be with his family. From Vermont, he called Ruit frequently and monitored the deteriorating conditions in the kingdom until his next scheduled trip to Nepal.

"Sanduk, can you hear me?"

"Hardly, Geoff. Can you repeat?"

"I said we've been watching news about the riots on TV. Jean's worried, and I'm wondering whether I should come or wait a bit until everything calms down."

"I don't think waiting will help."

"If you say it's safe, I'll be there in a few days."

"I'm not saying it's safe."

"Well, do you think it's stupid for me to come?"

"I wouldn't say that either. We have lot of work to do."

Despite the State Department bulletin warning all Americans to stay away from Nepal, except for those with "essential business," Tabin returned to Tribhuvan airport in the winter of 2002. He noticed the changes before he'd even deplaned. The runways were ringed by machine-gun nests. Soldiers in the green camouflage uniform of the national army tracked the Airbus as it taxied past their positions. On the drive to Tilganga, Tabin saw sandbagged fighting posts at every busy intersection, and he wondered if he'd made a mistake. But once he reached the hospital, he found the heightened sense of mission intoxicating. "Ruit was at his best," Tabin says. "Rallying the troops. Reminding them he never said their jobs would be easy, and I knew I'd made the right decision to return."

Tilganga employees had taken risks traveling the countryside, where they'd treated the mounting number of casualties on both sides of the escalating war. During one especially daring mission, Khem Gurung drove a jeep to a Maoist military post, parked it under a tree to hide it from the government's new helicopter gunships that were rocketing the area, and removed shrapnel, as calmly as he could while the explosions continued, from the local rebel commander's eyes.

Ruit was delighted that Tabin had the courage to come join them. He was particularly pleased when Tabin told him that the HCP had received a pledge from American donors and they could soon expect $110,000 with which to buy Tilganga higher-quality surgical microscopes.

"Marvelous news, Geoff, really," Ruit said. "At least America will be sending some technologies to Nepal that help rather than hurt."

"For the first few years, I'd been running the HCP like a family business," Tabin says. "Buying surgical supplies with my own salary and hitting up relatives like my uncle Seymour when I needed a microscope for projects in Pakistan or Sikkim."

With Reeta's help, Tabin had also launched an internationally accredited three-year surgical residency program at Tilganga, so that foreign doctors could receive comprehensive training in Kathmandu, rather than flying in for a month or two at a time. Tabin's dream of turning Tilganga into a training center, fully equipped to unleash an army of surgeons who'd mastered Ruit's technique on the developing world, was slowly becoming a reality.

But with the country he'd come to love in a state of war, the stakes had been raised; he had to move faster. Tabin needed to wage a fundraising campaign for the HCP with the same ferocity that Ruit's team fought to serve their country's most vulnerable citizens. When he returned home, he decided, he would hire a small American staff, people with the time to turn his piecemeal campaign into a professional organization.

The royal massacre and the growing Maoist insurgency may have made work in Nepal more difficult, but it had also opened a few important doors for the HCP. Media outlets suddenly found Nepal sexy. For years, Tabin had been trying to convince American journalists to cover the quest he was on with Ruit. But now that Nepal was a war zone, more of his emails and phone calls to editors, producers, and reporters in Washington and New York were being answered. Some media outlets even began contacting him. National Geographic Television had been inquiring about filming Ruit's work for years. But the present political crisis gave the green light to Lisa Ling, who hosted a series for National Geographic, to accompany Ruit and Tabin on an upcoming trek to an HCP-funded eye camp in Mustang and shoot a documentary about their work. Tabin discussed Ling's request with Ruit, and he agreed that the exposure such a film might provide could mean a dramatic uptick in donations.

Before the film crew arrived, Ruit received a request from another high Maoist official for emergency treatment. "By then, we'd worked out a system of security when they came to Tilganga," Ruit says. "I'd ask them to wear a certain color cap, red or blue, and be escorted by young ladies in pink kurta pajamas, so I'd know who they were. And I'd always have them arrive at the end of the day, so they wouldn't be exposed to too many prying eyes."

While the Maoists' secretary of trade unions waited on a plastic chair, with a patch over an infected eye wound and wearing a blue baseball cap as instructed, Ruit saw two thickly built men step into the waiting room and scan the patients. "They were obviously army guys, wearing civilian clothes," Ruit says. One of them dialed a number on his cellphone, and the mobile the secretary was nervously toying with began to ring. The men grabbed Ruit's patient by both arms and walked him out to their waiting vehicle.

"The arrest was big news," Ruit says. "It was in all the papers that he'd been caught in my clinic, and a few days later, a big boss from the army came to see me. He threatened that he'd shut Tilganga if I didn't stop treating Maoists. I told him very clearly, 'I'm a doctor. I treat everybody. I treat thieves and saints equally, and I'll continue to do so.' I'd come to the level where I didn't get scared by threats. I was confident in my abilities and that my work was correct. Maybe too confident."

In the days after the arrest, Ruit began to worry about whether the sensational news splashed across the front pages of the local papers would interfere with Tilganga's reputation as a neutral medical facility, uncorrupted by either the government or the Maoists. "The army was threatening me and calling me a traitor," Ruit says. "And I knew I'd be suspected by the Maoists after that, that some would think I'd played a part in helping the army with their arrest."

Ruit had spent years earning a reputation in Kathmandu that rose above politics. His greatest worry was how the arrest would affect his staff's ability to operate in rural areas, where the number of checkpoints, both military and Maoist, had proliferated since King Gyanendra had announced his decision to crack down on the uprising.

Ruit tied white silk *katas* around both of the sideview mirrors and threaded one through the grille for an extra measure of luck. Tilganga had acquired the aging city bus because it was capable of carrying thirty passengers and far more medical equipment than Hilda; the staffers christened it "Lady of Sight," painted it bright blue, and pushed it hard. The scale of their work in rural areas had expanded dramatically since the days when Ruit, Rex, and a few others could haul all they'd need for a few days' work in a single Land Cruiser.

Ruit, Tabin, and six support staff rode together toward Mustang to meet Khem Gurung's advance team and the National Geographic crew who were flying to the trailhead. The mood in the Lady of Sight wasn't especially somber, but the war was clearly on everyone's mind. Red hammers and sickles were spray-painted on the walls of nearly every town they passed, on banks, on government buildings, and even on police posts, many of which were pocked with bullet holes or scrawled with the slogan "Burn the old house down." Posters of the Maoist leader Prachanda, a man who looked more like a mild professor of literature than a revolutionary, were plastered the length of the route to their trailhead.

At first, Tabin was anxious about the Maoists, but after the bus had been waved through six or seven of their checkpoints without incident, he relaxed. When he got out and shouldered his backpack, he stopped thinking about the Maoists at all. "Once we were hiking, I was just happy to be trekking in the hills I considered my second home," he says. "Ruit set a blistering pace. I was still in pretty incredible shape in those days, and Lisa struggled, at first, to stay with us, but she was tough and eventually she got used to the altitude."

As they crossed high passes heading for Upper Mustang, Ling was amazed by how far Ruit and Tabin were willing to travel to reach their patients. "A steep, unforgiving landscape holds anyone without sight hostage," she said in her voice-over, "but Dr. Ruit knows that for many, Kathmandu is too far to travel, and so eight to ten times a year, he makes house calls."

Monks Ruit had recruited preceded the team on their trek, chanting, "The eye doctors are coming, bring your blind to Kagbeni." And in Kagbeni, the village where they set up their surgical center in a dirt-floored schoolhouse at 9,500 feet, Ling grew nearly too emotional to speak on camera while she watched patients' sight restored. A sixty-two-year-old woman named Tsering was so incredulous after Ruit removed her bandages that her laughter and tears spilled forth simultaneously. Ling took a picture of her with a Polaroid, and when Tsering saw herself she was surprised, but hardly upset, by how many wrinkles had appeared on her face in the years since she'd lost her vision.

Ling's cameraman cut in close on Ruit while she asked him why he was willing to work so hard and travel so far to restore sight. Ruit stared up at the stark crenulations of Mustang's mountains before speaking. "What I really believe is life is very short and what you can do in that period you must do. We have now got a system where we feel that we can [get close to] ninety-eight percent of exceptionally good vision with our patients immediately after surgery. If you can do that to hundreds of patients, I think walking for five or ten days is worth it, isn't it? It can change their life. It can change the life of their family. And for them this world is going to be totally different."

Ling and her crew left by chartered helicopter, flying away with footage Ruit and Tabin hoped would coax considerable donations from National Geographic's viewers. On the five-day trek back they had ample time to discuss the challenges facing the HCP. Money was the key to much of what they hoped to do, of course, but so was convincing officials in other countries of their work's merit. Ruit had made much progress toward obtaining permission to operate in China, a country with an alarming shortage of well-trained ophthalmologists in rural areas, but they conferred about who might be most capable of breaking down the walls China's bureaucrats still maintained to keep foreign doctors at bay.

Mostly, they discussed ways to spread the word of what they'd been able to achieve: a model, easily replicated, capable of curing much of the preventable blindness on earth. Videotaped evidence flown away in a helicopter might help. But to go global, they had to target a group more influential than any film's general audience; they had to take their dispatches from the field directly to their peers in international ophthalmology. Hiking down toward rebel checkpoints, on a rugged trail in one of the poorest nations on earth, their minds churning in concert with their legs, Geoff Tabin and Sanduk Ruit debated how, exactly, to launch their own revolution.

CHAPTER 20

Ravishing Beautiful Flowers

In medicine, we focus on that 2 percent improvement, that little refinement in equipment and technology, much as, I imagine, the space program does. But too often we ignore the 90 percent of people who need our services. That's the importance of the work Tabin and Ruit are doing. They're outsiders delivering a message many in my profession don't want to hear. That we have a duty to all of the world's patients.
—Dr. David Chang

In 2004, for the first time in the nation's history, there were more cataract surgeries performed in Nepal than new cases of cataracts reported. Politicians tried to meet—and be photographed with—the doctor identified with the turnaround, hoping to align themselves with one of the few inarguably positive stories to come out of the country in a time of war. Ruit refused most of these entreaties, careful not to allow himself to be used as a political pawn.

During 2003 and 2004, at the peak of the violence of the People's War, Ruit and Nabin Rai traveled the length of Nepal, sparking new projects and partnerships. They met with regional Maoist leaders and local politicians the rebels considered the least corrupt, and together they identified the best sites to serve the maximum number of rural patients. In towns where hospitals existed, such as Dhangadhi, on Nepal's western border, and at Janakpur, in south-central Nepal bordering India, Ruit pressed administrators to update their ophthalmic departments and to send staff to Tilganga for in-depth training. Across the length of the mid-hills, at seven regional hubs where passable roads remained more rumor than fact, Ruit directed the growing funds he had at his disposal toward the construction of seven community eye clinics, where technicians could prescribe glasses, treat all but the most serious trauma, and send patients with more severe problems to Tilganga.

Constructing such a comprehensive network during wartime, when Nepal's government had retreated to the safe bunker of urban centers, where they struggled to provide even basic services such as electricity and trash collection, was the work of Sanduk Ruit in his role as social architect, thumbing his nose at his country's corrupt leadership. He protested the state of his nation with actions rather than words. "Why, if we are able to do so much with such meager resources," the successes he piled up seemed to be saying, "are you, with all the mechanisms of governance, able to do so little for your people?"

One of the engines driving all this development was a battered cardboard box under the desk in Geoff Tabin's clinical office at the University of Vermont. This box contained all the financial records, travel receipts, tax forms, and grant applications that made the HCP economically viable. Tabin tried to support the HCP's expansion by applying for USAID grants, but peeling his way through the layers of bureaucracy ate up so much of his time that in 2003 he finally hired his first full-time American employee.

Tabin asked Emily Newick, who had a freshly minted master's degree in public health from Dartmouth, to turn the contents of the cardboard box into the administrative framework of an official charity. "I walked into Geoff's little ten-by-ten office after I'd accepted the job," Newick says, "and I asked to see all of the HCP's files. Geoff just pulled that box out from under his desk, and I thought, 'What have I gotten myself into?'"

Tabin hired the HCP's second full-time employee two months later. Job Heintz, a Vermont lawyer, had the tenacity to plow through the stacks of forms the U.S. government piled between charitable organizations' aspirations and the financial resources USAID offered. He also had patience and skill enough to dissect the technical language that left so many other grant seekers ineffectually spinning their wheels.

"At first, Job and I would just sort of hang around Geoff's office and cram ourselves between his piles of climbing gear, tennis racquets, and dirty laundry a few days a week," Newick says. "He'd rush in from surgery in his scrubs, or jog in after clinical rounds in his white lab coat, spoon his lunch from one of the open jars of Skippy peanut butter scattered around the office, and we'd talk as much HCP business as we could before he'd rush off again. The rest of the time Job and I worked from our home offices, where we could get the HCP organized, free from the Tabin chaos."

By the end of 2003, the HCP's files had migrated from the box to proper filing cabinets in Newick's and Heintz's homes. They designed and launched a website, hired a part-time accountant, and submitted revised financial records to the IRS. Newick built a database of silicon, rather than cardboard, to hold a file of their donors' addresses. Heintz sought out other grants that might be available to the HCP and directed his legal skills toward picking the locks of the USAID coffers that held one of the HCP's most important sources of funding.

When Lisa Ling's documentary *Miracle Doctors* aired, on September 28, 2003, it focused on the dedication of Ruit and Tabin and the worthiness of their cause. But the National Geographic editors had also tarted up the final cut with gruesome footage of Nepal at war. Images of the corpses of the royals borne through the streets to their funeral pyres and dead government soldiers in bloody fatigues being carried out of the hills, slung from poles on the shoulders of their comrades, painted Nepal as a country so mired in anarchy and violence that it conveyed a sense of despair neither Ruit nor Tabin felt. The flood of donations they expected after its broadcast never arrived, and the HCP continued to struggle for funding.

The USAID grants were expected to be spent primarily on infrastructure and matched with money the HCP raised from other sources. While building clinics, buying microscopes, and upgrading operating theaters was important, those funds were largely unavailable for what

Tabin had come to see as the heart of the HCP's mission: training a battalion of surgeons and technical staff who could build on Ruit's innovations by transferring them to medical facilities throughout the developing world.

"Ruit and I have been talking for a while now," Tabin told Newick and Heintz at a strategy session soon after they'd organized the HCP as a small, efficient charity, "and we think it's time to expand Tilganga from an outpatient hospital into a world-class training center."

"How much bigger do you want Tilganga to be?" Heintz asked.

"Ideally," Tabin said, "the Tilganga *Institute* would be about three times the size of the current hospital and have classrooms, a lecture hall, and offices for twenty-five surgical fellows to use during their training."

Heintz began mentally calculating the mountains of paperwork he'd have to scale, and the countless donors he'd have to contact, to start turning Ruit and Tabin's latest vision into a brick-and-mortar building. To build anything close to the facility Tabin envisioned, they'd need something like $10 million. "Well," he said, "we better start raising more money."

Newick remembers trying not to let her shock show. "You have to love Geoff to work with him," she says, "because he pushes so hard. He doesn't believe in limits. Which can be both good and bad. We had just turned the HCP from a stack of paper in a cardboard box to a tiny professional organization, and now he wanted to make a quantum leap from that to trying to cure all the preventable blindness on earth."

Heintz spent much of 2005 alternately talking to USAID officials and buried in the forms he had to finesse and submit. By the end of the year, the HCP had managed to land $700,000 in USAID grants toward building a new Tilganga, to augment the just over $1 million they'd raised from individual and institutional donors. The following year Heintz coaxed an additional $700,000 from USAID, and HCP's other donors delivered nearly $2 million more.

The fund-raising for Tilganga's expansion was on track, but to make it more than a building, to re-create it as a center for battling world blindness, Ruit and Tabin would have to come in from the medical wilderness. By 2005, they'd either built clinics or provided tools and training to the staffs of ophthalmic facilities in Pakistan, China, Tibet, northern India, Thailand, Vietnam, and North Korea. In Bhutan, Kunzang Getshen had made the most of Mark Haynes Daniell's money and established a network of village clinics capable of diagnosing eye diseases in their early stages and sending patients to Thimphu's National Referral Hospital for treatment by a growing staff of Tilganga-trained ophthalmologists. Despite these accomplishments, the HCP's biggest obstacle was the suspicion, still entrenched in the international medical establishment, that outliers like Ruit and Tabin might have achieved some success on the ragged frontiers of eye care but their methods were still too scattershot, unsafe, and untested to be applied beyond the handful of remote communities where they worked.

"If you're trying to change a model of how care should be delivered in international health, you can't do it on your own," says David Chang, a prominent California ophthalmologist. "You need powerful allies."

In February 2005, after meeting Chang at an ophthalmic convention in San Francisco, Tabin asked him to become one. He believed that Chang, one of America's most respected ophthalmologists, renowned for his leading-edge cataract surgical techniques, could be not only a potentially powerful ally but the ideal spokesman to publicize the HCP's mission, providing he could be converted. What Tabin wanted was for Chang to come to Nepal and conduct a clinical trial, operating alongside Ruit, so they could compare and publish their results.

Chang, a tall, eloquent American of Chinese descent who effortlessly commands lecture halls full of surgeons who gather to hear him describe the latest technical advances in ophthalmology, would be the perfect messenger to tell the medical establishment about the revolution Ruit was leading. All Tabin had to do was convince one of the busiest academic surgeons in the nation to carve a week-long hole in his schedule and fly halfway around the world to do someone he hardly knew a favor.

On a May morning in 2005 Chang slumped in Hilda's backseat, trying to shake his jet lag, as they passed mounds of smoldering trash and children scavenging through them for something to sell or eat. He didn't know where Dr. Ruit planned to operate, but he remembers hoping it would be considerably cleaner than what he could see out his window.

They climbed out of the Kathmandu Valley, into a pine forest a thousand feet above the motorbike exhaust, diesel fumes, and incessant barking of the capital's thirty-five thousand feral dogs. The Pullahari Monastery straddled a ridge with a distant view of the city and, on clear days, the snow peaks of the Himalaya. The property the Third Jamgon Kongtrul had bought was so lushly beautiful, so removed from its surroundings that the monastery's grounds crew had been obliged to put up discreet signs discouraging day-trippers from picnicking, so that the meditations of the 230 monks in residence wouldn't be disturbed.

Pullahari, the name the Third Jamgon Kongtrul chose before he died, means "ravishing beautiful flowers" in Pali, the language of the oldest surviving Buddhist scriptures, and it was the Rinpoche's hope that this forest sanctuary would be fertile soil for an exchange of Eastern and Western philosophies, that the wisdom cultivated here could bloom in forms surpassing the site's physical beauty.

Ruit had certainly hoped so, too, when he'd chosen Pullahari to host his trial.

Tenzin Yongdu, one of the monks living at Pullahari, perfectly exemplifies the fusion of East and West the Jamgon Kongtrul believed would flower on this ridgetop. When I visited the spot where Chang and Ruit faced off, Yongdu gave me a tour of the grounds. Biologists estimate that there are nearly seven thousand species of flowering plants in Nepal, and it appeared that most of them had taken root in the soil surrounding Pullahari, luring a visitor's eyes from the sacred buildings to sprays of orange, magenta, and crimson blossoms mimicking the colors of the quietly strolling monks' robes.

The monastery's main structure, the imposing Rigpe Dorje Institute, stands apart, even in such a landscape. It rises from a grand ground-floor shrine room that's been painstakingly adorned with grinning skulls and wildly colored murals painted by master artisans, depicting each stage in the endless cycle of samsara, the Buddhist wheel of life. Then it narrows, like clarified thought, past simple, wood-lined spaces devoted to study, and tapers to a modest residence on the roof, topped with slim golden spires.

Tenzin Yongdu, a white-haired, blue-eyed monk formerly named Harold Rolls, had retired to Pullahari after working as an architect in New York and Vermont, when the monastery was still a simple cluster of whitewashed dormitories. He'd taken a Buddhist name and prepared to spend his remaining days living a quietly contemplative life. But his fellow monks had other plans for him; they wanted him to design the building the former Jamgon Kongtrul had hoped would become Pullahari's beating heart. "They started in on me," Yongdu says, "after they found out I had been an architect. They were wildly excited, talking about the sacred geometry that should guide the building's design. I told them I had no idea what they were talking about. Then they all started laughing and slapping me on the back. 'Even better,' one of them said. 'Divine inspiration!'"

Rather than trying to re-create the classical monasteries of Tibet, Yongdu settled on something more modern, a design he felt reflected the Rinpoche's intentions. "I've learned to sacrifice my ego but not my intelligence," Yongdu says. "And I tried to summon all the intelligence an old man had left. I wanted the building to be a launching pad for thought, not removed from the world but viewing it clearly, like the Rinpoche did. That's why I made it spacious and bright, why I wrapped it in windows, and why I made the library and classrooms the soul of the structure, so it would be a place of engagement, not escape."

When Chang drove through Pullahari's gate, he was relieved to see how orderly and manicured the monastery's grounds were. But he was intimidated by the prospect of performing surgery there. "I was going, 'Wow, we're not in a hospital, we're in the middle of nowhere,'" Chang says. "It's sort of like if I went over to your house and we started operating on you in your living room."

"I may have had some spiritual home field advantages," Ruit says. "So I tried to do everything possible to make David's operating theater feel homely."

Chang had convinced AMO, the manufacturer of the Sovereign Whitestar model phacoemulsification machine he used in his California practice, to ship the same $100,000 ultrasound device to Nepal. He would use it during the clinical trial and, with AMO's blessings, donate it afterward to Tilganga. Ruit had entrusted a technically sophisticated engineer he'd hired, Ajeev Thapa, to disassemble the $52,000 Zeiss microscope the HCP had purchased, a five-hundred-pound piece of equipment similar to the scope Chang used in California, and transport it up to Pullahari, where Chang found it perfectly calibrated next to his familiar phaco machine, in a large classroom converted to an operating theater on the second floor of the Rigpe Dorje Institute.

Ruit had also enlisted the monks of Pullahari to serve as orderlies. They had sterilized each surface in the classrooms where they ordinarily gathered to study rolls of Buddhist scripture and empty their minds of the white noise of modern life, making the marble floors and wooden walls gleam like the center of the cloudless sky their meditative practice trained them to visualize.

"The way Ruit incorporates civilians, if you will, into his work is incredible," Chang says. "We had these armies of monks helping us, which I can only liken to eager Boy Scouts. They were so hardworking and helpful. And I needed that help because a trial like we were attempting had never been done before."

The gold standard in medical research is a randomized trial. In practice, this means that rather than collecting data from work that's already been completed, for the most credible results, the reseacher designs an experiment from scratch and randomizes the flow of the patients, so there's no possibility of infecting the results with bias. Tilganga's screeners had gathered 108 patients with mature cataracts;

they waited, eyelashes trimmed, eyes sterilized, in the monastery library, among sacred scrolls and classics of Himalayan literature that the literate among them would be able to read, once again, if the surgeries were successful.

After the Tilganga staff anesthetized them and gave them a retrobulbar block, an injection temporarily paralyzing the muscles that control movement of the eye, monks drew black or white Ping-Pong balls randomly out of a plastic bucket and sent the patients, depending on which color of ball had been picked, to Chang's or Ruit's operating room.

"Right away, I was pressed to the limit of my ability," Chang says. "At home, the cataracts we're operating on are much less advanced. As a cataract matures, it hardens from the texture of Styrofoam to something more like mahogany, and it's much more difficult to remove. In the U.S., you might see one case this tough a year." Chang activated the ultrasonic tip of his phaco device, trying to balance the force it took to carve apart the calcified nucleus of his patient's diseased lens with the delicacy required not to traumatize the surrounding tissue.

Meanwhile, Ruit had finished his first case and started on the second.

"In America," Chang says, "we usually operate one or two days a week, get a lot of rest the night before, and make sure we don't drink coffee that morning so our hands are steady. Then many ophthalmologists do four or five cataract surgeries a day, tops. A lot of us dread that one difficult case we know we have coming up in two weeks, so we have plenty of time to plan for and worry about it. But each of these cases was that one worst case. And it was an assembly line; they just kept coming!"

In his operating room, Ruit sat comfortably on his stool, humming a Bollywood tune, his bare feet fine-tuning the focus of the $9,200 portable Zeiss microscope he now took on trips to the field. The surgical instruments he needed for his manual procedure—the speculum, scissors, forceps, crescent blade, and irrigating cannula he used for hydrodissection of cataracts, which he'd had manufactured to his specifications in India—cost just under $80 for a complete, reusable set.

"How are you doing, David—do you need anything?" Tabin asked, looking in on Chang after he'd watched Ruit complete his fourth surgery while two monks guided his fifth patient to his table.

"I'm fine," Chang said, keeping his eyes trained on the inner capsule of his first patient's eye, where his phaco machine's ultrasonic probe had nearly finished pulverizing the opaque lens. "How many has Ruit done?"

"Ruit's speed was incredible," Chang says. "But I was pretty sure that my patients would have better results. Pretty soon, I began picking up my pace and finished a few cases I felt pretty good about. It was sort of like being a contestant on *Iron Chef*. You have a limited time, people scurrying around and watching, and a camera over your shoulder while you're . . . cutting up the beef."

Tabin darted back and forth between the operating rooms, making sure the patient selection was truly randomized and that every step of the assembly line was running smoothly. He leaned in to watch Chang, admiring the expertise with which he pulverized every crumb of hardened tissue before inserting a late-model foldable lens with the sort of grace and speed Tabin associated with Ruit. "Do you have any questions, David?" Tabin asked. "Anything I can do for you?"

"When do I get to use the toilet?"

"Waaayell," Tabin said, laughing, "that depends who you ask."

When Chang returned, he stretched his back and strolled over to observe Ruit. Then he began revising his opinion about who would prevail, once all the postoperative data was collected. "I was open-mouthed, watching him work," Chang says. "You just don't see something like that every day in my profession. That combination of efficiency, grace, and speed. After that, I wasn't sure who'd win the day, but I realized that Ruit was just a master, master surgeon."

After their second day of surgery, Chang, Tabin, and Ruit sat on a west-facing terrace, watching the sun set over the mid-hills.

"Tired, David?" Ruit asked.

"Oh, a bit," Chang said. Actually, he felt like he'd barely survived a day of hand-to-hand combat.

Early the next morning, Khem Gurung led the Tilganga staff as they prepared patients for their postoperative exams in a red sandstone amphitheater facing the shrine hall. There was no worry about disturbing the monks, who had been up before first light, completing their prayers at the time they considered the most spiritually charged portion of the day, when darkness gives way to the faint glow of dawn. They stood on the balconies of their dormitories, their scarlet robes burning in the low-angled sun, as bright as the blooms in Pullahari's gardens.

Ruit let his staff remove the patients' bandages while he hung back and contemplated the magnitude of what he'd just been able to prove. He was certain that he'd held his own against one of the West's finest surgeons. "We photographed and noted the degree of trauma in the eyes of each case," Ruit says. "I was quite sure that both David and I had done a laudable job. We wouldn't be able to compare our results precisely until our staff did follow-up examinations. But I suspected our trial would prove that David Chang, with his latest machines, had done well. But no better than I, with just a few needles and knives."

In the summer of 2005, when Tabin returned to Burlington, he began packing up his office, placing framed photos from Asian cataract camps into cardboard boxes. John Frymoyer, the dean who had first championed Tabin, had left the University of Vermont. His successor, Dr. Joseph Warshaw, had also been a firm supporter of Tabin's, until he'd been diagnosed with terminal multiple myeloma. But the team that took over the medical school after Warshaw's departure "micromanaged my practice and limited my time away," Tabin says. "Every time I came back from a trip I felt a little bit less welcome. It was death by a thousand cuts."

The cut Tabin found intolerable had come several months earlier. He'd returned from another trip to Nepal, walked into his office, and found a memo on his desk that enraged him. "It was this long, officious list of things I was no longer allowed to do, like make HCP-related calls from my office phone or use university copying machines, printers, and secretarial staff to prepare HCP materials," Tabin says. "That memo made it clear I needed to find a new home for the HCP. Jean and I had a great community in Burlington, and we loved our house, but I knew if the HCP was going to survive, I had to find an institution that would support my international work."

Before leaving Vermont for the trial at Pullahari, Tabin began searching for other jobs, and when the University of Utah's John A. Moran Eye Center presented him with an ideal opportunity, Tabin seized it. Dr. Randy Olson, the Moran's director, had grasped, instantly, the importance of Tabin's international work and the luster his presence could add to a facility already considered one of America's leading eye-care centers.

"Geoff was doing entire surgeries for less than we spend to drape a single patient," Olson says. "I'd always been told there would be more people going blind from cataracts than there would be surgeries available, but Geoff was proving that didn't need to be the case. Most American doctors working in the third world were still stuck on the old model: do twenty surgeries, make your trip into a little vacation, and leave complications behind. He and Ruit had created a whole new paradigm."

Olson offered both Jean and Geoff places on the University of Utah faculty and promised to create the sort of position for Tabin that he had fantasized about—director of the Division of International Ophthalmology. His salary would be considerably lower than those of his colleagues who worked year-round at the Moran, but his trips overseas would no longer be considered unpaid leave. They would be the heart and soul of his job. And as a sweetener to the offer that Tabin already found impossible to resist, Mormon-dominated Salt Lake City was populated by another spiritual community whose zeal he shared: mountaineers, obsessed with scaling the rugged peaks that ringed the metropolitan area.

By 2006, Ruit was facing fundamental changes, too: His success in reducing the number of Nepal's rural blind was making him famous. That year, he was named the recipient of the Ramon Magsaysay Award, often referred to as Asia's Nobel Peace Prize. The citation praised Ruit for refusing to accept "the absence of medical care [that] condemns [people] to darkness." In 2007, Asian *Reader's Digest*, the continent's largest publication, anointed Ruit its "Asian of the Year." "In the last 23 years," the magazine wrote, "Dr. Sanduk Ruit has personally conducted nearly 70,000 cataract surgeries, often saving more than 100 people a day from blindness. . . . As Ruit spreads new techniques to . . . many hundreds of others, hope grows that one of the great public health challenges of the 21st century can be overcome."

These accolades didn't go unnoticed in Nepal, whose appearance in the international press was often limited to reports of new atrocities in the ongoing war between the government and the Maoists. By 2006, 12,800 people had died in Nepal's civil war, and more than 150,000 had become refugees in their own country, fleeing from the worst spasms of violence.

International monitors like Human Rights Watch alleged that thousands of captured Maoist fighters were "disappeared" by government forces. The same monitoring groups also reported an organized reign of terror directed against supporters of the government in the Maoist-controlled countryside, where rebels, sometimes leading squads of child soldiers they'd pressed into service, would overrun police posts, killing or kidnapping whomever they found inside.

Ruit says that the country's competing powers, the Maoists and the Congress Party, each asked him to serve as their minister of health. He rebuffed both, telling them he preferred to remain where he was most useful, working where a powerful politician and a subsistence farmer received exactly the same standard of care in his clinic.

There was one life-changing move that Ruit felt compelled to make, for his family. Lisa Ling, before departing for Mustang, had filmed Ruit in his apartment. "Where do you think the most famous doctor in Nepal would live?" she asked as her cameras panned around the Ruits' dingy apartment. Ruit was pleased that Ling's focus on his modest home showed how he'd shunned the corruption that afflicted so many influential Nepalese, but Nanda was embarrassed by the film's implication that they lived one step above the poverty of Kathmandu's streets.

Each day, Ruit's elderly parents left their apartment in the center of town and transferred between three buses so they could make a morning pilgrimage to Swayambhunath. Ruit found their daily, traffic-choked journeys increasingly intolerable. For years, Ruit's relatives, who had preceded him to Kathmandu from Olangchungola and had built a successful business selling Tibetan antiques and carpets to collectors in the West, had offered to help Ruit find and furnish a house of his own, in a better location.

Ruit's family was proud of its most famous member and felt it was improper for a doctor of such renown to continue living like a student. "He could work anywhere in the world, but he chose to stay here for his parents and the people of his country," says his cousin Tenzing Ukyab. "One day Kasang was in a bad crash, when a three-wheeler she'd transferred to from a bus on her way to Swayambhunath smashed into a transport vehicle and turned over. Sanduk had to stitch up his own mother's face where it was torn." Ukyab told Ruit that enough was enough, that it was time to move. If *he* was reluctant to accept his family's help, then he should do it for his parents' sake. Let them live near the temple they revered. Neither Tabin nor Ruit had ever drawn a salary from the HCP. And Ruit says his wages at Tilganga, combined with work he did after hours in his private clinic, amounted to only $32,000 a year. So it was with real trepidation that Ruit decided to use an uncomfortable portion of his savings to purchase a house commensurate with his standing in Nepalese society. "For all he's done here, the Nepalese government should have built him a palace, but they're goons who can't take care of their own people," Ukyab says. "We were delighted after so many years of encouraging him that he finally agreed to move."

Ruit bought a house near the base of the hilltop temple that would allow Sonam and Kasang to make their daily pilgrimage by foot. It was a three-thousand-square-foot brick structure with a prayer room on the second floor and a window framing the golden spire of Swayambhunath. Inside the house's gated courtyard, a riot of purple bougainvillea blossoms climbed the brick walls.

The place seemed palatial to Ruit, especially after twenty years in a tiny apartment. But seeing the way Nanda's eyes shone at the prospect of moving up so dramatically in Kathmandu society pleased him. He took out a mortgage that made him as anxious as his father had been when the family had first moved to Kathmandu, and accepted his cousins' offer to fill the large, echoing building with comfortable furniture. Ruit hung the Ramon Magsaysay and the Asian of the Year awards on the walls of his expansive new living room, and allowed himself a flicker of pride for the way he'd been able to steer his family's fortunes. No one could doubt any longer that he was well matched with a beautiful Newari woman from Kathmandu's upper class. He'd managed to install his parents safely upstairs in their last home, a place they'd never have to leave, as they'd been forced to flee Olangchungola. What other blessings, he wondered, would this chapter of his life bring?

As his stature in Nepal grew, Ruit continued turning down offers to endorse any particular faction of his country's political leadership. But there was one invitation to visit with a part-time politician that Ruit was happy to accept. So happy, in fact, that he brought his parents with him.

"This is the woman who brought such a beacon of light into the world?" the man who'd summoned Ruit said. "Let me look at her!"

Kasang lowered her eyes shyly, unable to meet the gaze of the person she considered no less than a living god.

"What about your father? Let me at least shake his hand for raising such a man!"

Sonam was too overcome to reach for the outstretched hands. It was improper to stand face-to-face with the supreme leader of Tibetan Buddhism. He fell to his knees on the thick carpet, averted his eyes, and bowed his head.

The Dalai Lama settled for placing his hands on the heads of both of Ruit's parents and chanting a blessing, wishing them long life and excellent health.

"Come, come, sit next to me, Dr. Ruit," he said, patting an overstuffed cushion beside him in the reception room of his offices in Dharmsala, India. Ruit felt his mind bending in disbelief and endeavored to straighten it out. Could it be possible that the man on earth he revered most was speaking to him with such informality, such intimacy? Had he come so far from Olangchungola, achieved so much, that His Holiness was equally interested in him?

"We have so much to talk about and so little time," the Dalai Lama said. "My secretaries will attempt to hurry us along. Come, come."

Tenzin Gyatso, the Fourteenth Dalai Lama, has often said that if his karma had not been to spend his life as a Buddhist monk, he would have chosen a career in science. "He had so many questions about how we achieved our results," Ruit says. "He knew all about the latest surgical innovations and asked how he could help bring them to all the far-flung regions of the Himalaya. I was surprised and humbled by the breadth of his knowledge, and I told His Holiness so."

"But *you* humble *me*, Dr. Ruit," the Dalai Lama said. "You humble me with your compassion. I'm just a simple Buddhist monk. I often wish I had some technical skills, so I could be of greater use."

Ruit was watching the mouth of the leader of Tibetan Buddhism, the head of state of the government of Tibet in exile, and trying to take in his words. But in a separate chamber of awareness beyond language, he felt his attention drawn to his hands, to the way the Dalai Lama cupped them in his while they spoke, to the way they seemed to transmit an electrical current. "His hands were so soft and warm, like they were speaking their own language, passing on some of his inner strength," Ruit remembers. "I don't know how to explain it, but I was just so happy. Happy to be summoned to this meeting. Happy to meet with a man I admired so much. Happy to see my parents' happiness in his presence. And happy for the confirmation he was giving me that I had chosen the correct path."

As promised, his secretaries leaned into the room after fifteen minutes, subtly glancing at their watches, but the Dalai Lama dismissed them with a brief shake of his head, sending them away once, and then again, until he'd repeated his offer to help Ruit in any way he could and conveyed the message of gratitude he'd invited Ruit to Dharmsala to deliver: "You know, there are many kinds of Buddhas among us," he said, pulling Kasang and Sonam up from the positions where they'd prostrated themselves on the carpet, looking at them directly. "Your son is a Buddha, too. He is our medical Buddha."

"I don't know how to explain it, except to say that His Holiness really brings the light," Ruit says. "After I left him, I felt so full of power I felt I could accomplish anything."

Ruit's colleagues in the medical community concurred. After nearly two years of editing and peer review, the results of Ruit and Chang's trial at Pullahari were published in the *American Journal of Ophthalmology*. The study documented the fact that one of the world's best and fastest phacoemulsification surgeons had taken nearly twice as long to operate on each patient as Ruit had. It also demonstrated that one day after surgery, 91 percent of Ruit's patients had normal vision, compared to 78 percent of Chang's, an essential difference for people who often walked home over difficult terrain soon after the operation. The data equalized after six months, when there was no significant difference in the visual outcome of Chang's and Ruit's patients: 98 percent of each group had excellent eyesight. The results of the surgery Ruit was doing in monasteries, schools, police posts, and veterinary clinics—which the study referred to as SICS, for small-incision extracapsular cataract surgery—was comparable to the outcome patients could expect in modern American hospitals.

"I really wanted to do the trial," Ruit says, "because some of our own colleagues that we had trained to do manual surgery were feeling inferior, like they couldn't keep up with the West, with their latest, greatest phaco machines. So we wanted to make it little more sexy. We wanted to see how we compared, best to best. The results of the surgery were strikingly similar. But our turnover time was much quicker. That's what our colleagues needed to know. And because of David's good heart, we were able very vocally to say that SICS is the best solution for high-volume developing world surgery."

After more than two decades of uphill struggle, Ruit's renegade philosophy of bringing the best care to the poorest people in the most remote places had been vindicated in peer-reviewed print. He had a fanatically dedicated partner in Tabin and a powerful new ally in Chang, one of the thought leaders of his industry.

"What impressed me the most was that there was a magic in Ruit's system," Chang says. "And Sanduk had developed it on his own, without academic support. I was really happy that our study confirmed what he'd been fighting for for so long. But I felt like it was just the first step. Statistics can seem dry and distant. I didn't think people understood yet the scope of the problem, the challenges people face in the developing world, and the courage they have to go on living despite obstacles that would stop Americans in their tracks. I came away feeling people had to know that there were heroes like Ruit and Tabin fighting to change the world. That this was a story that needed to be told."

CHAPTER 21

Clear Vision for Life

In time past, wrapped up in clinging blindness,
I lingered in the den of confusion.
—Milarepa

I stepped out of the taxi after the driver finally found Ruit and Tabin's Hong Kong hotel. We'd been circling backstreets for twenty minutes before we'd located their modest lodgings: a narrow tower standing above a narrow street that specialized in the sale of toilets. Most of the doctors attending the World Ophthalmology Congress were staying in brand-name five-stars, connected by elevated, climate-controlled walkways to the Hong Kong Convention and Exhibition Centre. But the codirectors of the HCP, whose frugality with donors' funds was too ingrained for them to even pay themselves salaries, weren't about to spend $300 or more a night for hotel rooms.

After Tabin had gotten his teeth into me, I'd been trying to unearth and piece together the information to tell this story. And since seeing Patali Nepali's sight restored by Ruit in Rasuwa, I'd begun traveling with Ruit and Tabin, trying to understand the forces that drove them. In June 2008 I joined them in Hong Kong, at a conference attended by thousands of their peers, to hear them make a case for why their approach to cataract surgery in remote areas of developing countries should become the global standard.

Walking toward the entrance, I saw Tabin through glass beaded with condensation, waving good-bye with his tennis racquet to a surgeon, an over-forty singles champion from Rhode Island whom he'd played a few sets with before the congress kicked off. Ruit sat in the far corner of the lobby, on a slender plastic chair that bowed beneath his weight, as inert as Tabin was animated, scowling as he edited a copy of the speech he planned to give the following morning. I pushed through the door, and Tabin's face shone with the delight he directed at friends and acquaintances alike.

"*Ni hao!*" he yelped, hugging me to his sweat-soaked workout gear.

Compared to week-long treks through the mid-hills, our twenty-minute walk the next morning through the superheated streets of Wan Chai was more of an annoyance than a hardship. But it was enough to ensure that our small delegation, which included Ruit, Tabin, and six members of Tilganga's staff, arrived sweating through our suits and saris.

We left the seething streets, where breakfast soups boiling in cauldrons added even more moisture to the air, and entered the bland, modern exhibition hall. In the whir of industrial-strength air-conditioning and the patter of slick-talking salespeople, we might have been in Phoenix or Houston. Ruit hurried ahead, nervous about a lecture he was due to give that would lay out his vision for combating cataract blindness worldwide. I walked with Tabin, and we slipped farther behind the fast-striding crowd every time he stopped to shout an enthusiastic greeting and hug a colleague he recognized.

We were about to board an escalator that would take us up to the exhibition floor and lecture halls when a well-dressed middle-aged Asian man fell to the floor and rolled onto his back, his chest heaving spasmodically. There were more than eleven thousand ophthalmic professionals attending the congress, and the majority of them were doctors. But the stream of purposeful walkers parted around the fallen man, everyone continuing on their way. Not Geoff Tabin. He dropped to his knees without hesitation and took the man's hand. "I'm a doctor," he said. "Can you understand what I'm saying?"

The man nodded.

"Can you breathe?"

He nodded again, then tried to sit up.

"Why don't you just take it easy for a minute," Tabin said, rubbing his shoulder so he would stay in place, and checking his pulse. Tabin squatted on his haunches, talking soothingly until a team of paramedics in neon-orange jumpsuits arrived. "I think he just had a panic attack," Tabin told them. "No chest pain and his resting pulse is normal."

We left him in the hands of the paramedics and stepped onto the escalator, now sure to be late for the beginning of Ruit's speech. I said, "I thought you guys weren't supposed to do that anymore, with the threat of lawsuits and everything."

Tabin looked at me like I'd just denied the existence of gravity. "That's just craziness," he said. "I've never hired a lawyer in my life. If lawyers can scare us away from helping people, then the world will really be out of whack."

We passed a lecture hall with a standing-room-only crowd. The signboard at the door said, LATEST EXCIMER LASER: VISX CUSTOMVUE VS. WAVELIGHT ALLEGRETTO. Knowing how nervous Ruit was when addressing large crowds, I hoped our late arrival wouldn't make him even more anxious. But when we walked through the door of room 309, I counted exactly eleven people, apart from an equal number of Tilganga employees and HCP supporters, scattered across a sea of a hundred empty chairs.

Tabin and Ruit had come to the conference with several boxes full of *Fighting Global Blindness: Improving World Vision Through Cataract Elimination*, the textbook they'd written as a blueprint to help others replicate their success in the field. It included step-by-step illustrations of Ruit's sutureless technique, lists of tools and materials needed to conduct cataract camps, and tips on the best way to organize medical teams planning to work in remote areas.

Tabin took a seat near the door, by the boxes of books, shaking his head. "Every leading cataract surgeon in the developing world is at this conference, and this is the turnout we get?" he said. "I guess they're here to play with the latest toys so they can go home, say they're familiar with the most modern equipment, and charge the most money possible for their services. Did you know that China has the largest population of untreated cataracts in the world? We're in Hong Kong, and I don't see a single Chinese policy maker or surgeon in this room."

I was used to seeing Ruit in command, but he looked meek at the podium, reading haltingly from a prepared script and barely glancing up at his audience. "We estimate that there are upward of sixty million people who are severely visually impaired by cataracts," he said. "And in many parts of the world, these people live very far from hospitals. International organizations that fly in for a week or two do more harm than good because they leave complications behind. You have to build trust with your patients not only by delivering excellent care but by being there to follow up when they need more."

I knew how passionate Ruit could be on this subject. I'd sat with him during long drives, listening to emotion choke his voice as he spoke about the epidemic of unnecessary blindness, and much of the world ophthalmic community's indifference to eradicating it. But there was no passion in his talk to room 309, only nerves, perhaps because the indifference of so many of his eleven thousand colleagues was so vividly displayed by the rows of empty seats. Still, Ruit soldiered on. "So what I'm really saying is this. You have to change your way of thinking. You have to change your concept. These are more difficult surgeries than hospital surgeries. You have to build a system and put it in place. You have to be more serious about training people in un-served areas and helping them put together high-quality teams who can attack cataracts with a production-line approach. We can teach you how to do this," he said, regaining a little of his composure, knowing how solid the ground on which he stood was. He'd played a central role in transforming eye care across his country and much of the surrounding region. He'd done the hard work, created the model, and perfected it. Now, with Tabin's and Chang's help, all he had left to change was his profession's attitude.

Ruit flipped to the key slide in his PowerPoint presentation; it showed two charts, side by side. The chart on the left documented the nearly 24,000 cataract surgeries performed in Nepal in 1994, the year Tilganga opened its doors—a time, he told the audience, when small-incision surgery was still rarely performed in his country's rural areas. The second chart displayed the latest data available, from 2007, showing that Nepalese surgeons, many of whom Ruit had trained, had performed 167,000 cataract surgeries. "And by 2007," Ruit said, "nearly hundred percent of those were high-quality microsurgery with IOL implantation."

The small audience broke into enthusiastic applause, and I could see the Ruit I knew trickling back into the awkward figure at the podium. He raised his eyes, finally, from his text and made eye contact with the rest of us. "When we first started working in Nepal," he said, "we faced lot of barriers. People told us it was too expensive to provide the best care to the poor. We've worked out how to get round most of that now. We have a model you can take to the underserved areas of the world. And we're here to help you."

Ruit's speech had been designed to address his profession's indifference to overcoming the global crisis of cataract blindness. The turnout had highlighted that indifference among far too many of his peers. But at least the eleven strangers in the room who'd listened intently had heard his call to action. Tilganga had been built on the trash-strewn site of a temporary parking lot for buses, I reminded myself. Surely revolutions had been started with fewer people.

The main exhibition hall of the 2008 World Ophthalmology Congress was dominated by flashy multimedia display booths built by pharmaceutical companies and medical equipment manufacturers. Doctors circulated through the booths, stuffing free samples into World Ophthalmology Congress tote bags they'd received at registration and gaping at infomercials made by the producers of half-million-dollar-plus excimer lasers, which boasted of the profits the doctors could earn by investing in next-generation technology.

I took the opportunity to try my untrained hands at a cataract surgery simulator. I pressed my eyes to the rubberized microscope eyepieces, like a submariner lining up a torpedo, and maneuvered a virtual phacoemulsification cutting tool toward a dense white cataract nesting at the center of an imaginary eyeball. Once I was in, I promptly made a mess of the cataract, pulverizing it with the application of far too high a burst of ultrasound waves, traumatizing the surrounding tissue, and guaranteeing that, had my virtual patient existed in the fragile world of flesh and blood, they'd never see out of that eye again. I confirmed, as I had after watching the North Korean doctors struggling to learn Ruit's technique in Rasuwa, that surgical artists like Chang and Ruit only made the procedures they've perfected look easy.

Tabin gave a talk to a crowd of seventy or so at the booth of Santen, a large Japanese pharmaceutical company he'd wooed, convincing the CEO of their American subsidiary to donate tens of thousands of dollars of medication and IOLs to support the HCP's work. Under a banner that read, SANTEN: A CLEAR VISION FOR LIFE, Tabin delivered much the same speech as Ruit had the previous day. But he spiced up his PowerPoint with photographs of his mountaineering years, and seeing a bearded, wild-haired version of the man at the podium hanging from the Kangshung Face of Everest, many of the passing doctors took a seat and listened to at least part of his presentation, until the topic changed back to preventing blindness.

David Chang drew a much larger crowd. Striding the wide stage that his sponsor Alcon, one of the goliaths of the ophthalmic industry, had constructed, Chang spoke engagingly into a wireless headset while a blizzard of images and animations bombarded the translucent panels he paced along. Here was a $2,000 laser-etched intraocular lens, custom-cut to cure a patient's particular astigmatism; there, a golfer grinning and giving a thumbs-up after his new Alcon lens allowed him to track his ball's flight.

Corporate mission accomplished, Chang concluded his presentation by calming the storm of multimedia and turning to speak simply to the crowd. "All these technical advances I've been talking about are worthy achievements," Chang said. "But tomorrow, Dr. Sanduk Ruit of Nepal—stand up, Sanduk, there you go—tomorrow, Dr. Ruit will be performing live surgery of the small-incision cataract technique he pioneered. If you go to one event at this conference, go to that. You have to see what Dr. Ruit is able to do with your own eyes to believe it."

Since I'd arrived in Hong Kong, Ruit had been especially prickly and unapproachable. He was willing to speak about the technical challenges of his work, but he fended off most of my personal questions. I tried picking my spots during meals, when he was most relaxed, with little luck. I attributed some of his reticence to the strain he felt from fighting for attention at the conference. I had come to believe that his story, twined with Tabin's, was even more extraordinary than I'd imagined that day in Rasuwa when I'd watched him surveying his patients from a rooftop and had decided to write it. If I was to do justice to the journey they were taking together, I had to get Ruit to reveal more. It had taken Tabin years to win Ruit's trust before they'd developed a close working relationship. I didn't have the luxury of that sort of time, so I asked Tabin for advice.

"Ruit's tough," he said, speed-walking toward the exhibition hall on the last muggy morning I'd spend at the conference. "There are no shortcuts with him. I'm afraid you're on your own."

We entered a theater that had been arranged for the live surgery. Organizers had removed sliding partitions so the space could be enlarged. Perhaps one thousand people filled the rows of movie-style seats, including close to one hundred of the Chinese surgeons Ruit hoped to convert to his system. I sat between Tabin and David Chang, but technical problems delayed the start of the program and Tabin left to pace the aisles of the theater, stopping to network whenever he recognized a face.

As I watched the screen, waiting for the show to begin, the room thrummed with the expectant atmosphere that fills an arena just before the opening tip of a basketball game. Instead of uniformed players, a live feed from a local hospital appeared on the screen, and a world-renowned surgeon strode into the frame, holding his sterile latex gloves stiffly in front of him as he approached his patient. He was the head of the ophthalmic department at a prestigious medical school and attempting the same SICS cataract surgery Ruit would shortly perform.

From the moment he made his first incision, I knew something was wrong. His movements seemed fitful and tentative. He severed a blood vessel, until the image projected three stories tall was streaked with crimson gore. Expert panelists sat on a podium in front of the screen, commenting in hushed voices like broadcasters at a golf tournament.

David Chang leaned toward me and whispered, "Surgery is stressful to begin with, but live surgery is off the charts. I've seen superb surgeons who can't handle the pressure and really blow it. He can hear the audience's reaction and everything critical the panelists are saying. That makes it even tougher."

The surgeon narrated his procedure as he struggled to control the bleeding he'd caused, and his voice, which had started out authoritative, began to quiver with the strain. He sawed with his blade to enlarge his wound, and again the audience gasped. "He's gone too deep and punctured the iris," Chang whispered. "That will take some time to repair."

Tabin wasn't able to remain as reserved.

"This is outrageous!" he said loudly, hopping up from the seat behind me where he'd momentarily come to rest. "I wouldn't let one of my first-year residents make a mess like this!" For the first time since I'd watched Ruit operate in Rasuwa, I began to feel truly queasy, observing the enormously enlarged metal tools probing the patient's thirty-foot-tall bloodied eye. I had seen my share of eye surgeries by then, somehow insulated from my natural squeamishness by the fact that though they might seem a bit gory, they were part of the process of improving a human life. But as I watched a surgery go wrong, and worried that a man's eye was being damaged, the insulation suddenly wore thin. I covered my face with my hands.

When I was finally able to peer through my fingers, Chang whispered that the surgeon had been able to coax the prolapsed section of iris back, so the patient was out of danger. Now he was cleaning up the mess he'd made and preparing to insert an artificial lens. The problem, Chang said, was that the conference had allotted an hour for the three surgeries and the first had already taken almost thirty minutes. He didn't know if Ruit would get his chance to operate.

The second person who appeared on the screen was a highly respected female surgeon. She, too, struggled under the pressure of live surgery, and though her work wasn't as bloody, it stretched on for twenty minutes. As the seconds slipped by and she fumbled with her tools, Tabin picked up the speed of his pacing in the aisle behind me.

"We're trying to convince this audience that manual small-incision surgery is a simple procedure that should be widely practiced," he nearly shouted. "And now she's making it look so hard she's scaring off half the surgeons in the room."

With ten minutes left in the program, I saw a familiar face appear larger than life, and a pair of dark eyes above a blue surgical mask, shining with confidence. "With proper training," Ruit said, "small-incision cataract surgery is a very simple procedure, the solution to cure the millions of patients in poor countries who need our services. This," he said, holding up a curved metal tool scored with fine lines like a file, "is a Simcoe cannula. To a cataract surgeon it's what a rifle is to an infantryman: the one essential tool."

An elderly female patient lay prepped on Ruit's table. His poise as he prepared to operate, as he faced a complex physical task to perform, rather than a simple speech to deliver, was absolute. Technicians played a short video highlighting Ruit's surgical innovations. At one point, I was confused, because he seemed to be operating out of order, sliding an artificial lens into the eye *before* removing the mature cataract, and at that moment, the surgeons in the audience applauded wildly. "That was brilliant," Chang whispered. "The integrity of the patient's eye was too fragile for Ruit to remove the cataract without it collapsing, so he put the IOL in first and used it to keep the shape of the eye intact while he removed the clouded tissue."

"Have you ever seen that done before?" I asked.

"Not in exactly that way," Chang said. "I would make the analogy to a pro golfer. When the ball is sitting on the fairway, we all know what to do. What really separates Tiger Woods from the rest of us is what happens when the ball flies into the trees. They have trick shots to get out of that. For the rest of us, when our ball goes there we go into a death spiral. That's what it is for a master surgeon. You have to have that mental toughness. You have to be able to react instantly and creatively."

The screen switched back to a live shot of the operating room. "Dr. Ruit, I'm afraid we only have five minutes before our feed is cut off," one of the panelists said.

"Five minutes? Have little bit of mercy! I'll see what I can manage," Ruit said, bending swiftly to his work. But I could sense the smile spreading behind his mask, could hear him humming faintly as he made his first incision, the tip of his blade creating a small opening, then widening his wound, propelling his tool forward with graceful side-to-side strokes, like a speed skater's blades cutting into a pristine oval of ice. In another moment, he had the scored tip of the cannula under the hardened cataract and was drawing it steadily through the funnel he had created, until the woman's eye was clear. In went the artificial lens where the cataract had exited, and, as it slid into his patient's eye, with its promise of lifelong clarity, I looked at my watch. The entire operation had taken just under five minutes.

The audience stood and applauded. Ruit removed his mask as the patient was wheeled away, and I didn't need to imagine his grin anymore. It was there for all of his peers to see, three stories high. He began to say something just as the feed was cut and the screen went dark. But his hands had spoken eloquently enough.

The knock on the door of my hotel room later that night interrupted me as I was writing furiously in my notebook. I put my pen down with some annoyance and answered it. Ruit stood there, holding a bottle of Johnnie Walker Green and two tumblers in his right hand. He sailed a DVD of the live surgery to me like a Frisbee with the left. "A souvenir," he said. I placed it on the desk beside my notebook.

"Now, my dear," Ruit said, putting his arm over my shoulder. "Why don't we have a drink and discuss some of those questions you've been pestering me with?"

CHAPTER 22

The Singing Bowls of
Swayambhunath

Still the world is wondrous large—seven seas from marge to marge—
And it holds a vast of various kinds of man;
And the wildest dreams of Kew are the facts of Khatmandu
—Rudyard Kipling

I hiked up through the dark, winding lanes of Kathmandu, from my hotel toward Swayambhunath, whose golden, spotlit stupa guided me in like a lighthouse. Street dogs snarled from construction sites, where they'd retreated for the night, and near-naked sadhus slept, curled against the cold, on the concrete floors of small roadside shrines. I arrived at the Armed Police Force base where Ruit and Tabin planned to play badminton and waited by the locked gate as instructed. I looked at my watch: 5:00 A.M., exactly.

An instant later Ruit and Tabin materialized out of the dark from the direction of Ruit's house. Ruit rattled the gate until a sleepy soldier answered it, but the soldier said that due to the upcoming elections, security on the base was heightened and the athletic facilities were closed to civilians.

Ruit had looked forward to throttling Tabin in my presence; he'd boasted the night before that he'd never lost a match to him. Now he sighed, adjusting the ski cap he wore tugged down over his ears, and cast about for another way to get his morning exercise before we left on a seven-hour drive to southern Nepal. "Shall we climb Swayambhu?" he asked.

I was pleased by the change of plans. I'd spent a week two decades earlier, laid up by amoebic dysentery, in a cheap Thamel guesthouse. I'd climbed up to Swayambhunath after I'd recuperated, and ever since, I'd thought of the hilltop temple, with its visual cacophony of shrines to competing gods, as a symbol of well-being. I hadn't had an opportunity to visit in years; my hours in Kathmandu were tied to Ruit's schedule.

Ruit chose a wooded route, bushwhacking up a steep slope on the back side of Swayambhu Hill, weaving through trees strung with prayer flags as monkeys chattered at us for disturbing their sleep. As we climbed, I remembered the advice Ruit had received from his father as a child: "When facing two paths, if you are strong enough, always choose the hardest one." Ruit was certainly strong enough. Though he was a decade older than me and overweight, I couldn't keep pace with his stride, so I jogged as I tried to keep him and Tabin in sight. We climbed to the temple mount but bypassed entirely the tikka-smeared shrines and golden stupas I'd hoped to see. Ruit was out for exercise, not inspiration. After cresting the hill, he didn't pause to admire the view of Kathmandu at dawn; he set a winding course through a grove of pines on our descent, steering us clear of every point of interest.

By the base of the temple's great staircase, several female vendors rose from the blankets where they'd been sleeping among their wares, trying for an early sale. They struck their hammered brass bowls like bells to get our attention, then dragged sandalwood sticks along the bowls' rims, making them sing mournful notes, long, wavering cries that rose and fell like the protests of petulant children, a sound that matched my mood precisely.

Rex Shore was at the wheel of Hilda. Keeping our tires on the muddy track took all the skill he had accumulated during his twenty years of driving in the former kingdom. Hilda's odometer had stopped working, and her white lace headrests had grayed with age, as had Shore's blond hair, but driver and vehicle were still a formidable team.

In Nepal, there were roads and rumors of roads. "The road is coming" was a phrase I heard often, as if new highways were descending from the hills of their own will, like tarmac-topped glaciers. More often than not, probing new routes that appeared on maps as confidence-inspiring solid lines revealed rutted, muddy tracks. Ruit was always attentive to news of roads that could cut the distance his surgical teams had to travel. We were headed south to an eye camp celebrating the opening of his second full-scale Nepalese hospital, in Hetauda, between the capital and the Indian border. The two paved roads between Kathmandu and Hetauda were so jammed with truck traffic and so frequently blocked by the political demonstrations known as *bandhs* that Ruit asked Shore to test a new shortcut that had just been bulldozed through the mountains. If the road proved passable, we could save a few hours. I had been assigned to the test vehicle while Ruit and Tabin took the traditional route in the comfortable new Land Cruiser, which the Tilganga staff had decided to nickname the White Elephant.

One of the most obvious by-products of Nepal's bad governance was the country's lack of roads that didn't force those traveling them to risk rearranging their internal organs. Only six thousand miles of tarmac existed throughout the entire country of widely scattered cities and settlements. Compare that with Switzerland, where, despite similar topography, legendary efficiency has led to forty-four thousand miles of paved roads in a country a quarter the size of Nepal.

I rode in the back of Hilda with Alan Crandall, a colleague of Tabin's at the Moran. Crandall, sixty, was sandy-haired and solidly built. Tabin had bonded with him immediately after discovering that Crandall was one of the rare American eye surgeons who shared his commitment to working in the developing world for more than a week at a time.

"Bump!" Shore shouted.

We bounced over a boulder, and both Crandall and I hit our heads on the roof. "Not the smoothest road," Crandall said in his laconic cowboy drawl. Growing up, he'd worked on his father's sheep ranch and quarterbacked Utah's state-championship high school football team. He had since endured several potentially debilitating knee and back surgeries. The latest had come after an injury he'd sustained in Ghana in 2006; he'd taken Tabin there to introduce him to the work he'd been doing in Africa. As one of the world's leading practitioners of phacoemulsification surgery, Crandall had been testing prototypes of phaco machines compact enough to transport to remote areas. The one he'd brought to Ghana was a scaled-down version of the machine he used in Utah, about the size and weight of a suitcase packed with books. While they'd been riding from a surgical camp, their bus had hit a fallen tree, blown a tire, and lunged into a ditch. Crandall's phaco machine had shot off a rack over his head and slammed into him, fracturing his neck. Crandall had flown home from Ghana after his work was done, phoned Utah during a layover to schedule an MRI for himself, and, despite excruciating pain, conducted a day of surgeries at the Moran before enduring spinal-fusion surgery.

"Talking to Alan," Tabin says, "you'd never know what a badass he is. A lot of elite surgeons have attitudes to match their abilities. But Alan just has this easygoing approach to life that I really admire."

"Bump!" Shore shouted again, and we braced our hands against the roof. He chain-smoked most of the way along the cliffside route to Hetauda, taking his hands from the wheel only long enough to light another reeking Nepali cigarette. "Can't say as I'd call this a bloody shortcut," Shore complained, six hours later, when we rolled back onto the paved road only a few minutes ahead of the White Elephant.

Hetauda was a small hill town near the confluence of the country's north–south and east–west road systems, an ideal gathering spot for patients who lived below, on the densely populated plains of the Terai. Its proximity to the Indian border had also turned it, and its neighbor Birganj, into smuggling and banking centers; wealth had accumulated in the hands of the corrupt few and made the towns regular targets of Maoist attacks.

After a decade of armed struggle, the Maoists had done what Ruit had originally suggested: sign a peace treaty and reinvent themselves as a political party. King Gyanendra's plan to preserve the monarchy by force had blown up in his face. In April 2008, Maoist candidates had dominated the national elections. Prime Minister G. P. Koirala was swept out of office, though not out of power; he continued to wield considerable influence behind the scenes.

Maoist leaders declared the king a relic of the country's feudal past, and on May 28, the Maoist-led government ordered him to vacate the palace within fifteen days. Gyanendra reluctantly handed over his diamond-and-ruby-encrusted crown and scepter. Then he and his entourage drove out of public life on June 11, 2008, through Narayanhity Palace's pink gates after dark, in a convoy of black Mercedes limousines, officially ending 239 years of Shah dynasty rule and Nepal's status as a kingdom.

Two months before we rolled into Hetauda, the Maoists had formed a ruling coalition in Nepal's parliament, allying themselves with more moderate political parties. They'd renamed the country the Federal Democratic Republic of Nepal and elevated the leader of their revolution, known by his nom de guerre, Prachanda, to head of state, making him the new republic's first prime minister.

Hetauda's dusty, unremarkable appearance was diminished, slightly, by attractive rows of dense green Ashoka trees, their lower trunks painted white, that lined its main road. The banks, fabric stores, and snack stands that formed Hetauda's core were little more than cubbies in the low-slung, hastily built shophouses that made up most of the settlement.

The new hospital stood in a neighborhood of muddy vacant lots half a mile outside Hetauda's commercial center. The land had been bought, and the construction and running costs of the hospital were largely financed, with HCP funds, as well as a donation of $200,000 from a Buddhist organization named All for Charity, based in Australia and Hong Kong, that had become enamored of Ruit's work after *Reader's Digest* named him Asian of the Year. The money appeared to have been well spent; the gleaming, three-story brick hospital looked like a newly constructed science building at an affluent American college. The only clue that it stood in one of the world's poorest countries was a multicolored tent, the sort you would find at a large Nepalese wedding, that had been set up, temporarily, in the hospital's courtyard to house the five hundred cataract patients Ruit, Tabin, and Crandall planned to operate on for the hospital's official inauguration.

I climbed out of Hilda like someone trying to readjust to level ground after riding a roller coaster. "Did you enjoy the drive?" Ruit asked with a wicked giggle, putting his arm around my shoulder. "How about you, Alan? Any nausea?"

"Nope," he said. "I even got a few hours of sleep."

The operating rooms of the Hetauda Community Eye Hospital were almost exact replicas of Tilganga, down to the floors of locally quarried marble and the green-tiled walls. Crandall and Ruit faced each other across the bigger of the rooms, closely observed by Kishore Pradhan, the young surgeon Ruit had chosen to run the hospital. Tabin went to work in a smaller OR next door, with a cheaper microscope. (In my travels with Tabin, I'd noticed that he always volunteered to operate at the most poorly equipped table wherever he went, ceding the better gear to his peers or the doctors he was training and relishing the challenge of making do with less.) On his first shift, Crandall was treated to eight hours of Lata Mangeshkar's greatest hits. Mangeshkar, whose startling birdlike voice had skittered across the soundtracks of more than a thousand Bollywood films, was one of Ruit's favorites. Tabin, in a separate room, had a selection of electric blues playing on the iPhone he placed on a shelf behind his head. I tried to be helpful, guiding patients to operating tables and leading them down the stairs to recovery rooms inside the tent.

I missed the arrival of the next woman to land on Crandall's table, since Tabin had called me into his room, asking me to cue up Coltrane on his iPhone. She was covered by a green surgical drape by the time I returned. One hand protruded beyond the draping, immobile as a corpse's, and I was struck by how different it looked from the hands of other patients. Regardless of their age, most of their hands and feet were scarred and callused from agricultural work. But this hand belonged to someone whose life so far had spared her hard manual labor. It was a young hand, with manicured nails painted pink.

I studied her chart and saw that her name was Kiran Kumari and she was twenty-two years old. Ruit saw me looking. "This young lady had an accident with a propane rice cooker," he said. "It exploded in her face while the grains were still hard and did lot of damage. The wounds have been untreated since then, and I advised the family to wait for Alan. They've brought her here from Kathmandu because he's very expert at this sort of surgery."

"What sort is that? The kind you make up on the fly?" Crandall said, studying Kumari's eyes through his microscope. "You know, I teach a course in Utah called 'Worst Case of the Year: What Would You Do?' This is that case. The explosion really fused the layers of her eye together, and I'm going to have to figure out a way to gently peel them apart."

"Thank you, Doctor," said a soft voice from beneath the green draping. Kumari was awake and would have to summon the courage to face a complicated surgery with only local anesthetic. Crandall sat utterly still as he dissected the paper-thin layers of Kumari's sclera and cornea and the inner capsule of her eye, excising the scarred tissue. He retreated into the silence I'd seen overtake Ruit and Tabin when their skills were pushed to their limits and remained there for most of the hour and a half that he operated. Occasionally Kumari whimpered softly with fear beneath the drape. During all that time, Crandall said only two things: "Okay, we better go with Plan B" and, thirty minutes later, "Well, looks like this might work."

After he removed her drape the young woman's lustrous-haired, high-cheekboned loveliness was apparent. Kumari means "living goddess" in Nepali, and, if her eyes healed properly, she would once again embody her name.

Unlike the surgeons, I could leave the operating rooms when I craved disinfectant-free air. I used those breaks to stand on the third-floor balcony and watch the crowd of patients stream inside the walled courtyard. When we'd arrived, there were only a few, but by midafternoon of our first day hundreds of the blind and their families had gathered, getting their eyes examined by technicians beneath a sign that read, GIFT OF SIGHT: FREE INTRAOCULAR LENS IMPLANTATION.

After completing more than one hundred surgeries that first afternoon, our team retired to our lodging, a large colonial-style structure called the Motel Avocado. All the members of Ruit's board of directors had driven down from Kathmandu to inaugurate their most ambitious project since Tilganga. For three hours, we stood on the hotel terrace, as it grew increasingly dark and cold, while waiters in apple-red V-neck sweaters passed platters of gristly wild boar bristling with toothpicks, unidentifiable fried tidbits, and curried meatballs made of goat. Vietnamese, Chinese, Thai, and North Korean surgeons who'd come to be trained in the Tilganga system joined the party, and sniffed suspiciously at the food. "I have instant noodle in my room," one of the Thai surgeons said to me, passing on a plate of goat meatballs. "I think I'll wait for them because . . . diarrhea."

I passed much of the evening with Graeme Lade, Australia's ambassador to Nepal, the latest diplomat from his country to support Tilganga. We were joined by another Australian, Virginia Sarah, the international outreach director for the Fred Hollows Foundation. The FHF had a new CEO, Brian Doolan, who was determined to make amends for the foundation having cut back their support of Ruit when he'd needed their help the most. "The break with Ruit happened before my time," Doolan told me. "But as far as I'm concerned, Tilganga's one of the crown jewels of international eye care, and we're going to give them all the support we can." Doolan's pledge wasn't just talk; the FHF had made a small contribution to help build the Hetauda hospital, and Virginia Sarah was in Nepal to figure out the most effective way for Hollows to help Ruit and Tabin in the future.

Ambassador Lade was unusually mild and introspective for a man in his position. "Ruit's taught me a lot about Nepal," he said. "He's explained that it's the simple quality-of-life advances that Nepalese people really need. You know, before I came here, I never thought I'd get excited by a toilet. But when we spend six or seven thousand dollars to put sanitary facilities in a village, you see how much pride and self-respect such a little thing brings to a community."

I wondered why there were no American officials present, particularly because so much of the funding for the HCP's string of successes had been donated by USAID. "I can't even get the American ambassador to answer my phone calls," Tabin explained.

Ruit overheard our conversation and said, irritably, "We don't have time to be knocking them, they should be knocking us. They have more to gain!"

"It is crazy," Tabin agreed, "because we're giving them the best humanitarian PR bang for the buck they'll ever get. That is, if they're smart enough to publicize it."

"Hey," said Alan Crandall, steering the conversation toward another subject close to Ruit's heart. "The Buddha was from somewhere around here, right? Was he born in India or Nepal?"

Ruit, who'd been chatting up his Chinese Australian donors, lunged into the middle of our conversation. "He was very much born here! Lot of people out of ignorance think Buddha was born in India. He received enlightenment there. I went also to India, for my education. But that makes me no less Nepalese. Lord Buddha was very much born in Nepal. Very, very much!"

After a jarring seven-hour drive, a day standing and watching surgery, and three hours of consuming Johnnie Walker with curried goat, I was beginning to wobble on my feet. "I think I'm very much about to be the sleeping Buddha," I said, turning toward my room.

Tabin clapped a firm hand on my shoulder and fixed me in place. "It's never dinner in Nepal until you see the rice," he said. "You wouldn't want to offend anyone, would you?"

At midnight, with a platter of mutton *biryani* soaking up some of the Johnnie Walker, I stumbled down the unlit hall of the hotel, past an open door through which I observed three Thai doctors cooking instant noodles over a propane stove by flashlight, and found my room by feel. I scratched at the dark door with my key until I located the lock. After a few moments of listening to my stomach wrestle with wild boar, whiskey, and goat meatballs, I collapsed into a deep and dreamless sleep, a sleep that seemed to have lasted only about fifteen minutes when Tabin banged on my door at 5:00 the next morning.

"I've been reading this book called *The Female Brain*," Tabin said. "The author's thesis is that most women believe they can change the men in their lives. Why do you think they think that?" We were walking, much too quickly for my precaffeinated body, toward the hospital. For someone with so little spare time, Tabin was remarkably well-read. At dawn, Hetauda's sidewalks were strewn with trash and sweepers were already at work separating the refuse into piles, so we walked in the street, where a wildly painted transport vehicle on its way to India roared past us only inches from Tabin's shoulder. "When I was a bachelor, women would say, 'Geoff's crazy, but once he has kids he won't run all over the world. He won't wake up at four-thirty to climb a peak with his skis before work just because eighteen inches of powder fell overnight.'"

A platoon of government soldiers in full camouflage were running, in formation, down the center of the street toward us. Though the Maoists now controlled the country, a few extremist factions of the rebels had broken away, refusing to accept the slow pace of change that could be achieved through a political process. They had detonated several small bombs in Hetauda, and the government had increased the number of soldiers stationed there, as a show of force.

I don't think Tabin even noticed the soldiers jogging past us. "I mean," he said, "I'm the same person I was before I married. I'm just slowing down a little. Now I have to wake up at four if I want to have time to reach a summit and ski before work, but that's the only difference."

I remembered something Cliff Tabin had said to me when I went to visit him in his genetics lab at Harvard Medical School, to discuss the little brother he obviously adored. "The thing about Geoff," he said, "is that he's always hungry. He's got a lot of mouths to feed. Mouths inside him." And I realized that no matter how many times Ruit advised him that "you can't do everything at once," Tabin wasn't ever likely to quit trying.

"Take my international work," Tabin said. "I'm going to be spending more time in Africa soon, and that's going to really—"

He was interrupted by the blaring horn of a long-distance express bus bearing down on us. I grabbed Tabin by the neck and spun him away from traffic, toward the curb.

"Wow," he said, looking at the grease stain the speeding bus had left on the shoulder of his hospital scrubs, without thanking me or appearing particularly shaken. "That would have been a broken arm. At least!"

We turned off the main road and passed a brick wall painted with an advertisement for Shaka Laka Boom instant noodles, a fire-blackened gasoline tanker with no tires, and a hand-lettered banner on the dirt lane leading to the hospital that read, HEARTLY WEL COME TO ALL DISTINGUISH GUEST AND PATIENTS.

"So I worry that with the time I'm going to be spending in Africa, things are going to get even weirder at home than they already are," Tabin said, his thoughts continuing to chug along at precisely the point where our conversation had been interrupted, as if he hadn't nearly been flattened by a bus moments earlier. I had a vision then of Tabin's brain, laid out like a railroad switching yard. I saw rows of parallel tracks too numerous to count, and the force that animated Tabin pushing each of those individual, unstoppable trains of thought along toward destinations only he could discern. "Every time I come home now after a long trip," he said, exaggerating for effect, "Jean has taken in a new three-legged cat or a traumatized llama. It's almost like she's punishing me."

Or surrounding herself with creatures that will give her what she wants, I thought: the reliable companionship her husband can't provide when he's on the road for several months each year.

"It's got to be tough on her when you're away so often," I said.

"She knew what she was getting into when she married me," Tabin said. "We have such a terrific time when we're together. I've got to figure out a way to make it work better. If you find an Internet café, can you send her an email while I'm in surgery? Tell her I'm fine but we've got five hundred cases and no Internet access, so I'll be out of touch. And tell her that I love her."

"Geoff," I asked, "why don't you just travel with a satellite phone?"

He didn't answer. It was too late; his switching yard had already rerouted his thoughts from friction at home to the challenges he faced as we entered the gates of the hospital. On the far side of the courtyard a stage had been constructed for the official opening ceremony. Between the stage and the crowd of patients recovering in the colorful tent, hundreds of new visually impaired arrivals sat on the freshly seeded lawn like plants requiring care and water before they'd be able to thrive. Their families looked up hopefully at Tabin as he speed-walked past in his scrubs.

We entered the tent, and I left him examining the first in a long line of postoperative patients. The handiwork of Tabin and two other surgeons was evident in the one hundred bandaged Nepalese resting on quilted blankets, each patched eye marked with one of the doctors' initials. I watched staff nurses removing the bandages. And I saw the patients, after their eyes adjusted to the tent's dim, carnival-colored light, searching for and finding the expectant faces of their families, where they leaned in from the tent's many doors to watch the transformation. Witnessing so much unmitigated joy never loses its power. It felt no less humbling and true the thirtieth time than it had felt the first morning in Rasuwa. If your hands were capable of such restoration, I wondered, wouldn't you be obliged to spend much of your life traveling to the world's worst pockets of blindness, too?

I noticed Kiran Kumari waiting for the nurses to remove her bandages. She sat cross-legged between her seventeen-year-old sister, Ranju, and her thirty-year-old brother, Bisheswer. Ranju was as beautiful as I hoped her sister would be once the bandages were removed. She had Kiran's long hair and prominent cheekbones. Bisheswer hovered protectively, worried about what he might see when his sister's eyes were revealed. Parbitra Gartaula, a young, newly hired nurse, slowly unwound the layers of gauze that covered Kiran's head, then peeled back her bandages as her siblings leaned in anxiously. When Kiran blinked, and her lovely, fully functional eyes turned to take in the faces of her brother and sister, all three siblings began to cry, though Bisheswer coughed and brushed away his tears, trying to mask his emotion.

"Thank you, Doctor," Bisheswer said to me. "You've given my sister back her future."

"I'm not a doctor," I said. I'd lost track of how many times since meeting Ruit and Tabin I had tried to explain my presence in places where a foreigner was presumed to have useful technical skills. I took a picture of Kiran and showed her a close-up of the eyes that Alan Crandall had repaired so elegantly.

"Now that you have your future back," I asked, "what will you do with it?"

Her brother answered for her: "Before her accident, she was doing social work. She was teaching the illiterate village women how to read and such. She hasn't been able to continue this work because of the damage to her eyes. So she will begin again."

Finally, Kiran spoke for herself. "Mainly, my brother worried that with my disfigurement I would never find a husband. Now," she said, smiling, "I will be marriageable."

After Ruit, Tabin, and Crandall completed 634 surgeries over the course of four days, we brought one patient back with us to Tilganga; his wounds required facilities not yet available in Hetauda. We stuck to the paved road on our return trip, which turned out to be a mistake. Halfway to Kathmandu, we hit a lineup of immobilized vehicles that stretched for miles toward a mountain pass. Ruit sent La La out to ask what was happening and sighed when he heard the news. "A bus driver hit and killed the young daughter of a digger who works at a rock quarry at the top of the hill," Ruit told us. "The quarry workers have blocked the road with their trucks and demanded the death of the driver before they'll allow traffic to pass."

We waited out a two-hour delay—with Tabin twitching impatiently beside me in the rump of the White Elephant—until the diggers downgraded the price of passage from death to a lump sum of rupees, and arrived in the capital just before midnight.

Early the next morning, I stood outside the door of Tilganga's eye bank, watching Tabin pace back and forth until its director arrived for work. The passenger we'd transported to the capital from Hetauda was a farmer turned Maoist soldier who'd been severely injured four years earlier by a bomb. He'd lost both forearms in the blast, which had also destroyed his left eye and traumatized his right so severely that he could only make out shadows. Tabin was hoping to repair the man's remaining eye, but he needed a cornea—or preferably two, in case he made a mistake—before he could operate. He was anxious to perform the surgery himself, and soon: He was due to fly home to Utah the following day, to spend Thanksgiving with his family.

At precisely 8:00 A.M., Shanka Twyna strolled toward Tabin, looking distinguished in a wool houndstooth sport jacket with leather elbow patches, and, moving slowly and deliberately, he unlocked the eye bank's door.

"Do you have my corneas?" Tabin asked breathlessly.

"Patience," Twyna said, smiling. "Let the donors die."

While Tabin paced, waiting to learn when the eye bank could expect a delivery of suitable tissue, I darted across four lanes of fast-moving traffic and down an embankment, past piles of funereal wood, to the Pashupatinath complex. I hoped to meet Krishna Thapa, the cremator Ruit had told me so much about. And I wanted to see the spot where corneas were harvested from corpses that could give the living second sight. Walking along the left bank of the Bagmati, I admired the collection of tiny, ornate brick temples built to honor Shiva. But to my right, the river was little more than a trickle of filthy, foaming water passing through embankments of trash. I'd visited the Indian equivalent of Pashupatinath, at Varanasi, and had left convinced that drinking from the holy Ganges, as I'd watched pilgrims do, would leave me fit for cremation, a victim of its tainted waters. The Bagmati made the sacred stretch of the Ganges look like a pristine mountain stream.

Krishna Thapa wasn't hard to find: All I had to do was walk toward the flames. He left his assistants to tend the embers of a traveler on the wheel of samsara and shook my hand warmly. He wore clean white homespun clothing and was as small as Ruit had described, with a radiance in his light brown eyes that I attributed to the thirty years he'd spent launching the departed toward their next life. Thapa said he hadn't received any donated tissue for days. Next to a funeral pyre two other Chhetri were building around the shrouded body of a young woman, Thapa unlocked a metal gate set into a stone wall and showed me the room where Tilganga's technicians would harvest the next set of corneas a grieving family agreed to donate.

It was warm inside, and constructed like a miniature operating room, with tan marble tile and a steel gurney for the patients. The door facing the river was warm to the touch when I helped Thapa shove it closed, and its base was imperfectly sealed, so that we stood among gray drifts of human ash. I turned to face the small man. "Do you enjoy your work?" I asked.

"Oh yes!" Thapa said. "We are able to be of great benefit to the dead. And now, thanks to Dr. Ruit, I'm able to make a small contribution to the living."

I could hear the whoosh of flames beyond the door as the funeral pyre was lit, and the room became steadily warmer as we spoke. "Do you fear dying?"

"Not at all," Thapa said. "I know what an ordinary thing it is to move on to other forms."

"So would you like to be cremated here?"

"Oh yes," Thapa said enthusiastically. "That is my fondest hope. This is my home."

Thapa was so hospitable that I asked the indelicate question I'd been too embarrassed to put to him at first: "Working so closely with so many of the dead, are you ever afraid of ghosts?" Thapa's face curled up in a sneer, dismissing what I presumed he considered a foolish question. He was right to be offended, I realized. Just because he worked in a setting that seemed macabre to an outsider, why should I assume he'd be superstitious?

He fingered the collection of beads, amulets, and fetishes on leather thongs that hung in the hollow of his throat, including a slim metal cylinder containing ashes from the funeral pyre of King Birendra. "I'm not afraid the ghosts at all," he said, lifting the charms toward me to display their power. "I have very, very strong protections."

Thapa gave me a souvenir, a set of the small, clear plastic disks, the size of press-on fingernails, that he places over the wounds where the dead's corneas have been excised, so that their bodies appear intact to their families. Then we pushed the hot, heavy door open together.

While her parents clung to each other and watched, flames licked out of the young woman's mouth, and as the clarified butter trickled down her cheeks, it dripped burning drops onto the kindling piled beneath her body. "Do you know how she died?" I asked.

"The leukemia," Thapa said, tsk-tsking. "Terrible. She was so young."

I couldn't take my eyes off the flames. They leapt from the base of the burning pyre toward one of her hands, which had fallen free of the shroud. The young woman's nails were painted the same glossy pink as Kiran Kumari's had been while I watched Alan Crandall cure her. I stared until the flames reached them and the polished nails ignited, flaring hotter than the surrounding flesh. Then I walked past Thapa's colleagues, who were sweeping the still-glowing embers of other departed souls into the Bagmati, crossed the river, and returned to the land of the living.

Tabin was amped up to attempt a procedure so cutting-edge it had never been tried at Tilganga: With a keratoprosthesis, an experimental artificial cornea he'd brought from Utah, he would try to repair a shrapnel-scarred eye by combining it with donated human tissue. While Tabin briefed Reeta on the technique, I sat in Tilganga's waiting room, speaking with his patient, a thirty-two-year-old man, through an interpreter. His Maoist comrade and minder, a skinny teenager wearing camouflage pants and a black ski cap, tried to look more menacing than he appeared.

"How were you injured?" I asked.

"I prepared a bomb," the patient said, "which I intended to fling at a police post. But it detonated in my hand while I was in the motion of throwing."

The man wore sunglasses. He removed them with the stumps of his arms, which had been amputated just below his elbows. His face was scarred from blast wounds, and the socket of his left eye was empty. His right eye appeared intact, if heavily traumatized.

"Do you regret what you did?"

His teenage minder interrupted before he could answer: "He is a martyr injured fighting corruption, fighting to set his people free. He can't work, so now the party is feeding him."

"Yes," I said, then turned my attention back to the patient. "But do you think it was worth it, losing your hands and eyes fighting for the cause?"

Though he was wearing comically oversized plaid pajama bottoms with the blue surgical smock the hospital staff had tied onto him, the man carried himself with quiet dignity. "Though I've lost my hands and my eyes, the citizens of my country have lost much more than that," he said. "We have many resources, but they've been stolen by the few. People are still hungry. They have no clothes. They lack education. I have three daughters. If they, and all the children of Nepal, achieve universal literacy, if the revolution is fulfilled, then I'll be happy about my sacrifice."

The surgery seemed gruelingly complex. Moving more patiently than I had imagined he could, Tabin sewed donated corneal tissue to the patient's traumatized eye, delicately carved a round crater at its center, and, with Reeta murmuring her support, snapped the clear circular keratoprosthesis into a titanium ring that would hold it centered over his patient's pupil, succeeding in reconstructing the man's eye. "I wonder if that's the first artificial cornea transplant ever done in Asia?" Tabin said, elated, after two hours of surgery.

The intricacies of the procedure were lost on Tabin's patient. The man was happy simply to see anything again, to be able to make out forms a day after the surgery. Twenty-four hours later, after Tabin had flown home for Thanksgiving, the man was already seeing well enough to count fingers across the length of an examination room. During the next day, as his eyesight steadily improved, the fervor of his revolutionary rhetoric diminished. He didn't speak about stolen resources or his glorious martyrdom the last time I talked to him before he returned to

Hetauda. "What I want most," he said, staring at me steadily with his one working eye, "is to see the faces of my daughters. And to tell them that education, not violence, is the path I hope for them to follow."

I planned to head home soon after Tabin had, but Ruit approached me during my last day in Nepal. "Some people are holding a ceremony for me next week," he said. "It's silly, really, lot of noise and pomp. But you might find it interesting." The ceremony, I learned from Nanda, was in fact a formal affair commemorating Ruit's career. It would be held in a recently restored palace in the royal city of Patan, which was being opened for the occasion. I emailed my travel agent and arranged to miss Thanksgiving with my family.

Almost from the moment I pushed Send on my computer, I was leveled by a bout of fever. We'd been eating wild boar, left over from the inauguration of Hetauda's hospital, for days. Whether that was the cause of my illness or not, the huge bristly hog heads that drifted in and out of my fever dreams for the next five days argued that it was. And those plaintive notes from the singing bowls formed the soundtrack to my illness, ringing in my ears like a case of tinnitus, like a wailing child who won't be calmed, like a never-ending test of my brain's Emergency Broadcast System, though I knew in my more lucid moments I was too far from Swayambhunath to hear them.

By the evening of the ceremony I was well enough to travel to Patan. I rode beside Ruit, who wore a sober new gray suit for the occasion. Nanda was turned out in a long, pale blue blouse embroidered with white flowers. Sagar, at university in Pokhara, remained at school, as his father surely would have, studying for his exams. The teenage Serabla and Satenla, abstaining from the formality of their elders, wore sweatshirts and jeans.

Before urban sprawl, Patan had once been separate from Kathmandu, and its Durbar, or Palace, Square, was one of the architectural wonders of Nepal. We parked beside the Krishna Mandir, a masterpiece of Newari craftsmanship. Its concoction of filigreed pavilions tapered four stories high, like a wedding cake sculpted of stone. Ruit climbed out into a throng of reporters and cameramen from Nepal's major television networks, who jammed their lenses so close, as the head of the welcoming committee pressed a thumbprint of red tikka paste to Ruit's forehead, that I feared they'd smear his symbolic third eye.

We were led past burning urns of clarified butter and through low brass doors into what had been the royal palace when Patan was a competing city-state. The building had been converted into a museum, and this was its first function since its restoration. After the Ruit women were shown to their places, every one of the hundreds of seats in the courtyard was filled. Ruit and Sonam were led to a low couch on an elevated stage by a welcoming committee of women in red and gold saris. They draped father and son with white silk *katas*. And Sonam and Sanduk tried not to laugh as the women slipped a traditional checkered cotton *topi* on Sonam but struggled to make a small matching hat balance on top of Ruit's oversized head; he took pity, pulled it off, and jammed it into his jacket pocket.

I paced the perimeter of the courtyard, taking pictures, gathering evidence of the day of vindication Ruit had worried would never come. We were in the neighborhood where Nanda had been raised, at the epicenter of the elite Newari world. Here, the heart of Kathmandu society had rejected Ruit's marriage to one of their own and dismissed his medical career until his work proved so visionary he could no longer be ignored.

An elite member of the Nepal Ophthalmic Society—an organization that had once denounced Ruit as irresponsible for operating in rural areas—presented him with a carved wood plaque so enormous it could fill most of a wall in the Ruits' new living room. The writer Jagdish Ghimire, the chairman of Tilganga's board, was due to speak next. He had recently survived a bout with cancer, but only after Tabin's protégé Matt Oliva used his connections to arrange a bone-marrow transplant for him in Bangkok. His speech was brief and emotionally charged. "I would argue," Ghimire said, "that the founding of Tilganga, and the construction of its world-class lens laboratory, is a historic development for Nepal on par with the recent transformation of our nation into a democratic republic."

The guests included many of the country's most famous writers, poets, musicians, and progressive politicians, several of whom took the opportunity to speak. But Ruit and the Tilganga staff said little. Sitting quietly in the last row, I saw Reeta Gurung, Nabin Rai, and Rabindra Shrestha, the core of the team that had launched Tilganga fourteen years earlier and had demonstrated the excellence Nepalese could achieve when they burnished their intelligence and refused, as Ruit had taught them, to be treated like children of a lesser god.

There was almost too much to look at in the courtyard of the former palace. There were jeweled and silk-swathed dancers, performing the elaborately choreographed specialties of each of Nepal's major ethnic groups, and pairs of men stuffed into hairy yak costumes, stamping across the stage between performances. But my eyes kept returning to a stationary spot in the swirling complexity of the hours-long ceremony: the face of Sonam Ruit. While Sanduk had to periodically leap up off the couch to accept one award after another and mumble a few words of thanks to former foes after they made lengthy speeches praising him, Sonam sat quietly by his side, beaming with a look of Buddha-like contentment. I couldn't understand the droning speeches in Nepali, but I could read Sonam's face clearly. The fifteen days of trekking to place his seven-year-old son in school; the equal distance over treacherous passes he'd traveled to return home; the abandonment of his ancestral village and his struggle to reinvent himself as a shopkeeper; the flight during wartime to the strange new world of the capital; the shunning by Nanda's family and much of Kathmandu society—it had all been worth it, this humble man was surely thinking, because it had all been part of the fate written on the surviving members of the Ruit family's foreheads, the inescapable karma that had delivered them all to this unforgettable day.

CHAPTER 23

Eye Contact

*At that first sight of the town I felt that living among such people
might change a man for the better. It had done me some good already,
I could tell. And I wanted to do something for them—my desire for this
was something fierce. "At least," I thought, "if I were a doctor,
I would operate on Willatale's eye." Oh yes, I know what cataract
operations are, and I had no intention of trying. But I felt singularly
ashamed of not being a doctor—or maybe it was shame at coming all this
way and then having so little to contribute. All the ingenuity and
development and coordination that it takes to bring a fellow so quickly
and so deep into the African interior! And then—he is the wrong fellow!
Thus I had once again the conviction that I filled a place in
existence which should be filled properly by someone else.*
—Saul Bellow, *Henderson the Rain King*

Quiha Zonal Hospital was a plain, prefabricated building. It sat on
the dusty plateau above the city of Mekele, along a wide, well-
paved road the Italians constructed before World War II, when they
tried, and failed, to colonize Ethiopia. Most days, the building blended
into the landscape of sun-bleached thornbushes and dishwater-colored
hills. But when we arrived in early 2009, the hospital, obscured by a
crush of bodies, looked more like I imagine it had in the mid-1980s,
when it was hastily built, by other Italians with better motives, to treat
the victims of Ethiopia's famine, a catastrophe that killed more than a
million.

Tabin's goal was to restore sight to as many as eight hundred people. In the days before our arrival, patients began traveling by bus, by

donkey cart, and on foot to reach the hospital. By 8:00 A.M. on January 10, it was already uncomfortably hot, and more than four hundred people ribboned the perimeter of the hospital, squeezed into every sliver of available shade. We'd arrived in northern Ethiopia on a pre-dawn flight from Addis Ababa, but any notion of sticking to our original plan—checking in to a hotel, showering, and leisurely fortifying ourselves with coffee—evaporated when Tabin made eye contact with the few of his patients who were still able to see. "We've got to . . . get to work," he said, and I could hear the expectations of hundreds of blind Ethiopians in his voice. Without Ruit by his side to organize and fine-tune the process, the fun-loving Tabin I'd often traveled with was nowhere in sight.

That spring I sat next to Tabin's parents in San Francisco's Ritz-Carlton Hotel, in a ballroom filled with men in well-tailored suits and elegantly turned-out society women, while their son received an award from the Dalai Lama, who was suffering from a cold. He had selected Tabin as one of his Unsung Heroes of Compassion, and before he'd presented the awards, he'd given a short speech. His Holiness's hoarse voice made the audience lean forward, hanging on his every word. "Don't pray to a god and ask him to do things," he told them. "Illogical! You should do it. 'Compassion' is an empty word unless it's put into action."

The writer Isabelle Allende read out the names of the honorees. Each of the orphanage builders, microcredit lenders, and housers of the homeless briskly shook the Dalai Lama's hand or bowed briefly and returned to their table. But when Geoff Tabin's time came, he took both of the Dalai Lama's hands in his and spoke quietly into his ear for two solid minutes. When he returned to the table and sat beside his parents, their faces shining proudly, I asked him what he'd said.

"I said, 'Now that you've become such a chick magnet, do you regret your choice to spend your life as a monk?'"

"Come on."

"No, I said, 'It's a shame that my partner Sanduk Ruit couldn't be here to share this award with me.' I told His Holiness that everything I've achieved, I've achieved because of my partnership with Ruit. I said that he deserves the award at least as much as me, and that it would have been more meaningful to have him honored by my side."

Tabin's mother, Johanna, listened attentively, her sharp intelligence fully intact at eighty-three. She seemed more proud of her son's humility than of the award he'd received. The Dalai Lama concluded the ceremony by warning the winners not to rest on their laurels but to continue exemplifying compassion in action: "If after you receive this, then relax, wrong!"

Tabin didn't need to worry. Relaxation wasn't in the irradiated DNA he'd inherited. He continued to recruit talented young doctors and was thrilled when he convinced a dedicated corneal specialist named Matt Oliva to join the HCP. Years earlier, Tabin had arranged for Oliva, currently a surgeon practicing in southern Oregon, to get advanced training at the All India Institute and do a fellowship with Hugh Taylor in Melbourne. Since 1998, when he'd first watched Ruit and Tabin in action at a surgical outreach in Kalimpong, Matt had been operating with them in the field, and he was beginning to lead his own HCP-sponsored cataract camps in Africa. "After I saw the speed, grace, and economy of their surgical system," Oliva says, "I realized they'd found the solution for third-world blindness. I told them I was in, all the way in."

"Most doctors are risk-averse overachievers," Tabin says. "Matt wasn't one of those. As a researcher for Johns Hopkins, he traveled all over Kenya and Tanzania, conducting the best survey of blindness ever done in East Africa. He's also become a specialist in creating eye banks, which has been incredibly helpful as the HCP continues to grow. Since Matt joined us, he's been willing to go wherever and do whatever it takes."

That's often meant answering the phone late at night, whenever Tabin has a flash of inspiration. "Even when he's doing something else," Matt told me, "Geoff's brain is always sifting through a sea of facts, looking for the little kernel that will make the HCP a bit more effective. I can't tell you how many times he's called me at midnight, from some concert, with reggae or whatever blaring in the background, to talk about some technical detail that will make our next trip to Africa more successful. It comes from a place of incredible compassion, but it can wear on people. He's got twice as much energy as anyone I've ever met. I don't think Geoff even knows what a freak of nature he is."

During 2008 and 2009 Tabin was expending that energy to flit around the globe so frequently, on so many working trips, that I had trouble deciding where and when to accompany him. After signing the HCP's first five-year agreement with the king of Bhutan, Tabin and Ruit had traveled to that country every year to operate, help Kunzang Getshen create a countrywide network of eye care, and oversee the training of a new crop of Bhutanese ophthalmologists. Rates of preventable blindness were dropping so steeply in the kingdom that Bhutan had signed a second five-year agreement, asking for the HCP's continuing assistance.

Tabin's Unsung Heroes award was also a misnomer, of sorts. Since he'd moved to Utah to head up the Division of International Ophthalmology at the Moran, Tabin's profile had been steadily rising, and his praises were increasingly being sung in the media.

The outdoor equipment company North Face, which had long donated gear to support Tabin's work, funded a film crew that accompanied him and Ruit to eye camps in the Everest area. Called *Light of the Himalaya*, the movie North Face made attracted outdoor-oriented supporters to a cause they could believe in. *Outside* magazine did a feature story on the HCP and the making of the film, which added new donors to the organization's growing database. And Lisa Ling remained so enamored with Ruit's work that she followed him to North Korea, documenting his sight-restoring surgeries as well as his ongoing training of doctors in the world's most isolated country for another National Geographic special. Producers framed the film as more of a glimpse inside the secretive nation than a documentary on Ruit's work. *Inside North Korea* was timed to air during the first ever bilateral meeting of U.S. and North Korean diplomats, when news of the country's nuclear menace was splashed all over the American media, and drew another wave of donors to the HCP.

The reason I found myself in Ethiopia with Tabin was that his work had attracted the attention of Jeffrey Sachs, a Columbia University economist and public health advocate. Sachs had written in his best-selling book *The End of Poverty* that "Africa's governance is poor because Africa is poor." He argued that with properly targeted investment and intelligent development, extreme poverty could be eradicated throughout Africa within twenty years. As a founder of the United Nations Millennium Villages Project, Sachs set out to prove his premise in 2005 by choosing several of the poorest villages across the continent and attempting to turn them into showpieces of sustainable development by radically improving their agricultural practices, educational institutions, and health care systems.

Two years later, Sachs's project had made significant progress, but he was under intense pressure from critics and competing development experts to show measurable improvements in the villagers' quality of life. And few improvements were as demonstrably transformative and cost-effective as restoring a blind person's sight. He approached Tabin and asked him if he could complete a survey of one of the villages—Bonsaaso, Ghana—for $25,000 of the money that Sachs had raised for the project.

"With that much money, I'll not only survey every person in Bonsaaso, I'll survey everybody in the surrounding area and cure every case of treatable blindness that I find," Tabin told him.

Then, in August 2007, with Huckleberry Holz, a surgical fellow studying with him at the Moran and four nurses and technicians from Tilganga led by Khem Gurung, Tabin did it. His team screened 4,600 people, performed 160 cataract surgeries, and prescribed 1,100 pairs of eyeglasses. Sachs was so enthusiastic about Tabin's results that he asked if he'd do the same in the other eleven Millennium Villages.

Tabin offered to go Sachs one better. "I said, 'Let's not just do an intervention. Let's transfer our knowledge, train local people, and create centers of ophthalmic excellence that can change eye care in Africa.'" To demonstrate the results a few well-trained surgeons could achieve, Tabin proposed holding the largest eye-surgery camp in Africa's history, in the place where blindness is perhaps most widespread on the continent: Ethiopia.

In December 2008, Tabin began calling me three or four times a day, trying to persuade me to come with him. He was particularly enthusiastic about the country, where he had held a small surgical outreach program the previous year. He raved about the beauty of northern Ethiopia. "Like Moab but more amazing," Tabin said. "We'll climb up to incredible rock churches carved into cliffs. We'll drink the best coffee in the world, go dancing every night, and push the fun-o-meter into the red."

At least he was right about the coffee.

Inside the unventilated halls of Quiha Zonal Hospital, with the sun beating down on the roof, we were pressed close to patients being prepped for surgery. There were eight foreigners: six medical professionals and two journalists, whose skills seemed suddenly vague. The photographer Ace Kvale, Tabin's friend and climbing partner, had come to document the work and, with Tabin, scale sandstone pinnacles in the desert north of Quiha. Between the front door and the operating room were three long corridors where Ethiopians in sweat-grimed white wool dhotis sat packed together on benches, clutching their *dulas*, long shepherd's staffs that curled at the top. They propped these in front of their sightless eyes like question marks.

"God!" said Ann Bagley, an ophthalmic technician from Salt Lake City, cupping one hand over her face and stumbling forward. "It smells like beef jerky." It couldn't have been more than a hundred yards from the door to the operating room, but negotiating that gauntlet, trying not to step on bare, callused feet, skirting assorted open wounds, inhaling the very essence of poverty while staring into all those blind eyes, was one of the longest walks I've ever taken.

In a utility closet transformed into a makeshift changing room, Tabin had already pulled on scrubs when the rest of the team arrived. He was joined by three other American medical professionals: Alan

Crandall; Alan's wife, Julie, an ophthalmic nurse; and Ann Bagley, Alan's sister. This small group had to summon a remarkable quantity of optimism; they had to believe they were able to help every member of the crowd, growing larger every moment, outside the door. Tabin's team was also tasked with training a dozen Ethiopian technicians and nurses, as well as Dr. Tilahun Kiros Meshesha, one of only two ophthalmologists available to more than six million residents of northern Ethiopia. Fortunately, the HCP had brought two secret weapons: Sarita Paudel, a veteran surgical nurse from Tilganga, and Bal Sunder Chansi, a driven young technician whom Ruit had chosen as Tilganga's training coordinator.

It was Chansi who would be in charge, determining how many surgeries to do a day and deciding when the doctors were too exhausted to continue. I asked him if it was possible to cure eight hundred patients in five days. He answered with the subcontinent's most distinctive gesture, the head waggle, a response that confirmed that he'd heard my question but was too wise to offer a definitive answer.

"All we can do is try," Chansi said, tying on a mask.

Hunched over a surgical microscope, with his iPhone blasting Howlin' Wolf through cheap speakers, Tabin worked his thirteenth case of the day. The patient, Lam Lam Berhar, was a fifty-five-year-old woman with large, milky cataracts obscuring both eyes and a case of trachoma, an infection that can cause the eyelashes to turn inward and scar the cornea, which had required a course of antibiotics before she could have surgery. Berhar had traveled a day on foot and eighty miles by bus from her village to reach the hospital. She said her husband was also blind but they could afford only a single bus fare. Berhar's vision had degraded to the point that she could make out only light and dark.

I asked how quickly trachoma leads to blindness. "Not as fast as masturbation," Tabin said, holding out his gloves for Sarita Paudel to rinse with a sterilizing solution.

With Paudel assisting, Tabin made an incision in each of Berhar's anesthetized eyes, using a diamond blade that had been built to Ruit's specifications. Delicately, he worked each cataract-clouded lens out of the tunnel he'd constructed through several layers of the eye and flicked it into a bucket by his feet. Next he inserted a synthetic lens manufactured at Tilganga in its place. The process took him ten minutes. "Think of the eye like a peanut M&M," Tabin explained, "with the candy shell as the outer chamber of the eye, the peanut as the lens, and chocolaty goo holding the peanut in place. My job is to take out the peanut, clean out the cortex, the chocolaty mess, and insert a new peanut, an artificial lens. It's the single most effective medical intervention on earth, a little miracle. Tomorrow, she should see twenty-twenty."

Chansi drove the doctors hard the first day. They broke once in the early afternoon to use the bathroom and swallow a protein bar each before they tied their surgical masks back on. At 9:00 P.M. after 114 surgeries, Chansi pulled the plug. We all wedged into a Nissan Patrol for the short drive to our hotel in the town of Mekele. I wondered just how much energy Tabin would have left for the dancing he'd promised. He slumped sideways and began to snore. At our grim hotel, most of us skipped dinner and fell asleep in our clothes.

At 7:00 A.M., the Patrol arrived to take us back to work. Before scrubbing in, the doctors inspected the results of the previous day's surgeries. The line of squatting patients with bandaged eyes stretched along one entire wall of the hospital, around a corner, and halfway down the side of the building. Local priests with long beards and flowing *gabis* circulated through the crowd, comforting anxious family members. They held carved wooden crosses in one hand and horsehair flyswatters in the other. Say what you will about the efficacy of the crosses, but the flyswatters looked righteously useful.

It was difficult, staring at the six or seven hundred people gathered at Quiha, not to feel that the Ethiopians had won the genetic lottery. Their café au lait complexions glowed in the early light. Women wore their hair in elaborately plaited *shorubas*, piled high over imperious foreheads. And the eyes of those who were able to see pinned you in place with striking intensity.

Tabin crouched in front of Lam Lam Berhar, peeled back her bandages, and shone his climber's headlamp into her eyes. Berhar, like many women in the second-oldest Christian country on earth, had a black Coptic cross tattooed in the center of her forehead. "Perfect," Tabin said. "Crystal clear." He waved at her. For a moment, Berhar's face remained perfectly blank. Then her hand fluttered up to touch the cross on her head and she focused on Tabin's grinning face. Berhar jumped to her feet, threw back her head, and ululated. Her cry was contagious. As the doctors moved down the line, dozens of other women who'd regained their sight stood and added their voices to the trilling chorus. Sometime in my life, I may hear a sound that expresses joy more purely. But I can't imagine when.

All day long buses and carts arrived at the hospital gate, unloading streams of the sightless. They walked unsteadily into the compound with staffs or were led forward, clutching the hem of a son or daughter's long, trailing dhoti. The crowd grew to well over a thousand souls. Families, unable to find solid shade, squatted in the latticed shadow of thornbushes. The swelling crowd illustrated the toll blindness took on a developing country: Not only were the functionally blind unable to support themselves, but those who cared for them were pulled from the workforce as well.

While Tabin operated, Dr. Meshesha practiced the small-incision technique he'd been perfecting since Tabin's last visit. In the 1990s, when China offered twenty of the country's brightest students scholarships, Meshesha jumped at the opportunity. Despite not knowing a word of Mandarin when he arrived, Meshesha completed an ophthalmic fellowship in a Chinese medium. When he returned to the region where he'd been born—Tigray, in northern Ethiopia—as only the area's second ophthalmologist, he realized he could spend the rest of his life operating as he'd been taught and hardly make a dent in a population suffering so much from preventable blindness.

After reading a medical paper Tabin wrote about Ruit's technique, Meshesha concluded that SICS offered the best chance to serve the greatest number of patients. But without access to Ruit's specialized tools, he had to improvise. Meshesha took a long, narrow-gauge needle and bent it to a shape that approximated the illustrations that accompanied Tabin's article. Then, with a tool that cost three cents, he taught himself to perform credible SICS surgery.

In 2006, Meshesha told Tabin what he'd achieved. "I was so amazed by his passion and the progress he'd made on his own that I arranged for him to spend six months with me at the Moran," Tabin says. "Now Tilahun is one of the finest cataract surgeons in sub-Saharan Africa." But no amount of talent could keep pace with the need of the millions of northern Ethiopians who required Meshesha's services. Nepal had a population of twenty-seven million, and its doctors did more than 170,000 cataract surgeries a year. "There are eighty-two million Ethiopians," Tabin said. "I bet Ethiopian docs did fifteen thousand cataract surgeries last year, tops. And most of those were in Addis [Ababa]. We need to create a system around Tilahun and get him more support, so he can get his numbers up."

On the lot next to Quiha hospital was a small general nursing school built by a Spanish charity that had run out of funds. It turned out a few ophthalmic technicians and nurses a year. The HCP planned to expand it into a full-scale ophthalmic training center, and to add facilities that could support two more surgeons at Quiha hospital.

In the meantime, Tabin followed Ruit's philosophy of asking all motivated staff members to test the limit of their abilities. When we first arrived and I met a nurse named Tekeste Negusse, I presumed he was Quiha's surgeon. A tall man in his mid-thirties with a trimmed mustache, Negusse carried himself with an air of authority. As one of the few medical professionals available during the 1998–2000 war between Eritrea and Ethiopia, he'd been pressed into service as a battlefield surgeon. Tigray had been pounded by Eritrean artillery and fighter jets. "Medically, my trial was by fire," Negusse told me as he watched Meshesha operate. "Despite the fact that I had only recently completed my training as a nurse, I had to do amputations, chest wounds, everything, because there were no other trained personnel at the front." Tabin, hearing of his history, suggested that Negusse learn small-incision surgery on the spot and operate on some of the simpler cases when Dr. Meshesha took his breaks.

"Tabin and Ruit are doing as much as anyone to improve the delivery of health care in the developing world," says Al Sommer, a former dean of the Johns Hopkins Bloomberg School of Public Health and honorary chairman of the HCP's advisory board. He likens the state of the American medical system, with its dependence on hospital emergency rooms rather than prevention, to the dysfunctional state of medicine in many of the African countries where he has worked. "With blindness," Sommer says, "it all comes down to numbers. Last I checked, there were about five hundred ophthalmologists in San Francisco. But how many are there in all of sub-Saharan Africa? Not many more than that I'd guess. If you're ever going to defeat cataract disease, there simply aren't enough doctors. You have to train nurses and technicians to do the surgery." He adds, "Ruit has made the process so simple, I don't see why it couldn't be done."

Between patients, Tabin stood up from his operating table in Quiha hospital, offering pointers and checking on the progress of Nurse Negusse's surgeries. "Not great," Tabin told me when I first asked about Negusse's results. Tabin felt he was treating the delicate tissue in the eye's inner capsule too roughly. But by our third day, Tabin had already revised his opinion. "He's doing much better now," he said. "And he has surprisingly good surgical hands!"

Alan Crandall handled the most complicated cases. They were generally children who had been born with cataracts or had suffered an injury to their eyes—from thornbushes, knives, or any of the other objects that frequently inflict wounds on subsistence farmers.

The titanium plate that stabilized Crandall's neck made hunching forward on a surgical stool uncomfortable, but with Ann and Julie assisting, he operated for fourteen hours on our second day, straightening up only to take a single bathroom break. First thing the third morning, he prepared to operate on a five-month-old. She had a tuft of curly hair on top of her head, huge eyes, and congenital cataracts that rendered them useless. To complicate matters, she also had acute glaucoma, high pressure in her eyes that could injure her optic nerves. Crandall had to not only remove the cataracts without creating scar tissue that would damage her growing eyes but construct tiny vents to release the pressure. He pressed his own eyes closed. His hands, in white latex gloves, rehearsed the movements he planned to make, like a ski racer reviewing the contours of a course before heading to the starting gate. "I've never seen him this nervous before," his wife, Julie, said.

"It's just that in the U.S., you have so many resources," Crandall said. "Here, there's no backup. If you fuck up, this beautiful little girl is blind forever. Her life is literally in your hands."

In this case, that was a good thing. Crandall operated with the encouraging calm of a veteran pilot bringing a damaged 747 in for a safe landing. "That went fine," he said after two and a half hours, his blue surgical gown striped with sweat, as the bandaged, unconscious girl was placed in her mother's arms. "I think we might have a small victory here."

Not all of the children whose families brought them to Quiha hospital were as lucky. Eleven-year-old Cherkos had been dropped at the hospital by his father, who'd told a nurse he'd be back for his son in a few days, after he'd climbed to a church hollowed out of a rocky cliff, consulted with Coptic priests, and completed his prayers for the boy's recovery.

Cherkos's homespun clothes were dirty and torn, his head had been shaved to ward off lice, and his left eye was severely traumatized. If I understood the medical technician who had stepped in to interpret correctly, a chisel he'd been holding had skipped off a rock he was helping his father split and had punctured the center of his eye, driving down through his iris. A village healer had bandaged it with a poultice of herbs, hastening the infection that killed much of the surrounding tissue. After I placed Cherkos on Tabin's table and told him the story, Tabin just shook his head. "At least he has vision in his other eye," he said. "There's nothing I can do for this one."

I led two twelve-year-old girls named Louam and Maharene to Crandall's table. They were friends from the same village north of Quiha, and both suffered from cataracts. The girls sat together as they waited for their surgeries, their hair braided identically and pinned in place with pink bands, holding hands and talking, excitedly, about being able to see. It was a straightforward matter for Crandall to repair Louam's eyes. But when he looked at Maharene under the microscope, he simply said, "Shit."

"Do you know what happened to her?" Crandall asked.

"Her parents said she had an accident with a knife while she was cutting firewood."

"Well, it must have been when she was very young. This girl's cataracts are traumatic, and it looks like the injury occurred a long time ago," Crandall said. "I'm not getting a response from her retinas. And her brain's unlikely to be able to process visual information after so long with no input. I can clean her eyes up and make her look better cosmetically, but . . . " His voice trailed off, and that was as close as I ever came to seeing the imperturbable Dr. Crandall cry.

I brought the bandaged girls out to their families after their surgeries. In the recovery room, I made myself look their parents in the eye, and through another interpreter, I passed on the prognosis for each of their daughters. Louam's mother was elated, her eyes shining with excitement. But it was the faces of Maharene's mother and father that stayed with me long after I left Ethiopia. They didn't look shattered so much as stoic, subsistence farmers in a poor country whose lives had taught them too many hard lessons. I hated to be the bearer of another.

That evening, we had a formal meal with the Tigray Region's minister of health and his staff, in an airless private room off the lobby of our hotel. For two hours, we sat trapped in oversized chairs, picking at the hotel's bland interpretation of continental cuisine, watching Tabin fidget in his seat, struggling to transition from experienced surgeon to fledgling diplomat. Waiters wandered in listlessly, delivering the beers we'd ordered thirty minutes earlier one or two at a time. When one placed a lukewarm bottle of local St. George lager in front of me, Tabin snatched it, drained a third of the bottle, and replaced it before his own beer arrived.

Tabin was hoping to make Quiha hospital and the attached nursing school one of the HCP's centers of excellence he'd talked about with Sachs. He outlined his ambitious plans to the minister, including expanding Quiha hospital, making it capable of supporting itself by charging a sliding scale for cataract surgeries, and offering Lasik surgery and an eyeglass boutique to the middle-class residents of Mekele.

"Implementation may take longer than you think," the minister said. "This is Africa."

"I don't accept that," Tabin replied with something resembling Ruit's steel in his voice. "There are people willing to work hard and people who aren't. The staff of Quiha hospital has been fantastic so far. They're willing to work hard."

The minister conceded the point. But perhaps to rectify the criticism he'd leveled at his continent, he pointed out that the American medical system was not without flaws. "America still leads the world in developing the latest technology. But Australia, Sweden, Great Britain—these are the places I really study. We can't learn much from your medical system because you don't actually have one, in my opinion. Your country has only a crisis-management system."

I realized the minister was making almost precisely the same point Al Sommer had in his office at Johns Hopkins. If the minister could see clearly how broken the American health care system had become from this distance, from the high desert of northern Ethiopia, why, I wondered, couldn't so many of our own politicians?

By the fourth afternoon of surgery in Quiha hospital, I could barely keep my eyes open. I wished I could draw some juice from the batteries that drove Tabin, but they powered him alone. Our driver and fixer was named Mulu Mohari, which he said meant "strong medicine." Mohari had short gray dreadlocks, wore mirrored aviator glasses day and night, and wound a dashing Palestinian-style kaffiyeh around his neck. "You look tired," he said. "The strongest medicine I know is our Ethiopian coffee. Come, come."

We drove north, past shouting boys playing foosball on tables placed at the side of the road. Mohari overtook a flock of sheep tended by a teenager wearing shorts and green rubber gum boots, then swerved around a donkey towing a handmade wooden cart rolling on car tires. Lashed upright to the cart, looking like a vision from an alternate universe, was a gleaming silver Westinghouse refrigerator.

We stopped in front of an unmarked cinder-block coffeehouse, and Mohari fetched a powder-blue plastic thermos from under his seat. Ethiopia claims to be the cradle of both humankind and coffee. Before entering that building, I thought my local baristas back in Oregon took the transformative power of roasted beans seriously. I learned that an Ethiopian coffee ceremony raises the preparation from art to spirituality.

A young girl spread freshly cut grass at our feet and set on our table a woven basket full of popcorn, coffee's traditional accompaniment in Ethiopia. The girl's mother sat in the corner, on a low stool, roasting green coffee beans over a charcoal brazier. When the beans were black and shining with aromatic oil, she held the pan under our noses and wafted the scent toward us with a reed fan. She then crushed the beans with a mortar and pestle, mixed the ground beans with water, and set a long-necked black clay *jebena* on the coals to brew. She served us the coffee in espresso cups filled to the brim, the brew splashing onto our saucers, a symbol of abundant hospitality.

Perhaps it was the guilt and pleasure I felt at stealing a moment while the others were still at the hospital, but I'd never had a more satisfying cup of coffee. I drank a second, feeling Mulu's strong medicine taking effect, fortifying me to go back. We filled the thermos and borrowed a dozen china cups for our colleagues.

By the time we returned, more than two thousand people were crowded into Quiha's compound. Women tended large earthen stoves, turning out yard after yard of the flat, spongy *injera* bread that is the staple of the Ethiopian diet. Hundreds sprawled on mats, sleeping or nibbling roasted barley they had brought in burlap sacks. At the center of each recovery room, buckets for the patients who couldn't find their way to the concrete squat toilets fouled the air.

Every time I stepped outside, trying to breathe, mothers held up babies with infected wounds and pressed them to me, or elderly men unbuttoned their shirts to show me tumors. I tried to explain that I couldn't help them, that I was just a journalist. I tried to convince myself that my writing would raise awareness to make more work like this possible. In the face of overwhelming need, storytelling felt like a poor excuse for my presence. I closed my notebook, rolled up my sleeves, and scrubbed my hands.

Tilganga's training coordinator sat outside the operating room, cataloging the numbers of cases completed and patients still waiting for surgery. I asked Chansi if, whenever he had a few moments free, he could teach me how to be helpful. He showed me how to change IV bottles and present surgical tools so they remained sterile. He demonstrated the correct way to carry patients onto the operating table, how to tape bandages over their eyes when the surgery was complete, and how to cross their hands in front of them so they'd follow confidently as I led them to the recovery rooms. No one would have mistaken me for a medical professional, but at least it was better than standing around and observing.

The first patient died that day: An elderly man scheduled to have surgery the following morning had a heart attack and collapsed on a bench in the courtyard. We heard his family wailing through the windows of the operating room. The second died soon after. The night before his surgery, a man in his forties who had traveled from his village near the Eritrean border slipped while walking to a bathroom in the middle of the night. He hit his head on the concrete floor of the toilet and bled to death before he was discovered.

"That's horrible," Tabin said the next morning when he heard the news, looking up from his operating table. But he sounded surprisingly matter-of-fact. When I asked him about it later, he said, "Blindness in a place like Ethiopia is often a death sentence. The life expectancy of blind people in the developing world is less than one-third that of people with sight."

Nearly every time I looked out through the screened windows of the hospital, which almost succeeded in keeping out the flies, I saw Cherkos standing alone on a boulder that gave him a clear view into the operating theater with his one working eye. At first I took his presence as a reproach, a reminder that we had failed him, and tried to ignore him. As the hours passed, as he watched us while waiting patiently for his father's return, I made a point of meeting his eye and forcing a smile onto my face. Whenever I had a moment free, I bought him drinks from the roadside stand at the hospital gate and passed him treats from the plastic tub full of power bars, cookies, and candy that Alan and Julie Crandall had brought from Utah. For Cherkos, we served as insufficient entertainment during the hours while he waited for his father. For me, he served as a reminder of the pitilessness of poverty, and the limits of modern medicine's ability to alleviate its symptoms. I never had a chance to say good-bye. One day when I looked out the window, the boulder Cherkos had stood on for so long was vacant.

We all got sick. The photographer Ace Kvale had stomach trouble. So did Julie Crandall, but she swallowed antibiotics and Imodium and stayed by her husband's side in the operating room. Chansi had a sore throat. Paudel was running a fever. Even Tabin, who typically barked, "*Fan-tastic!*" whenever anyone asked how he was doing, admitted that he felt only "pretty average." I began coughing so strenuously that I pulled a muscle in my chest. But we knew our ailments were temporary and our time here brief. We could afford a plane ticket home to another world.

By the fifth evening the team had completed 699 surgeries, but more patients kept arriving. We had planned to head north the next morning, to relax for a few days at an Italian-run ecolodge where the food and wine were reputed to be the best in Ethiopia. From there we were going to visit the U.N. Millennium Village of Koraro, explore the nearby red-rock wilderness, and climb to churches hollowed out of stone pinnacles.

Tabin broke the news on the drive back to the hotel. "I'm going to stay here until we're done," he said. "This is their only chance to see." I realized that, despite his protestations, Tabin's philosophy of trying to do everything at once no longer applied when blind patients required his services. He had packed a pair of climbing shoes, and the sandstone towers to our north beckoned, but Tabin didn't budge. Despite the fact that Ruit was probably sound asleep on another continent, I couldn't help feeling his approving presence.

By the measure of my own disappointment, though, I learned an uncomfortable truth. I was overwhelmed by the heat and dust and suffering, by the impossibility of grasping a moment of privacy anywhere on the hospital's teeming grounds, by the limitless need of the patients flowing through the hospital's rusted gates in a never-ending stream. I wanted to flee, to find a decent meal or a comfortable bed. But shamed by Tabin's dedication, I stayed. We all stayed.

On our sixth day, I worked beside Tabin from dawn to dusk. I managed flow, taking care to always have someone prepped at the end of his operating table so I could slide them into place the moment I finished bandaging the previous patient. Mohari made frequent deliveries of his strong medicine, and we found an agreeable rhythm that sped the surgeries along, accompanied by Tabin's electric blues. Just after 10:00 P.M. I dripped antibiotic drops into the eyes of Tabin's last patient, a frail, emaciated woman who was far too easy to lift onto the operating table. When he was done, I pressed surgical tape over a gauze patch, smoothing it to the woman's forehead and cheekbone. Tabin and I both noted the number I wrote on her bandage with green marker: 82. She was Tabin's eighty-second patient, a record for him in a single day.

He pulled his gloves off, tilted his head back toward the screened window, and, trilling his tongue in imitation of his patients, ululated. To me, his warbling cry sounded like someone being electrocuted. The Ethiopians recognized it for what it was: wild delight. Across the hospital compound, we heard a gentle musical response echo from women resting on reed mats in the various recovery rooms, drowsing on benches beneath homespun blankets, or curled under thornbushes with their families. "Yes, we're in agreement," the echo seemed to say. "What's happening here is cause for celebration."

By the middle of the eighth day, the compound finally began emptying out. Buses and carts drove patients away. People who'd arrived clutching feebly at the hem of a relative's robe walked confidently, without assistance, toward their homes. I bandaged patient number 907 and, with a shock, saw that no one else was waiting and we would all be leaving soon, too. Most of us would return to our own countries, to sleep as much as our families would allow while we nursed our minor ailments.

Not Geoff Tabin. He was feeling "fantastic" again and had scheduled a tennis match with one of Ethiopia's top players on his return to Addis Ababa. Two weeks later, after a few days with his family in Utah, he would climb back into his eternal long-haul seat and travel to Nigeria, where he would lead another high-volume surgical camp. Tabin's HCP colleague Matt Oliva would arrive in Ethiopia eight months after we left, to help expand an eye bank in Addis and run a surgical outreach with Dr. Meshesha, which would cure another 598 people.

But while I stood in the stilled operating room, that was all in the future. At that moment there was only Quiha Zonal Hospital and a single hard-won lesson: The overwhelming need of the crowd outside the door made some people, certain rare individuals like Tabin, not only stronger but better. As I walked our last patient out into the blinding sunlight, into the quiet courtyard where for more than a week hundreds of patients had crouched and cried and ululated with joy, I realized we had all found hidden reserves in ourselves that Geoff Tabin had known about all along. And we had become better, too.

CHAPTER 24

The Road Is Coming

There are only two mistakes one can make along the road to truth:
not going all the way, and not taking the first step.
—Siddhartha Gautama, the Buddha

Any remaining worries Ruit had about whether the Maoists trusted him and any lingering resentments he harbored about the indifference American diplomats had shown his work for two decades were put to rest on April 30, 2009. That day, America's ambassador to Nepal, Nancy Powell, along with Nepal's prime minister, the former Maoist rebel commander known as Prachanda, arrived to inaugurate the new Tilganga Institute of Ophthalmology.

Ambassador Powell, a career diplomat, had been posted to Ghana just before the attacks of 9/11. In their scorched-earth aftermath, she accepted the offer to serve as ambassador to Pakistan, managing what had arguably become America's most challenging diplomatic posting from 2002 to 2004. Adding a tour of duty in Nepal to her distinguished foreign-service career, Ambassador Powell was more attuned to the value of promoting humanitarian aid than some of her predecessors. She gave a speech formally opening the new facility, which she called "a combination of the best of American intentions and Nepalese ingenuity."

Tabin, along with the HCP's Job Heintz and Emily Newick, stood off to the side of the stage while the VIPs made their speeches, surveying what their five-year fund-raising campaign had made possible. Uphill from Tilganga's original building, a new five-story, 110,000-square-foot brick hospital stood, connected to its predecessor by an elevated blue walkway that curved between the buildings, like a sanitary version of the Stream of Sesame Seeds that had given the site its name. The series of USAID grants that Heintz wrote, submitted, rewrote, and resubmitted generated almost $3 million for the project. Tabin made personal appeals to his most important supporters, and more than six million additional dollars rolled in to complete the construction, and equip the facility, from both private donors and foundations like Fred Hollows.

In 1994, the year Tilganga was founded, the hospital and its outreach teams screened 22,290 people for eye disease and completed 1,728 surgeries. In 2009, the new Tilganga and its mobile surgical units would screen 275,430 people and provide 16,603 surgeries. On the third floor, a library, lecture hall, and a suite of offices gave Tilganga the capacity to house and train twenty-eight surgical fellows at once, realizing Tabin's vision of Tilganga as a formidable incubator for teaching young ophthalmologists the techniques Ruit had pioneered. Four additional operating rooms below meant Tilganga could enlarge its staff, perform more than two hundred surgeries a day, and care for patients in a twenty-five-bed recovery ward.

Tabin had also convinced the London Vision Clinic, one of the world's foremost Lasik surgery training centers, to partner with Tilganga. The LVC had donated two late-model Zeiss lasers and was training the Nepali surgeon who would operate them. Once the Lasik suite was functional, Tilganga could cover a significant portion of its operating costs by charging Nepalese of means $500 a surgery, less than they'd been paying for a plane ticket to a facility of similar quality in Singapore.

Before the formal speeches began, Ruit walked hand in hand with the prime minister, giving the man who'd fought so unflinchingly for the rights of their country's poor a tour of the spacious new facility that was now so well prepared to treat them. Ruit, wearing a sober black jacket and a plain black *topi* tailored not only to fit his enormous head but to match the prime minister's own hat, sat on a specially placed couch, surrounded by the prime minister's security detail, and observed one of Tilganga's brightest surgical stars, Dr. Govinda Paudyal, at work in one of the institute's sparkling new operating theaters. Paudyal had become Tilganga's speediest cataract surgeon; he had set Tilganga's record the previous year, when he'd completed 204 cataract surgeries in a single day, during an outreach he led in Uttar Pradesh, India. As the prime minister watched, Paudyal whipped through several cases to demonstrate Tilganga's increased capacity, removing diseased cataracts and inserting artificial lenses in three minutes, less time than it would take to walk from the new hospital building to the laboratory where the first-world-quality IOLs had been manufactured by an entirely Nepalese staff.

Heintz stood watching the head of the new Tilganga Institute and the nation's leader, two former rebels who had risen to improbable heights, chatting happily on the far side of a piece of plate glass that had been installed so large groups of students could observe surgeries that transformed the lives of Nepal's citizens, regardless of caste, class, or social standing.

"This is one hell of a dance," Heintz remembers thinking. "I was struck that we'd actually achieved the goal we'd set. We built and equipped the place, and we did it all in a period of civil war, total chaos, limited leadership from the local government, and almost no support from the U.S. embassy. And I was thinking, mostly, about the ripples that would reach around the world from the powerful factory we'd built for good."

Ruit had a new headquarters in a state-of-the-art medical facility on the hill above the lot where pilgrims' buses once parked, and a new title, medical director of the Tilganga Institute of Ophthalmology. But just like Tabin after receiving his award from the Dalai Lama, he was in no danger of relaxing and savoring his accomplishments. Shortly after the inauguration, Ruit set out on one of the most ambitious surgical outreach expeditions he'd ever undertaken: a three-week trip across much of the eastern Himalaya, stopping to operate at four separate eye camps in Bhutan, Kalimpong, and Sikkim.

Along with failing to govern effectively, Nepal's leaders had also failed to complete the long-planned road from Kathmandu to the country's eastern border. The current route, which swerved south to the plains, took twenty hours of driving. Ruit had heard another "road coming" rumor; this one said that if it didn't rain and the rivers ran low, it might be possible to head east and, navigating a tangle of dirt tracks and dry riverbeds, reach a stretch of pavement that had recently been poured from far-eastern Nepal to the Indian border.

We set off before first light. In the countryside, oxcarts still outnumbered motorized vehicles, and thousands of small, fiery red chilies left to dry on tin roofs glowed as the sun's first rays ignited them, like coals too hot to touch. Just before we turned off on a dirt road, we rolled by a large billboard that read, in English, for maximum prestige: VISION SUPER-DELUXE WHISKEY — MANAGE YOUR DREAMS! It seemed an odd brand name for a drink that could get you blind drunk. I pondered this unimportant mystery drowsily as we followed the south bank of the Kosi River, the White Elephant lumbering gently along, rocking me back to sleep. When I opened my eyes we were in the middle of the river, with water rising so high along both sides of the Land Cruiser that we cut a wake. Manbhadur, another of Tilganga's professional drivers, was at the wheel, and he looked perfectly relaxed, as if he were at the helm of a pleasure craft, rather than a Toyota with an exhaust system that could easily flood.

We bumped up onto the riverbank, and Khem Gurung and Manbhadur, riding side by side in the front seat, slapped their hands together in victory as we turned onto two tire tracks cut through a floodplain of reeds. We didn't see another vehicle for hours, which was fortunate, since the narrow "road" we were traveling on was little more than an elevated dike between flooded rice paddies. The gauge on the White Elephant's dashboard said the outdoor temperature was ninety-five degrees. We drove with the windows closed to keep out the dust, and with the air-conditioning off to save gas. Ruit didn't care much about comfort, but his time was valuable. He could fly to Bhutan in two hours while his staff brought the supplies he needed for surgery by land. I asked why he didn't. "Well, as you know," Ruit said, "I'm not so fond of flying. And these trips give me lot of time to think straight and plot out the future."

"What are you plotting now?"

"I was considering how best to adapt phaco for work in the bush. It's the coming thing. There's no use denying it. SICS is still the best solution in most cases. But people will think they're getting second-rate surgery if we can't offer phaco to them, even in the villages. So I'm wondering just how much we can push the manufacturers to make the machines smaller. If we can get them down to about the size of a brief-case, that should do."

"Aren't phaco machines too expensive?"

"Not if we can get the volume really up. My goal on this trip is to work out how to do ninety to one hundred phaco surgeries a day, so we can transfer that process to Thailand and China and such. That's not being done anywhere in the world. And I'm going to establish this. In urban China now, surgeons are doing twenty a day. Maximum. If we can do hundred a day in the places we'll be working, which is much harder, I'm sure we can pull it out anywhere."

Woozy with heat, I'd mistaken Ruit's silence for relaxation. As with Tabin, I suspected, there was a switching yard up there in Ruit's over-sized head, with trains of thought running, day and night, on multiple tracks, chugging toward destinations a decade in the future.

Eight hours after we left Kathmandu, we saw the new road switch-backing down from a spur of Himalayan foothills. On pavement, we made better time toward India, but still cut only two hours off the twenty the other route would have taken.

At the Indian border post the following morning, an agitated, ener-getic man with close-cropped graying hair was waiting for us. "Come, come, come!" Kunzang Getshen said, steering us through a mob to the jeep he'd brought down from Bhutan. Manbhadur remained with the White Elephant while customs officials slowly unloaded crates of med-ical gear strapped to its roof rack and scattered their contents on the ground. We hoped we'd see him in time for surgery the next morning. Indian police with long truncheons began beating the food vendors whose carts blocked our vehicle until they moved their *paan* and samosa carts out of our way. "This is India, a mad, mad mess of a country," Getshen said apologetically. "Courteousness won't get you far."

As we rolled toward Bhutan in the jeep, Getshen greeted Ruit warmly. Since he and Tabin had helped pry open the door to the kingdom, Ruit had driven through it each year, performing eye surgery and checking on the progress of the Bhutanese staff who'd come to Tilganga for training. In many ways, Getshen's history mirrored Ruit's own. He'd been born into a traditional Buddhist family in a small mountain kingdom, and his relatives had debated whether to send family members abroad to receive an education. "At that time, we had no electricity, no services, and scarcely any schools in my country," Getshen said. "To pass on messages to the outside world, we relied on strong men who would run for days from the capital to the nearest telegraph office in India. Many Bhutanese believed that if we came down out of the mountains to seek an education in India, we'd die of malaria, cholera, and other lowland diseases."

As Sonam Ruit had, Getshen's grandfather consulted the birds. "He went to the mountaintop to pray and put out buckwheat cakes for the crows," Getshen said. "But they didn't touch them. So he was opposed to sending any of us out. But my father insisted. He was in the first group to leave, walking all the way to Kalimpong. And when he didn't die, and returned after taking his exams in Darjeeling, he paved the road for the rest of us."

We sped across the flat Indian plain, past the wrecks of head-on collisions that had been picked clean of salable parts, and by a series of billboards urging drivers to control themselves. SPEED THRILLS AND ALSO KILLS was followed, a few miles later, by LIFE IS SHORT. DON'T MAKE IT SHORTER, which was topped, just as the mountains of Bhutan came into view, by IF YOU ARE MARRIED, DIVORCE SPEED!

We were enveloped by the lush, rolling landscape of a large tea plantation, and, slouching in my seat, I thought it looked like we were fording another river, with green waves of new growth cresting and lapping at our windows. "We used to have a lot of lands like this," Getshen said. "A lot! But the British chased us up the slope in colonial times and took them. Now our nation begins at the base of those mountains. It's a tragedy," he said, grimacing to emphasize his point, before his default sunny expression returned. "But it's what we have."

The ornate gate to Bhutan looked otherworldly after the trash-filled streets of Jaigaon, the settlement on the Indian side of the border. Serpents and dragons crawled up its freshly painted pillars toward a plinth topped with a slim golden spire. "My father designed this town," Getshen said. "Before we were pushed to the base of the hills, there was nothing here. My king made him something like the magistrate of this region and told him, 'We need a place for the people who've lost their farmlands and have to live here, so draw it up and build it,' and he did. We lived here during the construction, but it's so *hot* down here." Getshen flashed his theatrical grimace. "I'm always relieved when I return to the mountains."

Getshen's father had done an exemplary job of city planning. Bhutanese wearing dress shoes and knee socks along with the traditional *ghos*, which looked like bathrobes, strolled uncrowded sidewalks. The streets of Phuntsholing were washed and swept; I couldn't see so much as a candy-bar wrapper blowing across the town's wide and orderly main boulevard, which canted up toward a vista of misty foothills. And the buildings that lined it had been designed in a similar high-Himalayan style, resembling the classical temples of Tibet.

Ruit's team operated for three days in Phuntsholing's large, newly built hospital. In Africa, fully a third of our patients had been children. Even in the surgical outreach camps I'd visited in rural Nepal, a significant portion of the patients were middle-aged or younger. But in Phuntsholing, nearly every patient was elderly. When I asked Ruit why, he said, "Because of our victory here. Kunzang can give you facts and figures when we reach Thimphu."

On the winding five-hour drive up to Thimphu, Bhutan's eight-thousand-foot-high capital, I rode between Getshen and one of the first protégés he and Tabin had selected for training at Tilganga, Dr. Dechen Wangmo. She was in her mid-thirties, wore her hair in a fashionable spiky crop cut, and spoke in the clipped cadences of the English-standard school she'd attended. Wangmo's husband had also risen through merit in Bhutanese society and now served as a lieutenant colonel in the Royal Bodyguard, where he was personally responsible for the king's safety. She was determined that their two daughters hit the books as hard as she had. "I don't want them to dillydally and waste their time obsessing about Western pop stars," she said.

At Thimphu's National Referral Hospital, a large, harmonious butter-yellow building that loomed above the center of the town, a fusion of Eastern timelessness and Western science, patient intake was remarkably orderly; the separate queues for royals, monks, nuns, and ordinary citizens all moved briskly. But in a courtyard outside the operating room where Ruit, Wangmo, and their peers would be performing eye surgery for local residents and treating complex cases transported from the most isolated villages of the kingdom, chaos reigned. Wangmo looked at the crowd of patients straining to cut the line and then cocked her head at me. "I always tell my daughters, 'Common sense is very wrongly named,'" she said. "Sense is, in reality, very uncommon."

"Okay!" she shouted to the crowd. "I don't know why you're jostling like cattle. Everyone here will be seen and attended to. We need a smart young person to help organize this mob." When no one answered, she singled out a shy-looking teenage boy in a bright green T-shirt who'd brought his grandfather in for surgery and was avoiding her gaze, his eyes fixed on his white tennis sneakers. "You!" she said. "Are you volunteering? You look like a sensible enough young man. I want you to tell all these people to take a seat on the benches we've thoughtfully provided. They're well shaded from the sun. It shouldn't be too much of a hardship for them to wait there. Nurse! This very good person will call out the names of the patients and bring them to you. You can manage that, can't you?" And without waiting for an answer, she pushed through the crowd to scrub in for surgery.

Yes, I thought, Tabin and Getshen had certainly chosen their troops well.

Inside Thimphu Hospital's operating room, Ruit was working with the same type of portable phaco machine that had fractured Alan Crandall's neck. He asked me to time his surgeries, and I told him they were averaging ten minutes each. "I've got to get quicker," he said, and retreated into the silence of extreme concentration.

The next morning, Getshen gave me a tour of his clinic while his staff screened candidates for the day's surgeries. "Before Dr. Geoff came here, I had a quieter sort of life," he said. "I had time for lunch, time to go out and play at archery if I liked. It was nice. But now it's always like a railway terminal in here, and I'm rarely able to leave."

In the nine years since the HCP had begun working in Bhutan, Getshen's staff had grown to include seven ophthalmologists and forty-nine technicians. With Tabin's help, Dechen Wangmo had traveled to the Moran, to do specialized training in pediatric ophthalmology before gaining invaluable experience in the high-volume crucible of Tilganga. Another Bhutanese ophthalmologist, Dr. Nor Tshering, had also traveled to Utah, where he'd worked as Tabin's fellow, learning the latest techniques in corneal surgery, before spending three months at Tilganga putting them into practice.

Along with fully outfitted surgical facilities in Phuntsholing and Thimphu, Bhutan now boasted two HCP-funded eye-care clinics in the country's isolated eastern provinces. Each year since the HCP had begun working in Bhutan, tens of thousands of the country's children had been screened for eye disease, first by teachers Getshen's staff of outreach workers had trained, then by technicians in regional eye centers. Since 2000, some 340,000 students had been screened for correctible eye conditions in a country with a total population of only 700,000, and HCP-trained staff had conducted more than 5,500 cataract surgeries. HCP-funded outreach workers also made sure that every child in Bhutan received enough vitamin A, to prevent the increased incidence of blindness that a deficiency can cause.

It had taken more than five years from the time Tabin signed his first working agreement with the royal government of Bhutan, but the country's eye-care system had been transformed. Mark Haynes Daniell had gotten his money's worth; Bhutan was a model of unmitigated success that the HCP could advertise when it sought future donors.

There was still one prominent failure in Bhutan, a single uncured patient whose condition was driving Dechen Wangmo crazy. "I wonder if you can help me," Wangmo asked me in a conspiratorial whisper one morning. "My own auntie is blinded by cataracts. She lives in Thimphu with my cousin, but he believes she's so old and frail there's no point putting her through the operation. I've tried everything. We've grown so accustomed to seeing old people with cataracts, it's difficult to convince Bhutanese anything should be done for them. I've told him, 'If you're so worried about transporting her a few miles to my hospital, I'll send a horse and carry her myself.' But he keeps refusing. You see, my cousin is a justice on our high court, and he can be quite stubborn. I wonder if you'd be willing to interview him, and perhaps, together, we can convince him to let his mother see again."

Wangmo telephoned her cousin to tell him I was eager to interview him, and the following morning the judge and his mother met us at Thimphu Hospital. He was a formidable-looking middle-aged man wearing a checkered *gho* and a neat salt-and-pepper mustache. I asked him a few cursory questions about Bhutan's recent transformation from an absolute monarchy into a parliamentary democracy, and he answered with the brisk forthrightness that had characterized most of my conversations with the Bhutanese. Then I turned my attention to his mother, sitting cross-legged on a hospital bed and shivering under a blanket.

She was certainly old. She had white hair shaved as short as a Bhutanese nun's and a deeply lined face. I asked my questions slowly and phrased them simply, not sure how responsive she would be. I'd underestimated how much fiery spirit still animated the old woman. "What's my life like now?" she said. "What life! They're kind to me, but my mind is shriveling up. Even when I'm in a room full of my family I feel alone. How would you like to live like that?

"I'll tell you what," she said, aiming her face directly at her son, who sat in a chair by the foot of her bed. "If you're wondering how long I'll be here, you won't have to wait much longer. No one wants to stay alive just to live like this. I'll die sooner if I stay blind!"

The judge had doubtless heard many closing arguments in his day, but I imagined few had hit so close to home. He gave consent for his mother's surgery.

Dechen Wangmo performed the operation herself. The next day, I joined her in a private hospital room as she unwound the bandages from her aunt's eyes while the woman sat up in bed. After a few minutes, her aunt blinked and shook her head, as if to clear the fog of so many years of blindness. "Can you see me, Auntie?" Wangmo asked. "Can you make out my face?"

The old woman placed her hand tenderly along her niece's cheekbone. "Your face looks fine, but what have you done to your hair?" she said, scowling. "I don't like it. It looks like you've got fronds growing out of your head."

I left Bhutan reluctantly—partly because I'd had a glimpse into a rarefied mountain kingdom, a place that was unspoiled, unlike many of its neighbors, a country where an enlightened monarch's policies made his people's "gross national happiness" paramount, but also because I knew we were climbing back into the White Elephant for another twelve hours.

Near the end of our long trip, as we were driven up the winding road to Kalimpong that the Third Jamgon Kongtrul had traveled down his final day, Ruit seemed strangely unconcerned by the blind turns and sheer drop-offs. "Are you really as calm as you look?" I asked. "Isn't this the sort of place you'd usually get out and walk for a while?"

"It's true. I'm not as frightened as I once was. And I'll show you why," he said, drawing his left hand out of his pocket and holding it out for me to study. I expected to see an amulet, a precious stone, or some sort of lucky charm, but all he displayed was his open palm. "On my last trip to Thailand, when I was leading an outreach with local doctors we'd trained up, they introduced me to a palmist. Look at my hand."

I didn't notice anything out of the ordinary, other than the fact that it still struck me as too large and powerful for the delicate surgeries I'd seen it perform.

"No, look at this line," he said, tracing a deep fold that ran perfectly straight across the width of his palm. "The palmist said that in all his years, he'd never seen such a thing. And it makes sense, because really, I'm the luckiest person alive. I had very serious trauma on both arms as a boy, but that didn't prevent me from becoming a surgeon. When my right arm was in a bamboo splint, I become a lefty. I'm ambidextrous, actually. And that's been very helpful during surgery. My work is too good to do for money, yet I get paid. With all the trips my staffs have taken on roads like this, no one has ever been seriously injured. Myself, I should have died a dozen times on the road or in the bush, but here I am. And no matter the gradient, if I stay on the straight path, I always get to the top of the mountain."

We reached the four-thousand-foot-high hill station of Kalimpong safely, and as the reddened tip of Kangchenjunga broke free from a bank of dark storm clouds, Ruit sighed at the sight of his home mountain. "One day, I'd like to make it all the way back," he said, "instead of circling and circling my homeland. But I know too well how far it is, and there's never enough time."

We turned off a bumpy dirt road into the smoothly paved parking lot of the Jamgon Kongtrul the Third Memorial Home, and a man with a shock of gray hair and a shaggy goatee ran down a flight of stairs. Thinlay Ngodup placed *katas* around our necks and welcomed us to the experiment in social planning he oversaw. Children spilled down the stairs to greet us, and Ruit ruffled the hair of ones he recognized from previous trips. "How many at the moment, Thinlay?" Ruit asked.

"Thirty-nine children. And we had round about forty old folks until we lost two last week," he said. The children led us to rooms they'd vacated for our stay and helped unload luggage and medical gear from our three vehicles. Even though we were in India, most of the children were Nepalese—survivors of the civil war who'd lost their parents in the fighting or refugees from the war zone whose parents had sent them somewhere they'd have a chance, a place they could get both an education and three meals a day.

The children seemed delighted to temporarily share quarters with the home's elderly residents, treating our arrival like an excuse for an extended sleepover party. As we were shown to our rooms, we passed open doorways and I saw several girls sitting in the laps of elderly women in Tibetan-style garb, who were brushing their hair or helping them with homework.

At the base of the hill, below the residential compound, the Jamgon Kongtrul's trust had constructed a smaller version of the original Tilganga and had hired a young surgeon in residence to run its operating theater. Sona Yonjo lived in an apartment with a panoramic view of Kalimpong's sloping hills with her husband, Saumya Sanyal, an ophthalmologist who worked out of a private clinic in Siliguri, on the Indian plain. Business was booming at the Jamgon Kongtrul Eye Centre. They'd recently installed a laser surgery suite, and Thinlay was trying to convince Sanyal to stop commuting and work with his wife as a full-time employee.

We joined Thinlay's staff under a striped plastic tarp that had been erected to serve as our mess tent during the four days we'd be at the center for surgery. Patients were already sitting on benches in the courtyard, though work wasn't scheduled to begin until the following morning. "The patients look as elderly as your residents," Ruit noted happily.

"Proof of our success," Thinlay said, filling our cups with hot, milky tea, which we sipped gratefully as the sun sank into a fog bank and the temperature plummeted. "We opened the eye hospital in 2005. We broke even in 2007. The last two years we've made a small profit. People here used to call cataracts 'pearl tikkas' and believed they were an honorable mark of aging. But we've changed their minds about that. Now we've cleared out many of the most serious cases in the region and we're catching up the young ones before they go blind."

I asked Dr. Yonjo why she was working at the eye center.

"Dr. Ruit's been coming for many years," she said. "At first he used to do six or seven hundred patients at a single camp. But the Indian government banned surgery outside hospitals, so the Jamgon Kongtrul's trust built this place, so they could carry on, according to the law. I was born in Kalimpong, but I trained downside and began working as a nurse. Dr. Ruit had a strong effect on me. He looks like one of my own uncles." Her face, with its Mongolian features, broke into a broad smile. "He speaks Nepali with an accent like we do. Mountain people face a lot of discrimination in India. The minority groups of this area are very proud of him, because he demonstrated we can rise as high as we want. So, after meeting him, I applied to medical school, and here I am," she said as if she could scarcely believe her good fortune, "resident ophthalmic surgeon in my hometown. People can't believe they can get this level of care in this terrain. I couldn't be happier. And it's all due to Dr. Ruit."

The next morning, the older students began their hour-long walk to the school the center ran off-site, while twenty-two of the younger ones climbed into the battered gray Indian jeep that would drive them there. It coughed and sputtered before its engine eventually caught. "That's our school bus and our hearse," Thinlay said. "Don't worry. We scrub it clean after the cremations. The children don't find it disturbing. We're an old-age home, after all. We have lots of funerals here, and they become very familiar with the cycle of life. I think it makes them better students. It gives them perspective."

The morning after a long day and evening of surgery, one of the home's brightest young residents knocked on my door at 6:00 A.M. I opened it, blinking in the bright sunshine, and saw a poised eleven-year-old girl wearing a red-and-white-striped turtleneck, her long, dark hair pulled back into a neat ponytail. I took a cup of milk tea from the tray Tsering Dolpo held shyly before her. And as I sipped the tea, I asked Tsering about herself. Her last name told me where she came from, as well as the violence she'd likely seen and survived during the People's War. She avoided all mention of the past but spoke effusively about her plans for the future. "Nowadays I'm the top student in the eighth class," she said. "I'm going to be a surgeon, like Dr. Yonjo."

Talking to Tsering, I understood clearly that Ruit's campaign was not simply about helping Himalayan people see better but allowing them to envision brighter futures in a region that often presented only the bleakest of prospects. Ruit had set in motion a formidable domino effect, his achievement inspiring not only the Jamgon Kongtrul Eye Centre's surgeon but the young people who saw her as proof that they, too, could rise as high as their ambition would carry them.

Tsering led me to the room she shared with six other girls and proudly showed off her personal space, the top bunk of a bed against the far wall of the room. There were two posters taped to the wall over her heavy pink comforter. One displayed an illustrated English alphabet, with an apple, a bee, and a cat standing beside brightly colored letters. The other showed a series of cartoons, titled "The Importance of Courtesy"; one panel contained a smiling child, who looked not unlike Tsering, holding a door open for an elderly woman.

As we were walking back toward my room on the terrace, through the compound's gardens, where pumpkins grew on vines that climbed onto bungalow roofs and ripe star fruit hung from trees, Tsering shouted, "Look!" I followed her finger toward a line of freshly washed green surgical drapes clipped to a rope, drying in the sun, then above and beyond them, where the broad summit ridges of Kangchenjunga hung from a perfectly clear sky, like a line of snow-white sheets.

After breakfast, I traveled an hour up to Lava, where the young Jamgon Kongtrul lived in a monastery abutting the town. I'd seen enough surgery by then to fill several books, and I wanted, instead, to seek out one of the sources of Ruit's inspiration.

Since the day I'd met him, Ruit had been telling me stories about the foresight of the Third Jamgon Kongtrul, the handsome young monk who'd secretly taken the ambitious surgeon's measure in Kathmandu before his followers donated the money to build Tilganga's first surgical center. Ruit spoke of his departed friend often, in the hushed tones he reserved for those he most admired. He talked about the Jamgon Kongtrul's wisdom, his refusal to stand on ceremony or pursue a cloistered meditative life, rather than working to relieve the poverty that surrounded him.

Ruit had been fortunate that, after the Jamgon Kongtrul's death, powerful allies like the Fred Hollows Foundation and the HCP had stepped forward to provide funding when he needed it most. But I sensed that, at his core, Ruit worried that all Westerners would one day fail him. If his scientist's mind didn't allow him to believe, unquestioningly, in reincarnation, his Walung heart hoped that the Fourth Jamgon Kongtrul, now fourteen, really *was* his dependable old friend returned to a new vessel, a well-funded force for good he could rely on for the rest of his career.

"I'm not *really* what you would call a true believer," Ruit had confided to me during our long drive to Kalimpong in the White Elephant. "Over the years, my religion has become eye care more than Buddhism. But I'm not prepared to rule out the possibility that my dear Rinpoche has returned. For such a young boy, he certainly seems to have remarkable bearing, you see?"

The Kagyu Thekchen Ling Monastery straddles a hilltop at seven thousand feet, just above the village of Lava. Like Pullahari, the monastery had been built in a landscape of sublime mountain scenery. But unlike the Jamgon Kongtrul's other residence, which seemed to float above the coarse realities of earthly life in the Kathmandu Valley, this one stood hard against the grit of the adjoining settlement. Only an iron gate separated the monastery's lush gardens and glittering buildings, freshly painted plum, cinnamon, and gold, from the sagging tin-roofed shophouses and cinder-block residences topped with TV aerials that constituted the town of Lava.

A sign near the entrance reminded guests that they were treading on sacred ground and should behave accordingly. VISITORS ARE KINDLY REQUESTED TO REFRAIN FROM ALL ANTI-SOCIAL BEHAVIOUR, it read. PLEASE DO NOT SMOKE, SPIT, SHOUT OR PLAY MUSIC WHILE VISITING THE MONASTERY. I wondered what sort of diversions there would be in this place for a fourteen-year-old boy, no matter how spiritually advanced he was reputed to be.

An aged monk gave me a tour of a prayer hall, where, behind the altar, hundreds of gilded Buddha statues sat in small compartments behind glass. Then I was shown to a reception room in the Rinpoche's living quarters and directed to sit on a Tibetan carpet a few feet from the Fourth Jamgon Kongtrul. He sat calmly before me in the lotus position, on a cushioned platform a few feet above my head. "He's grown so tall and his feet are already size nine or ten!" Ruit had told me

proudly that morning, charting his Rinpoche's journey toward man-
hood.

His feet were indeed large, but the most prominent aspect of his
appearance was his ears. They were enormous, and brought to mind
classical depictions of the Buddha. I shuffled forward on my knees to
receive a blessing, and the Jamgon Kongtrul held a golden statue of the
Buddha to my head before sprinkling blessed water onto my hair from
a horsehair brush. As the droplets ran down my scalp, I felt torn, as I
imagine Ruit did, by the twinned perspectives from which I regarded
him: as a skeptical journalist and as a human hoping for a glimpse of
deeper meaning, something beneath the uninspiring surface of daily
life.

After I scooted back to a seated position a yard or so from the
Rinpoche's feet, I took out my notebook. I directed the first question
to the fourteen-year-old boy, rather than the reincarnation of a living
god. I'd heard he was a devotee of video games, so I said, "You can't
study all the time, Your Eminence. What do you do for fun?"

"Well, I was previously very fond of PlayStation," he said in flawless
English. "But I'm putting childish things aside now and assuming my
responsibilities."

I wondered how he dealt with the hopes thousands had invested in
him, and I asked him to describe a typical day. "I wake up at four-
thirty," he said, "to begin my prostrations." Then he accounted for his
entire schedule, in half-hour increments: He described his courses in
Buddhist philosophy and scripture, the time set aside each morning for
meditation, the hour each day he studied ancient Tibetan grammar,
and the time reserved for meeting with advisers about humanitarian
projects like a medical clinic in Lava and the Kalimpong eye hospital
his charitable trust funded, all before his nonnegotiable bedtime of
9:00 P.M.

I asked him which of his duties he enjoyed most, and he answered
without hesitation.

"Debate," he said. "Three times a day I'm obliged to argue the fine
points of Buddhist philosophy with my senior lamas. One of us stands
and questions the other, who remains seated, according to tradition.

Then we reverse roles. I relish those opportunities, and if I may be immodest, I can say that I'm not bad at debate. I'm practicing for a competition that will soon be held at Bodh Gaya, the site of the Buddha's awakening."

I thanked the Rinpoche for his time and wished him luck at the debate, though I doubted he'd need it. Ruit, I felt, had been right to put his faith in this boy, who was, at the very least, wise beyond his years and, at most, something much harder to describe with the black-and-white language of logic. Escorted down a series of steep staircases by two of the 110 monks in flowing red robes who called the monastery home, toward the harsh reality of life on the other side of the iron gate, I looked back up, past gardens of carefully tended flowers, toward the Jamgon Kongtrul's residence.

I saw him standing, framed by a gilded window on the topmost floor, studying me as I left. Even at that distance, I could make out the surprising scale of his ears. I thought about all the Buddhas behind glass in the prayer hall beneath him and considered whether he ever felt as isolated and compartmentalized. I tried to imagine what it would be like to be plucked from your family's home in a country across the mountains and planted, however comfortably, in this well-appointed hothouse of Buddhist faith. How lonely would the rest of his journey be, I wondered, as he traveled the road from fourteen to full adulthood?

Visiting with postsurgical patients before we left Kalimpong, I noticed the shrunken noses and gnarled fingers of many of the elderly, indicating that leprosy had still not been eradicated from the surrounding forests. Suru Mundu, who lived in the woods between Kalimpong and Sikkim, had been particularly ravaged by the disease. At seventy-two, his sun-blackened face seemed to fold in on itself, and his fingers were so warped that I imagined what agony his work must have been, before he went blind. "I worked at the river, when the tide was low, carrying big rocks up to the bank and breaking them into chips for roadwork," Mundu said. "A year and a half ago, my eyes shut all of a sudden. I didn't know I could have them cured here for free, or I would have come sooner. The last year has been very hard."

Mundu sat beside his wife. Both were so thin they appeared skeletal. Mundu hardly seemed affected by the fact that his cataracts had been removed and his vision returned. But when Thinlay told him that he and his wife were welcome to stay at the hospital for a few days and eat as much as they liked, his face split into a grin that displayed his remaining teeth, and the Mundus hugged each other in relief. "After a few days, when their bellies are full and they've had time to think," Thinlay said, "I'm going to ask if they'd like to come live here. As you know, we have a few new vacancies."

The final night of our long road trip together, after Ruit and Yonjo had done 134 surgeries in Kalimpong, and after three more days we'd spent across a river valley in the neighboring Indian state of Sikkim, during which Ruit and Dr. B. P. Dhakal had performed another 150, we gathered for dinner at the colonial-era bungalow where Ruit was staying, along with a group of his Chinese Australian donors.

While we ate, with Ruit prodding and teasing them to answer, Gilbert Leung, who'd been shooting video the entire trip for a presentation he was preparing for a fund-raiser in Hong Kong, and Rosana Pittiyapongpat, a Thai surgeon who'd been training in Ruit's technique at each of the places we'd stopped, admitted that they had agreed to marry. Ruit promised to organize a traditional Nepalese wedding for them when the medical caravan passed through Hetauda—they had first met at the hospital there—on the drive back to Kathmandu. They accepted his offer with obvious delight. Their engagement was further evidence of what I was coming to see as the most impressive aspect of Ruit's career: He'd not only pioneered and refined a surgical technique but had woven a strand of personal relationships, spanning the Himalaya and beyond, bringing people together in a shared quest to improve others' lives.

After the meal, politicians came to make speeches in front of the local press, and medical administrators presented each of us with enormous framed certificates commemorating our visit. Ruit kept his remarks customarily brief, praising the efforts of his team and the strides the local staff had made since he'd first come to Sikkim. Dr. Dhakal, the ophthalmic consultant for the Sikkim State Health Service, didn't hold back his praise. During the fifteen years since Ruit had started operating in his isolated corner of the Himalaya, Dhakal had come to see his friend Sanduk as something more than a mentor. He seemed to view Ruit—as the Dalai Lama did—more like a medical Buddha. Dhakal spoke emotionally and at length about the isolation and poverty Sikkim had once faced and how dramatically Ruit's frequent visits had upgraded not only his own surgical skills but the local population's quality of life. "My excellent friend Dr. Sanduk Ruit," he concluded, "is a true *illuminary.*"

Technically, the word may not have existed in English. But I could think of no better way to describe what the boy from Olangchungola had become.

CHAPTER 25

This Is Rwanda

People can be made bad, and they can be taught to be good.
—President Paul Kagame

John Nkurikiye met us at the airport, wearing the green camouflage combat fatigues of the Rwandan Defence Force. I hadn't realized that he was still a soldier, but we hadn't talked about much beyond his medical aspirations when I'd met him at the Moran. In Utah, he'd seemed bright, witty, and a bit meek for a surgeon. He'd been out of his element, I realized, watching Major Nkurikiye stride across Kigali International in his combat boots, his bright eyes fastened on the Styrofoam box plastered with stickers that Geoff Tabin carried casually under his arm.

"How many were you able to bring?" he asked.

"Eighteen fresh and two preserved."

"Eighteen fresh!" Nkurikiye said. "Good, good. We have a lot of customers who'd like to see."

On our drive into the capital we passed several billboards that featured a photo of Nkurikiye, in a white lab coat and a green military beret, squinting to examine a young woman through a slit lamp. The billboards commemorated Army Week, a period of public service during which Rwanda's armed forces put aside their defense duties and worked on humanitarian projects across the country. Alongside Nkurikiye's image, the billboards showed soldiers digging trenches for clean-water projects and distributing sacks of high-yield seeds to farmers from the rear hatch of a military transport helicopter.

Looking out the windows, as we entered the city with Nkurikiye at the wheel of his worn SUV, I was struck by the recently built glass-and-steel structures topping the many hills that made up central Kigali, and the late-model vehicles gliding through a series of traffic circles planted with flowering shrubs. Kigali had a coffee shop in a mall modeled after Starbucks that offered complimentary Wi-Fi. Fifteen years after enduring the worst rampage of mass murder in modern history, Kigali didn't look like the survivor of anything; it seemed like a model of affluence and intelligent development. But scars were still visible, if you knew where to look.

Nkurikiye pointed to the bullet holes that pocked the façades of the national parliament building and the Mille Collines hotel, the infamous setting of the film *Hotel Rwanda*, as he drove us toward our lodgings, a newly built boutique hotel that featured an expansive view of Kigali's hills from its terrace café and a pool with a swim-up bar.

While we were waiting to check in, I browsed a rack of pamphlets. Next to brochures touting trips to visit Rwanda's endangered mountain gorillas I saw a pamphlet advertising the city's top tourist attraction, the Kigali Genocide Memorial Centre. It noted that the complex featured "artfully arranged exhibits explaining Rwanda's recent history, mass graves containing the remains of more than two hundred and fifty thousand victims, and a fully equipped gift shop." After I put it back, I noticed deep scars in the scalp, forehead, and neck of the maid who was polishing the marble floors of the reception area.

Tabin was clearly growing as a leader in his own right, capable of assembling teams of technicians and supporters in Africa, similar to the way Ruit organized them across the eastern Himalaya. Following the path Alan Crandall had paved, the HCP was building an eye hospital and ophthalmic training center in Ghana, and with the HCP's help, Dr. Meshesha was turning Quiha Zonal Hospital into one of Africa's best eye-care facilities. Tabin had even greater hopes for Major Nkurikiye. I recalled the phrase he'd used the first morning we'd sped down I-80 in his truck, when I'd eavesdropped on his daily call with Ruit: "I think John could be the person to really anchor eye care in Africa,"

he'd said. And I remembered the moment over weak coffee in the Moran's café when Nkurikiye had told me he hoped, one day, to be the "Ruit of Rwanda." For Tabin, more was riding on this trip to Rwanda than simply repairing patients' eyes. As Ruit had done to him, he planned to put Nkurikiye to the test.

Tabin seemed elated that the logistics he'd organized hadn't hit any road bumps and that we'd all arrived with our gear intact. At the hotel's reception desk, holding the box of corneas, he tapped his feet with anticipation. Ace Kvale and his friend Michael Brown, the filmmaker who'd shot *Light of the Himalaya*, had brought still and movie cameras along to document Tabin's work for future HCP fund-raisers. Bal Sunder Chansi, the logistical specialist who'd directed our effort in Quiha hospital, and a scrub nurse named Soba Sharma had come from Tilganga to manage a cataract camp we planned to conduct in the countryside. And Tabin had invited Laura Cohen and Chaz Langelier, two American medical students who would help Chansi screen five thousand potential patients in the U.N. Millennium Village of Mayange and the surrounding communities.

They were joined by Tabin's twenty-four-year-old daughter, Emilia, who had just been accepted by Stanford's medical school. She was here to watch her father work and get experience in the field before classes started in the fall.

Check-in took nearly an hour, since we arrived at the same time as another large group of Americans. Andrew Palau, the fresh young face of the Oregon-based Palau ministry, which his father had founded, and his wife, Wendy, had come to Kigali with an armada of doctors, nurses, sound and light technicians, and a pack of teenage skateboarders with bright pink and platinum-blond faux-'hawk hairdos. They had arranged to hold a combination skateboarding exhibition, free health clinic, and evangelical prayer meeting in the national soccer stadium.

Missionaries, medical groups, agricultural experts, and, now, even skateboarders for Jesus. A varied influx of individuals aiming to make the world a better place, in the ways they considered most effective, had invaded Rwanda since the genocide. I believed it was an invasion motivated by the guilt of a world that had failed to step in when Rwandans had needed them most, to put a stop to the slaughter. Despite their initial unwillingness to become involved, it was hard to fault the fact that many of the international community's charities had since opened offices in Kigali, investors had arrived en masse, and the city that was inarguably the most dangerous place in the world in 1994 had, by the time we arrived, become one of the safest and most orderly in all of Africa.

Dr. Paul Farmer, the international public health advocate most famous for his work in Haiti, and the subject of Tracy Kidder's powerful book *Mountains Beyond Mountains*, had opened a branch of his Partners in Health NGO in Kigali. It was Farmer who'd introduced Nkurikiye to Tabin, calling him, according to Tabin, "one of the most dedicated doctors I know of in Africa." And it was on our first day at Kigali's King Faisal Hospital, where Nkurikiye directs the Department of Ophthalmology, that I saw that dedication in action.

In his operating room, even though he was wearing scrubs rather than fatigues, there was still something military about Dr. Nkurikiye's bearing. He ordered his staff into their positions in a low voice, and they leapt to their places, eager to please him. I tried to recall who his manner reminded me of, and when he tied his mask on and bent over his first case, I realized it was Ruit.

Tabin operated at another table. He was only ten feet away, but with the nurses, technicians, photographers, and filmmakers, plus a local television crew who'd come to report on the surgery, the room was too crowded for the doctors to talk to each other while they worked. "This is really a mixed blessing," Tabin said. "I put in a request for all available corneas just before I left. I expected to get four or five. But eighteen! I've never had so many at once, and we can't waste them. I'd planned to sit with John while he did the cases, but now there's no time."

When I first met him in Utah, Nkurikiye had already watched Tabin perform corneal transplants for three months at the Moran, but American medical practices forbade him from operating. At Tilganga, he'd done a handful of his own surgeries but had mostly watched Reeta work. Now he had a young woman on his table who'd traveled to South Africa for a corneal transplant that had since failed. He had a chance to better the work of the most accomplished surgeons on the African continent, and he was delighted to perform such an advanced procedure in his own operating room.

At first, watching the two doctors, you'd think Tabin was the novice. But that was due to the crisis developing on his table. A sixteen-year-old girl named Claudine Cyuzuzo had been prepped for surgery with an injection of anesthesia, and Tabin had begun to operate. After he had cut away half of the corneal tissue he needed to remove, Cyuzuzo began writhing and wailing with pain. "I need help!" Tabin shouted. "I need everyone in the room focusing on this case only! Can we convert to general? Can we get her a better local block? Her eye is open and she could lose her lens. We need to do something! Right . . . this . . . second."

Emilia was frozen by her father's side, her blue eyes wide as the situation threatened to spiral out of control. A Rwandan anesthesiologist rushed across the room with a needle and plunged it into the side of the girl's eye socket. Within minutes, her thrashing calmed, her wailing quieted, and Tabin went back to work.

"Well, that was quite exciting for a few seconds," Tabin said, "but now we're out of danger." He removed the rest of the opaque center of the cornea and asked his daughter to bring him one of the donated tissues. Emilia brought her father a cylindrical plastic container and struggled to unscrew the top. The cornea, about the size of a contact lens but with ragged edges, floated in pink preservative. After Tabin removed it delicately with a forceps, I looked at the container's label. It said that the donor was a fifty-two-year-old female from Birmingham, Alabama, who had died three days earlier of lung cancer.

For me, no mission of the space shuttle or probe beaming back photos from the cold edge of the solar system could overshadow this incredible, and incredibly rapid, transfer of resources—the journey this flap of tissue had made from the American South to east-central Africa. Because of recent advances in medicine and the generosity of an anonymous American woman facing her own premature mortality, a blind sixteen-year-old girl in Kigali would have a chance to compile a lifetime of visual memories.

Tabin called me over to examine the graft as he tied his last suture. I looked through the eyepiece and saw the neat circle of black stitches, magnified so it looked like a helicopter landing pad. "It looks clean and tight," I said. "Not that I'd really know."

"It's perfect," Tabin said. "I really, really like my wound edges. This young lady's going to see just fantastic!"

Nkurikiye had successfully finished his first case and started on a second when his voice rose with uncharacteristic concern. "Geoff! Could you come take a look at this?"

Tabin threaded his way across the crowded room, holding his gloved hands aloft, careful to keep them sterile.

"I think I might have stitched this one on upside down," Nkurikiye explained.

"That's easy to do," Tabin said. "What happened?"

"I may have turned the tissue over after I removed it from the solution. I don't think so, but I can't be certain."

"You always have to keep the orientation," Tabin said. "Once you've turned it over, it's hard to tell which side is up." While Tabin looked through the lens of the microscope, I studied the patient's chart. She was thirty-six, her name was Yvonne Uwamungu, and her intake form listed her as an elementary school teacher.

"You can tell which side is up by looking for faint Descemet folds beneath the surface," Tabin said. "I'm pretty sure you've placed the cornea correctly. Nice suturing, by the way."

"Yes, I also believe I saw folds. That is why I had the confidence to continue."

"Well, we'll know for sure when we look at her tomorrow. Her eye will either be much clearer or much cloudier."

"Yes," Nkurikiye said. "That is my hope and my fear."

For one hundred days in 1994, John Nkurikiye, a junior medical officer with the Rwandan Patriotic Front, experienced more hope and fear than any human could be expected to endure. Though that year's genocide made headlines around the world, the Rwandans' colonial masters had left them with a legacy of inequity that had led to regular outbursts of violence little known outside Rwanda for much of the twentieth century. Belgium, employing a brutal divide-and-conquer strategy that would make the most oppressive British colonial officer blush, had drawn an artificial line through Rwandan society to create an aristocratic class, indebted to their colonial overlords, and a peasant class that the elite were ordered to control.

"Do you know how they did it?" Nkurikiye asked me, over dinner at an open-air Chinese restaurant clinging to the side of one of Kigali's hills. "Look at those lights below us. Can you tell which belong to the homes of Hutu or Tutsi? That's what it was like before the Belgians. We lived together peacefully, intermarried, and even we had trouble telling each other apart. But the Belgians made it simple. In 1933 they passed a law declaring that every Rwandan who owned ten cows or more was a Tutsi and the rest were Hutus. They issued identity cards to make it official, gave Tutsis greater rights and privileges, and planted the seeds of the slaughters to come. So you see why I hesitated to answer in Utah when you asked me what I was. By Belgian classification, I'm a Tutsi. But in actuality, I'm a Rwandan. Full stop."

In 1959, as Belgium prepared to grant Rwanda independence, it switched allegiances, elevating Hutu politicians to positions of authority and turning the prevailing power structure on its head. Hutu militias, in a campaign they called the "wind of destruction," began systematically massacring Tutsis. More than twenty thousand were killed, and hundreds of thousands fled to neighboring countries. Nkurikiye's family settled in a refugee camp in neighboring Burundi. "We were really second-class citizens in Burundi," he remembers. "We hadn't access to land ownership or professional careers. Primary education was provided. But we had to jump over a high post if we wanted a secondary education."

I remembered something a Burundian engineer I'd sat next to on the flight from Brussels had said about the Rwandan refugees in his country. "When I was growing up," he said, "Rwandans were not even second-class citizens. They were poor people you would see digging ditches and doing odd jobs. My friends and I would mock each other's clothes, if they were inferior, by saying, 'Look at you! You're dressed like a Rwandan!'"

Nkurikiye, like Ruit, forged an unlikely path to higher education through sheer brainpower. As a standout student in the Muramba refugee camp, he was one of a handful of children allowed to continue their formal education. Through secondary school and university in Burundi, he topped every standardized test he was allowed to take and won a scholarship to medical school. In 1990, the Rwandan Patriotic Front, the Tutsi-led government in exile, launched a guerrilla war against the Hutu-dominated Kigali government from bases across the border in Uganda, and Dr. Nkurikiye volunteered to move north and join them.

In April 1994, his unit was camped just north of the border, on high alert because the leader of the rebel army, Paul Kagame, didn't trust a power-sharing agreement the U.N. had just helped broker. French troops reinforced the Hutu-led military and had repeatedly helped them repel what they considered an invasion of a francophone nation by an anglophone power, never mind that the invaders were largely French-speaking Rwandan refugees.

At 8:20 P.M. on April 6, 1994, as the presidential jet, a light Dassault Falcon carrying Rwanda's head of state, Juvénal Habyarimana, who supported the peace agreement, began its final approach to Kigali International, a surface-to-air missile struck its left wing, followed by another that streaked up out of the darkness and shattered its tail. The plane crashed into the garden of the presidential palace and burst into a fireball. Who fired the missiles has remained a matter of debate. But whoever murdered Rwanda's president also killed any hopes he'd had for peace.

"We'd been hearing rumors for months that Hutu militias were stockpiling weapons and preparing to attack Tutsis across Rwanda," Nkurikiye remembers. In Rwanda, where Tutsis are generally thought of as taller than Hutus, terror spread throughout the Tutsi population when Radio Télévision Libre des Mille Collines, a station run by the extremist Hutu Power movement, began broadcasting ominous orders that all patriotic Rwandans should prepare to "cut the tall trees." Invoices collected after the genocide document that Hutu businessmen had imported 581,000 machetes into Rwanda during a two-year period before the massacre.

"The killings started as soon as the plane crashed," Nkurikiye says.

"Almost immediately, we began receiving phone calls from Tutsis and Hutu moderates saying, 'We are being killed,'" recalls the man who served as Nkurikiye's senior officer, Charles Kayonga, currently commander of Rwanda's Defence Force. "Sometimes even, we would be on the phone, hear them being killed, and the line would go dead."

Nkurikiye's battalion was one of the first Rwandan Patriotic Front forces ordered to fight its way to Kigali, to support the six hundred RPF soldiers, VIPs, and prospective government ministers who had traveled to Kigali for the peace talks and were trapped in the parliament building. If the battalion reached the capital, it would be tasked with protecting them, then trying to put an end to the killing. "We marched for five days," Nkurikiye remembers, "mostly at night to elude Hutu forces. And on the fifth day we came under heavy fire, fighting through the streets of Kigali, where we saw some terrible things. And those of us that survived established a perimeter around the parliament building and my hospital."

Nkurikiye told his story over several days. In short bursts. Like single magazines emptied all at once from an automatic weapon. His voice was emotionless as I asked him to reload and recount events he'd spent fifteen years trying to forget.

"As more of our RPF troops arrived, our mission was to go out each night and fight from one island of security to another, trying to join them together. We were able to secure a perimeter that included the hospital, the soccer stadium, and the parliament and then link them with a corridor to the north, so we could hand off people and supplies," Nkurikiye says.

Radio announcers urged the mobs armed with machetes on, advising them to strike their victims "at the level of the ear," to inflict maximum carnage. They broadcast the locations of churches, medical clinics, schools, and government buildings—supposedly safe havens— where the people they called *inyenzi*, or "cockroaches," were hiding.

"While the international community abandoned us, and talked and talked for months about whether the genocide was an internal matter, just a natural outgrowth of ancient tribal feuds, and the French led the argument against military intervention, we listened to the radio all day long and our soldiers fought through ambushes and roadblocks and raced the militia to these locations. We pulled two hundred and fifty people out of St. Paul's Church, whose priest had abandoned his congregation and told the murderers where they were. We sent squads out every day and brought the distressed and the wounded we found back through our perimeter." Eventually, Nkurikiye says, more than eight thousand Tutsis and moderate Hutus found sanctuary on the hospital's grounds.

There was no room for them in the wards.

Nkurikiye oversaw the triage and treatment of the wounded. "The first injuries I encountered were something you can't believe," Nkurikiye says. "A young woman with a spear still thrust through her abdomen. People who had been clubbed by *masu*, sticks studded with nails. Children whose arms and legs had been hacked off with—" He stopped himself. "You know, you can only be surprised for so long. Every day for three months I saw and tried to treat every kind of injury a gun, a blade, or a blunt object can inflict on a human body. But I don't want to talk any more about that. I'd rather discuss how we can heal my country."

Nkurikiye and the RPF forces managed to hold their positions and save the lives of more than one hundred thousand people, who waited out the hundred days within their perimeter, until Kigali fell to RPF forces on July 4 and the bulk of the *génocidaires'* fighting force was driven west, to refugee camps across the country's borders.

There is no questioning the bravery of Paul Rusesabagina, who sheltered more than twelve hundred potential genocide victims at the hotel he managed and became the hero of a Hollywood film. But listening to Nkurikiye's story, I wondered why the bravery of John Nkurikiye, Charles Kayonga, and their brothers in the RPF, many of whom died during the process of saving one hundred thousand lives, is scarcely known outside Rwanda. Perhaps the country inspires selective blindness. It certainly does among too many of its current citizens, who have no choice but to live alongside the men and women who murdered their families.

When we returned to King Faisal Hospital the second morning, I saw through new eyes the building that had saved so many. It had been renamed after the leader of Nkurikiye's rebel force, Paul Kagame, had become president and had appealed for help in rebuilding his nation. In 1995 the Saudi government had paid to renovate the three-story concrete facility, which had been hit by bullets, rocket-propelled grenades, and a tsunami of human suffering.

Dr. Nkurikiye had no time to talk about history. He was making it. While the hospital had been undergoing renovation, he, too, had received an upgrade, completing an ophthalmic residency in South Africa. Now he had to inspect postoperative patients who'd received the first corneal transplants he'd ever attempted in Rwanda, and for the first time since we'd arrived, he was visibly nervous.

Tabin joined him at the slit lamp as they studied twenty-seven-year-old Theresa Murakatete, the first woman Nkurikiye had operated on the previous day. "Centration is excellent. Wound edges excellent. This looks perfect," Tabin said as they moved on to Nkurikiye's second patient. Nkurikiye couldn't bring himself to look as Tabin bent to examine Yvonne Uwamungu, the woman whose cornea, he feared, he'd stitched on inside out.

"John," Tabin said, "you'll be happy to know that this woman's eye looks much clearer today. Congratulations, my friend. This is an excellent transplant!"

The director of the hospital's Department of Ophthalmology grinned with relief. "I'm not unhappy," he said.

With the remaining corneas quickly losing their viability, Tabin and Nkurikiye worked straight through until evening. "You know," Tabin said to me as he settled back on his own surgical stool, "the cornea really is a remarkable tissue. There's nothing else like it in the body. The really fascinating thing is its composition. It's made up of five thin layers, and they're very difficult to work with. If I can dissect one or two layers and graft on a new cornea, there's almost no way the body will reject it. But if I remove all five layers, then the odds of rejection skyrocket. With this woman on my table, whose chart says she's rejected a cornea before, I'm going to try to do a very, very fine dissection."

Tabin was soon walled off within his own world. Nkurikiye came over between patients to watch.

"How's the dissection coming?" I asked after an uncharacteristic fifteen minutes of silence from Tabin.

"Very, very well!" both surgeons answered, in stereo.

By 8:00 P.M., only one patient remained, and I asked Nkurikiye how he'd chosen from a long list of people waiting for the limited supply of tissue. "Those who are struggling or have stopped work or study are the first priority," he said. "My last patient was crying in the ward for three hours because she was at the end of the line and I'd told her the chance was only fifty-fifty. If I had damaged one of the corneas, she would have been heartbroken. But fortunately I didn't do so badly today, and I was able to complete her transplant."

They had exhausted the supply of fresh corneas, and Tabin decided to attempt a final transplant with the two corneas preserved in glycerin. For safety's sake he needed both—one for the first attempt at surgery, the other as a backup in case of complications.

"These may be a neat solution for remote areas, because they last for months, but it's much harder to work with them," Tabin told me. "Imagine the difference between sewing through a piece of cloth and a plastic Frisbee and you have an idea of what it's like to suture a preserved cornea. If I pull this off, I'm going to write about it and follow up on the results. I bet it would be one of the first successful glycerin transplants in Africa."

The patient's name was Francis Kiiza, and I was glad he couldn't hear Tabin discuss his surgery's degree of difficulty; he was in another room, receiving his injections. Kiiza was thirty-four, with a wife and three children. He'd been waiting years for a donated cornea, he told me while Tabin paused to allow his anesthesia to take effect. "I am a teacher of maths," he said, "at one of Rwanda's best schools, Sonrise High, which is supported by the Anglican churches of Little Rock, in Arkansas. Maybe you have visited them?"

I told him I hadn't.

"Ah," he said. "A pity. Such righteous people. Well, as you can imagine, I have to make a lot of marks each day in my profession. So many papers to correct. And I have to write extensively on the chalkboard. In recent years, I've had to stand so close to the board that my nose was essentially touching it. In addition, I could no longer see my students well enough to supervise them, so I've had to quit working, temporarily, while my wife attempts to support us."

I asked how he had known to come to Nkurikiye's hospital.

"At first I was sure the Lord would lead me to a solution," Kiiza said. "My wife helped me research corneal transplants on the Internet, and I was referred to hospitals in India who said they could manage the job. But that would have cost three thousand American dollars, which I was in no position, as a teacher, to pay. So I fasted and I prayed. Finally I simply gave up and surrendered. But then a friend of mine, who is a doctor of bones at this hospital, told me, 'I have good news for you. American doctors are coming with corneas. Do what you can, Francis, to avail yourselves of their services!' "

When Tabin examined his work through a slit lamp two days later, he pronounced Kiiza's surgery an unqualified success. We were due to leave the next morning to hold a surgical camp in the countryside, near the U.N. Millennium Village of Mayange, and I asked Tabin if Kiiza was in condition to travel, since I wanted to hire him as my interpreter. Tabin said his graft was secure, so I availed myself of Francis's memorable facility with English. He sat beside me during our drive. He was large, solidly built, and wore a matching two-piece tan safari suit. Our convoy traveled south through the countryside, through a rolling ocher-and-green landscape of family vegetable plots and small stone farmhouses built atop rounded hills that reminded me of Tuscany, if I didn't look too closely. "It's beautiful here," I said.

"I'll have to rely on your judgment," Francis said. "I can see that we are crossing what appears to be a river, and I'm able to see some flashes of vegetation, but nothing more."

"Dr. Tabin told me it will be two or three weeks until your new cornea is working well."

Kiiza held up the business card Tabin had given him, pressed it close to the wraparound sunglasses we'd bought him to protect his eyes, and scanned the small print with some difficulty.

"Doc . . . tor . . . Geoff . . . rey . . . Ta . . . bin," he sounded out, tasting Tabin's name for implications. "Tell me, what was this doctor paid to perform my surgery?"

"Nothing. He volunteers his time to work in Africa and Asia."

"Mmmm," Kiiza said, a low growl that I came to recognize as an expression of his deepest sense of approval. "In the hands of such a man, my hopes increase accordingly."

We coasted downhill, past of grove of glossy banana trees, then through a coffee plantation, the dense bushes planted in hard-to-discern rows that played tricks with my eyes, appearing first random and then regularly spaced. In a ditch along the roadside, a crew of workers in pink shorts and shirts were picking up scraps of trash in a landscape so peacefully bucolic it was hard to believe that anything horrible had happened here only a few years earlier.

Nkurikiye leaned back toward me from the front seat. "Here," he said, as we crossed another bridge over a lazy brown river. "You asked me if I'd ever been wounded. Only once, and it wasn't much. But it happened right here. We were chasing the *génocidaires* across this bridge, and they fired their light French artillery, trying to slow us with one-hundred-and-twenty-millimeter shells. I took shrapnel in both legs, had to leave my unit and get treatment in Kigali for two weeks."

The Nyamata District Hospital was a modest collection of low brick buildings, with covered walkways connecting them to shelter patients from the sun. The facility had been built, in part, by USAID, and the center of healing stood in contrast to a former Catholic church nearby, where twenty-five hundred of the parishioners who'd come seeking safety had been slaughtered. The church had been left in its ravaged condition and converted into a memorial, like so many of Rwanda's houses of worship.

The hospital was at the center of a group of small villages largely populated by genocide survivors and returning refugees. Several hundred patients were waiting for us as we unpacked, and, as in Ethiopia, I was struck by how many of them were children. Chansi had arrived early to organize the operating room and patient flow, and everything was in perfect readiness for the doctors to begin surgery. Tabin wanted to calibrate the keratometers, instruments that measure the curvature of a patient's eyes and calculate what power lenses the patient will need. He asked Nkurikiye to sit in front of one of the devices, so he could drip a mild numbing agent onto his eye and test the machines by measuring him. Tabin picked up the wrong bottle and squeezed a drop of dilating solution in Nkurikiye's right eye. "Oh, shit!" he shouted, realizing his mistake.

Within moments, Nkurikiye's right pupil was comically enlarged, and he could only see out of his left. "It figures," Nkurikiye said, taking the potential crisis in stride. "I often have to give four or five drops to my patients. But with a single drop I'm perfectly dilated."

"How long does it last?" I asked.

"About five hours," he said. "But I don't have that long with so many waiting. I've done over four thousand cataract surgeries with two eyes. Now we'll see what I can do with one."

We were standing on a shaded terrace where the patients had lined up on benches. The old clutched their canes, teenagers squinted at me with what degree of vision I couldn't tell, and mothers in flowered cotton-print head wraps held babies with ghostly white cataracts, tied to their backs with colorful cloth slings. I felt a ripple of tension pass through the crowd, and several people began speaking in low voices. A group of nine men and women wearing bright pink shirts and shorts, trailed by a guard with an M16, arrived and looked for a place to sit. It was a hot day, and there was plenty of room on the shaded benches, but they moved to the middle of a lawn between buildings and took seats on the grass, fully exposed to the sun.

"Do you know who they are?" Nkurikiye asked me. "Those people are convicted genocide killers. They've been brought here from prison. So we can cure them." Nkurikiye spoke in the flat, emotionless voice he'd used when recounting the events of his one hundred days, and if he thought it was improper for them to be treated along with the rest of his patients, he gave no indication.

Looking at the prisoners, watching them avoid making eye contact with the rest of the patients, I asked the question I'd been reluctant to put to Nkurikiye since I'd met him: "Did you lose any family members during the genocide?"

"At least eighteen," he said, "perhaps more," and walked inside to scrub in.

It's difficult to say, with precision, how many Rwandans perished in the genocide. Many of the dead have never been accounted for. A practice common among Hutu militias was to simply throw young children down wells, rather than waste ammunition or the energy it took to swing a machete. Mass graves are still being unearthed. Gang rapes of Tutsi women were organized so that they were purposefully violated by HIV-positive men, their victims gradually adding to the total death count, year after year. Most chroniclers of the carnage, like Human Rights Watch, the U.N., and the Rwandan government, put the number between eight hundred thousand and a million, or approximately one-tenth of the entire population.

No organized effort at extermination had ever killed so many people in such a short period of time—not the Nazis, not the Khmer Rouge. Paul Kagame's government struggled to find a mechanism capable of producing reconciliation, of delivering justice to the victims and punishment to the perpetrators. With so many Rwandans implicated in the murders, no standard legal system could suffice. Kagame championed the creation of the *gacaca*, a type of village court modeled on the traditional Rwandan tribunal that settled disputes over land or livestock. Every village in Rwanda held *gacaca* proceedings, where survivors identified the murderers among them and killers were encouraged to confess their crimes. Ordinary killers who confessed to being swept up in mob violence were often released without punishment or received short jail terms. Those identified as leaders of the militias or as particularly enthusiastic and prolific murderers were sentenced to longer terms in prison and ordered to wear pink clothing to emphasize their shame.

Philip Gourevitch, whose *We Wish to Inform You That Tomorrow We Will Be Killed with Our Families* paints a devastating portrait of a country coming to terms with its temporary insanity, interviewed Kagame about the *gacaca* for a piece in *The New Yorker* more than a decade after the massacre. "Not the victims, not the perpetrators, nobody will tell you he is happy with the *gacaca*," Kagame told Gourevitch. That's how, the president said, he knew the system was fair. "*Gacaca*," Kagame said, "gives us something to build on."

With Kiiza translating, I spoke with the patients waiting for surgery. He put them at ease, telling them he'd been blind himself a few days earlier and had been cured by the doctors on the other side of the swinging doors they would soon pass through. Sezikeye Athanase said proudly that he was eighty-four and still strong enough to have walked to Nyamata from his home, three hours away. He'd dressed up for his surgery in a baggy suit jacket and a broad-brimmed hat that would have shaded his eyes from the sun, if that had been necessary. Like many of the patients I spoke with, I noticed that he divided his life into the time "before" and the time "after," without ever saying the word "genocide."

"Before, I also had some problems with my eyes, but doctors were able to repair them, and I could see reasonably well," he told me. During the first chaotic days of the genocide, he and his wife had been separated from their children. They lost four—three boys and a girl. "I don't know what happened to them," he said. "I only heard they'd been taken away to Congo, where they were killed. After, when I found out, my eyes stopped working almost immediately, as if they didn't want to see anymore."

Athanase had a remarkably sunny disposition for a man who'd survived so much, and I asked him why. "My wife convinced me we can't spend the rest of our lives blindly suffering," he said. "That's why I'm here. I'm ready to see again."

So was Eminante Uzamukunda.

"Come, you must talk to this girl," Kiiza said, hurrying me along. "She's very intelligent." I picked up her chart. It listed her age as eighteen and her profession as "student, interrupted." She had close-cropped hair, a wide face with sculpted cheekbones, and wore a torn T-shirt and a sun-faded wrapper. She slumped so low in her seat that, at first, I presumed she was unusually short. Next to her sat a ravaged woman who could only be her mother; she offered a preview of what Eminante would look like after twenty more years of poverty.

"The girl is able to be of no help at home," her mother said. "She can't cook or care for the other children. She just sits inside all day."

I asked Eminante how long she'd been sitting at home, and she said, in a voice so soft Kiiza had to ask her to speak up, "Some years. Since I left school. My eyes were decreasing in capacity for a long time. But when I became blind my mother said school is too expensive for someone who can't see, so I went home."

I had expected to hear that she'd lost her sight recently. But she had been sitting in her home, without stimulation, while her siblings continued attending classes, for several years. I asked what she missed most about school.

"Drawing," she said. "And reading. I miss reading so much. Sometimes my sister reads to me, but we're very poor. Everyone is obliged to work at our house, and there isn't much time for books." I asked the cost of a year's tuition. "Oh, a lot," Eminante said, naming a number of Rwandan francs that equaled eight dollars.

We all worked until after dark for the next four days, drove away in our convoy, and ate dinner together in open-air restaurants atop Kigali's hills. Nkurikiye wore a bright yellow dashiki to one meal and a handsome dark brown version to another, explaining that members of Rwanda's military were forbidden from appearing in uniform at any place that served alcohol, to avoid any implication of corruption. We had Indian food one evening, Italian the next, and we returned to the Chinese restaurant, Nkurikiye's favorite, the following night. The cost of any one of those meals could have sent Eminante and all of her siblings to school for at least a year.

I dealt with my discomfort about what Fred Hollows would have called "the disequity" by trying to be helpful in the operating room, by performing the small tasks Chansi had taught me. One day while I was walking a patient into surgery, I saw two large, muscular men in U.S. Army camouflage standing in the hallway, jotting down notes. The American military had begun to take an interest in Tabin's work, hoping he could help its forces do a better job of organizing their humanitarian medical outreach, and these two officers had been sent from a base in Djibouti to observe Tabin's methodology. I found them scrubs and surgical masks and led them into the operating room so they could look more closely. They were clearly moved by what they saw inside. The soldiers left with their notebooks filled and numerous compliments about the efficient assembly-line surgery they'd witnessed.

After a shaky start at King Faisal, Tabin's daughter Emilia threw herself wholeheartedly into making sure the OR ran smoothly. She worked closely with her father, leading patients to and from his table and double- and triple-checking their charts to make sure Tabin had lenses of the correct power to implant. Emilia had been a champion Nordic skier and a standout student of the liberal arts at the University of Vermont, but a visit to Nepal—and the opportunity to watch Ruit at work—had changed the course of her life, as it had changed her father's. "You know," she told me, "I never had any interest in medicine until I saw cataract patients in Nepal after surgery. If I have a chance to do something like that, I think it will be a pretty satisfying life."

As he operated on each of his patients, John Nkurikiye certainly seemed satisfied. He worked with confidence and unusual grace. The signs at Nyamata hospital were in French, and the door to the recovery room read, RÉANIMATION. I preferred to read it as English, because the hunched and withdrawn patients we brought there came back to lives full of possibility. I had just placed Eminante on a hospital bed, making sure her head was comfortably propped up on a pillow, when Kiiza burst into the reanimation room. "Quickly," he said. "Dr. John is asking to see you!"

I jogged to Nkurikiye's table. He was concentrating and not yet able to talk. I glanced over at Tabin, whose patient had deep slash marks on her legs. Half of her left foot had been cut cleanly off, on a diagonal. I looked away and watched Nkurikiye work until he was ready for me. He preferred a variation on Ruit's technique, inserting a fine steel probe shaped like a tiny spoon and drawing out the cataract by cupping this tool under the diseased lens.

After he'd delivered it, he took extra care to clear up every single scrap of cortex, the filmy residue left after a cataract is removed, which I'd seen some developing-world doctors ignore; I couldn't find a speck left when Nkurikiye slid one of Tilganga's high-quality artificial lenses into his patient's eye.

When he was done, Nkurikiye drew aside the corner of the green surgical drape so I could see what lay beneath. His muscular patient was clothed in a pink prison uniform. "This is one of the people we were discussing," he said, and for the first time since we'd talked about the genocide, Dr. Nkurikiye's voice was pregnant with emotion. "You know what he is, and yet I am treating him. So, you can see that this is our relationship. This is our reality. This is Rwanda."

Since I'd been writing about Ruit and Tabin, the incomparable moment each morning when a patient's bandages were removed and they were again able to see had made whatever hardships we'd encountered while traveling seem worthwhile. The emotions that ceremonial procedure released convinced me, each time I witnessed it, that Tabin and Ruit had chosen their careers wisely. But in Rwanda, only fifteen years "after," emotions were still held close, like hands of cards people didn't want others to see. When we removed the bandages of the patients at Nyamata hospital, they hardly reacted at all. Sezikeye Athanase blinked, and his face remained blank. When I showed him a photo of himself, he studied it briefly, then said, "I need a new hat." A middle-aged man whose name was certainly not Buddy, though that's what it said on the chest pocket of his cast-off work shirt from Standard Compressor, in Lubbock, Texas, looked straight through me when he was finally able to see well, after five years of making out only shadows, and didn't say a word.

Eminante was an exception. When Tabin pulled the patches from her eyes, she giggled at his foreign face and manic behavior. While he held up two fingers and asked her to count them, she had a hard time stopping her laughter long enough to answer. As she looked at the stained T-shirt she wore with a cartoon image of Tigger the Tiger, at her mother's lined face, at me, leaning in to take her photo, she grinned and grinned, like a girl unwrapping one unexpected present after another.

That afternoon I drove home with Eminante and her mother in Nkurikiye's SUV. During the mile or two we traveled, neither of them could stop laughing at the experience of riding in a motorized vehicle. Their small house was made of mud daubed onto a frame of cut branches, and the clothes of Eminante's six siblings were streaked with the red clay soil of their village. Leading us to meet the rest of her family, Eminante bent to greet a gentle dog lying in the shade at the side of the house with his legs in the air. She stroked his belly, rose, and touched each of her siblings' faces, in turn, with her fingertips, then pressed her palms against the solid walls of her home, as if she were still seeing with her hands rather than her eyes.

Her seventeen-year-old sister, Muteteli, who could have been her twin, studied us suspiciously. Their yard was fenced off by a hedge built of braided thornbushes. An outdoor kitchen, little more than an open fire pit topped with thatch, stood among a straggly grove of banana trees. There was no electricity, no furniture, and little to see inside the home. Eminante showed us the raised platform, built of mud, where the entire family slept. I noticed sacks of rice and beans stored in the rafters, to keep them from the rats. As we walked through a narrow passageway to the house's second room, Eminante stopped, in midstride, and opened her mouth.

Hanging from a rope, attached by clothespins, were several of her sister's pictures. They were simple sketches of village scenes—a mother nursing an infant, a woman with a child tied to her back working in her garden, a girl in a bright purple dress dancing ecstatically—done with crayon on lined notebook paper. Eminante held each tenderly in turn and stared and stared at them. She had been living in monotonous darkness for far too long, and now art had returned to Eminante Uzamukunda's life.

"I want to see if I can still draw," she said.

As her sister went to look for paper and crayons, we said good-bye and left Eminante to her reanimation.

Before we left Nyamata, I sat with Edward Macumi, the patient Nkurikiye had called me in to see. He told me he was fifty-eight and came from Butare, in the south of Rwanda, but he'd been incarcerated near Nyamata, which was inconvenient for his family to visit.

I asked him why he was in prison. "I didn't kill anyone," he said. "I was with some people who killed, but I did not." He said he'd been sentenced to fifteen years by the *gacaca* and forced to do difficult agricultural work, even though his eyesight was poor. When I asked how it made him feel that the man who'd restored his vision was a Tutsi, he changed the subject. He asked me if I was able to get his sentence shortened, if I had a spare set of clothes I could lend him, if I could arrange for him to be transferred to a prison closer to his family. I said I could not. Concluding that I was of no further use, he looked away from me and shut off like a light. "It's an injustice," he was muttering as I left him, "an injustice."

"Are you ready to go?" Nkurikiye asked. "I'm sure that you're as tired as myself." Over the course of three long days, he and Tabin had completed 263 surgeries. They still had to check on the progress of their corneal transplant patients and meet with government officials about the eye center Nkurikiye hoped to build, before we'd be leaving the country.

"What did he say?" Nkurikiye asked on our drive back to Kigali, after we left the bridge where he'd been wounded in our rearview mirror.

"That he hadn't killed anyone."

"Ha ha! He said that? I'm sure he did it. It was difficult not to do it. For your own sake. The groups got carried away and became like animals."

"On the subject of the genocide," Kiiza said, "I've been thrice to see the *gacaca*, and I think it is fair. The people said something animalistic came over them and begged forgiveness. In a way, I think all of Rwanda went crazy. What are you going to do, kill everyone? I've seen many perpetrators become good people and do good things. In the end, we must have mercy."

President Kagame was in America, on his first official state visit to meet President Obama. We drove in a convoy of Land Cruisers stamped with the seal of the Rwandan Defence Force to meet with the country's second-in-command, Prime Minister Bernard Makuza. Nkurikiye had changed outfits once again, and arrived in his gray dress uniform with red epaulets and a green beret.

Tabin had also made an attempt to dress up for the occasion. His hair was neatly combed in the front, but wild in the back where he'd slept on it. He wore his usual pressed khakis, along with a new, sharply creased blue oxford shirt that he'd pulled out of its plastic wrapping for the occasion. The prime minister, wearing a well-tailored double-breasted suit, was waiting for us in the driveway, along with General Charles Kayonga, commander of the Rwandan Defence Force. Makuza made a brief statement to television reporters who'd come to cover the meeting. Tabin was asked to speak next. Just as he was walking toward the cameras, I noticed, snatched at, and missed a plastic label stuck to his collar that he'd neglected to remove. It said, 16 1/2 BY 32.

In Prime Minister Makuza's elegantly appointed office, we sat on overstuffed chairs, surrounded by oil paintings of the Rwandan countryside. Tabin sat next to Makuza and launched into an impassioned speech without preliminaries. "I know that you have many offers of medical aid," Tabin said. "But most of them are missionary groups who're only here for a few weeks and often create more problems than they solve, because they leave their patients without care when they go home. John Nkurikiye is the best-trained ophthalmologist in sub-Saharan Africa. I'd like to duplicate our model from Nepal in Rwanda and make this a center of excellence for African eye care. With your support, my organization wants to help John build a world-class eye hospital and training facility here, run by Rwandans, to serve Rwandans, that will change eye care not only in your country but across East Africa."

Tabin was growing into his role as diplomat, with only a glitch or two in his professional comportment. I looked down and noticed his feet, tapping impatiently on the thick cream-colored carpet as he talked. He wore red Adidas trail-running shoes and mountain-biking socks that barely covered his ankles. But that didn't seem to distract the country's leaders from hearing the heart of his message: that they had a precious resource in Nkurikiye and he needed support. Tabin had learned not only the means of restoring sight from Ruit but also the ability to inspire visions of excellence in others.

Tabin urged the prime minister to visit King Faisal Hospital the following morning and inspect the outcome of the modern corneal transplants Nkurikiye had performed. As we were leaving, General Kayonga pulled me aside and spoke with none of Nkurikiye's reserve: "John was selfless and exemplary when he was under my command. But now he has a chance to be something bigger. My own brother was tortured and killed by the militias to try to break my spirit. But they failed. And if we allow Rwanda to be remembered as an island of evil in the center of Africa, we will have failed, too. There must be a reason for what we've endured. We must build something superior to what was here before the genocide. I guarantee you'll get our full support. Because John can help us make Rwanda an example of how to be better."

The next morning, Prime Minister Makuza arrived at the ophthalmic clinic at King Faisal Hospital without an escort, to inspect Nkurikiye's work; he'd driven his own jeep on a Saturday morning instead of playing the round of golf he had planned. Kigali's TV reporters got wind of his presence and swarmed into the hospital soon after.

Makuza watched a video of a surgery that Tabin showed him on his laptop, then walked along a row of eighteen seated patients, bending over, looking into their repaired eyes, and listening to their stories. The nineteenth patient was too enthusiastic to remain in his seat. Francis Kiiza had woken Nkurikiye at six, screaming into the phone with joy, saying he could finally see clearly. Kiiza pulled Nkurikiye to his side, clasped the prime minister by both shoulders, and began the sort of uninterruptible soliloquy I associated with Tabin. The television cameras closed in, assuring that his testimony would be heard nationwide. "You know, Mr. Prime Minister, loss of sight means loss of life! I had surrendered to remaining in the darkness before I came here. But now I have my life back. More operations like Dr. John is doing will help many more people like me survive!"

After we left, Nkurikiye had an architect draw up plans for the center, modeled on Tilganga, that he hoped to open in Kigali. Six months later, as I was packing for another trip to Nepal, I received an email from Rwanda. Tabin had returned to Kigali in the interim, bearing a fresh box of corneas, and successfully sutured one onto Francis Kiiza's other eye. The report I received from Tabin said that the preserved cornea he had initially taken so much pride in transplanting was looking "faaaaantastic!"

"You are always on my heart and in my prayers," Kiiza wrote me, "because I never expected to see again and He knows what you did for me. Dr. John is so good to me, and my sight has fully recovered. I am sending you a photograph of me in action." I scrolled down to study it: Francis in a tweed jacket and dress pants writing an equation far too complex for me to understand on a blackboard, while his students looked attentively toward him. "I am planning to enroll in a master's program and hope to be a head of school someday," he continued. "You should know that my life has been entirely transformed. May sweet Jesus watch over you in your travels," he wrote. "And," he added, in a sentiment that Tabin seemed to have stitched into him, along with his sutures, "remember to have fun!"

When I'd met Cliff Tabin in his lab at Harvard, he had expressed concern that his little brother might be wasting his time in Africa. "I'm worried that Geoff's diluting his efforts," he said, which sounded, to my ears, much like Ruit's warning against trying to do everything at once. "I don't know if he can succeed in Africa. It all depends on getting the right partners. And I don't know if Geoff will ever meet his African Ruit."

I thought about the eighteen or more family members John Nkurikiye had lost, and I looked at the eighteen seated patients, reanimated by a doctor's unusual dedication. Cliff Tabin of Harvard Medical School was among the brightest minds in American medicine, but on one point, at least, he was dead wrong. His little brother wasn't wasting his time roaming Africa, searching for a partner capable of helping him transform the eye care of an entire continent. He'd already found him.

CHAPTER 26

Hands, Eyes, Heart

*And now here is my secret, a very simple secret. It is only with the heart
that one can see rightly; what is essential is invisible to the eye.*
—Antoine de Saint-Exupéry

"You should have died sooner!" the dignified middle-aged Nepalese man shouted at the elderly corpse. "You should have left us long ago!" The manager and uniformed bellboys in the lobby of the Kathmandu Guest House seemed shocked by the display of emotion. A reasonable-looking local citizen was yelling at a television broadcasting the funeral procession of G. P. Koirala, the leader who had dominated Nepal's politics for decades. "Now," the man said more quietly, conscious of how his outburst had silenced the bustling lobby, "at least we'll have a chance."

Most of the official obituaries running in the press praised Koirala as a statesman who'd hastened the demise of Nepal's monarchy, brokered a peace agreement with the Maoists, and led Nepal's march toward democracy. Ruit, like many other Nepalese, saw things differently. To him, Koirala was a formerly idealistic politician who'd become far too comfortable in his role as kingpin of the nepotistic clique that ensured power never strayed too far from Kathmandu's elite.

The coalition of Koirala supporters in the new Nepalese government had thwarted the efforts of Maoist prime minister Prachanda to integrate his former soldiers into Nepal's military, forcing him out of office in protest just days after he'd cut the ribbon of the new Tilganga Institute. And with his resignation, Ruit feared, went much of the country's hope for corruption-free leadership and rapid improvement in the lives of Nepal's poor. "Koirala had a chance to change everything," Ruit whispered to me, "to steer this country up. But instead he drove it down."

We were standing in the lobby of my hotel while bellmen dragged my hastily packed bags toward the door, and Ruit and I tore ourselves away from the televised images of riots that had replaced the funeral procession. We were about to set out on the trip I'd convinced him to take to his homeland in the country's far northeast. But with the sudden power vacuum, ugly street demonstrations were breaking out. Maoists were threatening violence and general strikes, and Ruit wanted me to stay at his home for a few days, where I'd be safer until we left Kathmandu.

I spent the morning organizing my trekking gear in Sagar's vacant bedroom, then hiked up the 365 stairs to Swayambhunath, where visitors walked clockwise, spinning the prayer wheels that circled the golden stupa to send their wishes fluttering out above the city's smog. I spun the wheels, too, praying for the ability to keep up with Ruit and Tabin on the trek over rough terrain we had planned. I'd injured my Achilles tendon just before leaving for Nepal, and though I'd wrapped my ankle in an Ace bandage and the pain seemed manageable, I didn't know how fast or how far I'd be able to walk.

After I returned to the Ruit home, a wave of jet lag swept over me. When I woke it was dark. I padded down the carpeted hallway and peered into the living room. It was mid-March and frigid in the house. Ruit, Nanda, Serabla, and Satenla were curled up together under a heavy quilt, wearing fleece coats and wool ski hats, leaning comfortably against one another and watching Koirala's cremation on TV, like a family warming itself by a campfire.

The Ruits had left their one-room apartment without heat or air-conditioning behind, but even though they had both settled in their luxurious new home by Swayambhunath, they weren't yet comfortable with the extravagance of turning a dial and heating such a large space when they had insulated clothes and body heat to ward off the chill.

Koirala, who'd died of respiratory failure at age eighty-five, was burning on the same exclusive upstream bier where the assassinated royal family had turned to ash. The flames leaping from his mouth seemed to shoot higher than those of the other bodies I'd seen burning at Pashupatinath. Perhaps the grade of clarified butter in his mouth burned hotter than most. Or maybe his departing spirit, so used to dominating Nepal's political conversation, was still straining to be heard, as the tiny white-clad figure of Krishna Thapa stood by, stoking the fire.

While I stared at the flames, I mourned a different loss; I thought of the news Khem Gurung had given me that morning. I'd just learned that Patali Nepali, the seamstress whose sight I'd seen returned the first time I'd watched Ruit work, had died. Patali had endured for a good six months after her operation, Khem told me, able to sew, support herself, and gaze at the faces of her family, before complications from the asthma she'd suffered from for years killed her. It was a harsh reminder that though restoring sight could be transformative, it couldn't eliminate all the factors that could destroy you in a poor country like Nepal.

Before we left on our trek, eighty-three-year-old Sonam Ruit asked us to wait in the foyer and dragged himself upstairs to his shrine room to fetch something he considered crucial for our journey. He returned, wheezing, and unwrapped a bolt of marigold-colored silk containing an antique bronze *vajra*. Chanting a *puja* for us, he placed white silk *katas* around our necks, then touched Sanduk's forehead, and mine, with the divine thunderbolt he'd carried for the half a century since he'd last seen Olangchungola.

"You know how dangerous those trails are," he told his son. "This will keep you safe."

The machete was wielded expertly. It hit the target again and again with a firm *thunk, thunk, thunk*, severing the limb into equal-sized portions. Ruit bought a bundle and handed a piece to his daughter Satenla. She began gnawing the sugarcane while the old Tamang woman at the end of the Mulghat Bridge wrapped the rest in newspaper.

I looked down over the rusted iron railing. By the bank of the Tamor, two men held a water buffalo's head upright by its nose ring while a third sharpened a long curving *kukri* against a wet river rock, then slashed it casually across the buffalo's throat. Blood pumped out of the dying animal's carotid artery in rhythm with its heartbeat, fountaining foamy pink into a bowl the executioner held, until the spurting slowed, stopped, and the buffalo's front legs collapsed into the water. Then the butchering began.

Each year, during the fall Dashain festival, Nepalese, propitiating their many gods, but especially the goddess Durga, destroyer of evil, conduct the world's most extensive ritualistic slaughter of animals. As many as half a million buffalo, goats, ducks, roosters, and pigeons are sacrificed to ensure luck for the coming year. The killings cause an outcry from the country's more outspoken Buddhist leaders, who suggest that if celebrants need to cut something up, they should substitute pumpkins. Year after year, the slaughter continues. We were traveling in March, during Little Dashain, altogether a much smaller affair. Still, on our drive to eastern Nepal, we'd passed sheets painted to resemble ornate Hindu temples dedicated to Durga erected on wooden frameworks in many small villages, and enough blood running in the gutters to make me glad I'd missed the main event.

We'd planned to drop off specialized surgical equipment at an eye hospital in the town of Janakpur, but Ruit, his ear pressed to his mobile phone, monitored the rioting along the route. He told Manbhadur to hold the White Elephant to an easterly course and give Janakpur a wide berth. "The Maoists are getting grumbly down there," he said.

We drove up a recently paved road into the hills, following the Tamor for a time, the river of Ruit's childhood, through foliage dried by drought, to Dhankuta, the town where Sonam had washed up when war and flooding had chased his family down from the heights of Olangchungola. Ruit was concerned that visiting the site of his family's saddest history might be too much for his youngest daughter. "Satenla's the most sensitive of my children," Ruit told me. "She's always been the most upset when I'm away working. She calls me every day and needs to know what I've had for lunch, what the weather's like, and how hard we're working. So now that she's thirteen I told her it was time to see all of this for herself."

Satenla, plugged in to her iPod, wasn't listening. But when we passed through Dhankuta and stopped on Hile's humble main street, in front of a row of tin-roofed shophouses, Ruit told his daughter to take out her earphones. We climbed out to have a closer look. "This is where we lived, Sat," he said, indicating a house indistinguishable from the others. It had a small hand-painted sign hanging out front that read, WELCOME TO FANCY SHOP, but it looked no fancier than its neighbors, all of which sold nearly identical stock: Chinese acrylic sweaters, toiletries, phone cards, and dust-covered bags of potato chips in flavors tailored to the subcontinent, like prawn curry and mutton masala.

With her long hair spilling over the shoulders of her silver Nike windbreaker and her spotless white skateboarder shoes planted cautiously on Hile's muddy road, Satenla looked at the shop like a tourist eying an ancient ruin, a relic from a history that wasn't hers. Ruit explained to his daughter that before a road came all the way to their home, he had to take a bus from college in Kathmandu to a trailhead in Dharan, sleep overnight on sacks of grain in a warehouse owned by his father's friend, then hike over two ranges of hills, setting out before breakfast and arriving, with luck, long after dinner. "What do you think, Sat?" Ruit asked. "Could you do a hike like that?"

Instead of answering, Satenla took out a pink diary she'd bought for the trip. On the title page she'd written, carefully, in English calligraphy, "Love is a bond between the hands, the eyes, and the heart." She scrawled a few notes; then, at Ruit's request, father and daughter posed while I took a photo of them with Ruit's camera. Another teenage girl tended shop, cracking seeds in her teeth as she stared enviously at the clean clothes of the city folk. I thought of Ruit's young sister Yang La spending her last days in this place, lying on a cot behind the counter, coughing into a bloody cloth, and rousing herself to a sitting position whenever a customer wanted to buy something.

Ruit was clearly on edge after visiting the home he hadn't been able to reach for the funeral while he took his exams. He was as turned in on himself as I'd ever seen him, his eyes focused not on the colonial-style bungalow where we began unpacking but back toward a time when he'd been a student, powerless to save his sister.

A fleet of sleek black SUVs pulled up outside, disgorging a group of politicians in business suits who were threatening to use their clout to bump us from our rooms. Ruit ran up a long flight of stone stairs and stepped between the guesthouse manager and the leader of the group. "Are you telling me these parasites are trying to take our rooms?" he shouted. "We've come here to cure people, and who are they? Politicians? What have they done for the people? Nothing! Now tell them to climb back into their cars and be on their way."

The chastened politicians slid back into their vehicles and rolled down the road while we waited for Tabin. He was due that evening, flying in at the last minute after celebrating the wedding of his eldest daughter, Livia. Tabin also had to leave earlier than Ruit wanted, to give a speech at the annual meeting of the American Society of Cataract and Refractive Surgery, where Alan Crandall was due to be sworn in as president. Immediately after that, Tabin planned to fly to the Caribbean and meet with U.S. general Lie-Ping Chang. General Chang had asked Tabin to critique the American military's humanitarian medical outreach around the world and help recast it in the model of the HCP. He wanted Tabin to advise him how to build permanent centers of excellence and train local medical professionals, rather than just docking hospital ships for a few weeks at the world's neediest ports and sailing away to leave patients behind with their problems and complications. Tabin blithely added the meeting to his lengthy to-do list and moved on to planning his next six or seven trips to Asia and Africa.

He drove up just before dark, a few hours after we arrived, with an American donor who wanted to see the HCP work he supported up close, lucky to have flown and missed the two-day drive that had brought us to Pakhribas, the town fifteen minutes farther into the hills than Dhankuta, where we planned to operate in a middle school. Tabin also arrived without his luggage, which had vanished somewhere between San Francisco and Kathmandu.

Tabin had spent the few hours he had in the capital running between the homes of his former Sherpa climbing partners, borrowing gear for our trek. He arrived with no waterproof clothing and none of his specialized surgical tools, only the foam Crocs clogs he wore during surgery and a pair of borrowed approach shoes a size too small, which smelled so pungently of foot rot that I asked him to leave them outside the door of the tiny room we shared.

"Well," Tabin said cheerfully, unzipping his borrowed duffel bag and spreading the rank, unwashed gear he'd gathered on his single bed, a foot away from mine. "I may not have any of the clothes I need for our trek, or the tools I need for surgery, but at least the shoes I have to walk in for weeks smell like a steaming pile of buffalo shit!"

The group gathered for dinner that night in the drab concrete commissary of the district department of forestry, across the road from our guesthouse. Ruit and Gurung had typed up complex itineraries, which they passed out while we waited for our lentils and rice. They had reserved three days for surgery in Pakhribas, then charted the distance we would march for three days toward the upper Tamor River and a surgical camp we planned to conduct at Sinwa, a small town at the confluence of two river valleys.

I took out my topographical map and traced the route. It looked like three exceptionally hard days of hiking to Sinwa, double the length of the stages most trekkers would attempt, then another three long days, after the surgery was finished, to climb up and visit Ruit's birthplace in Olangchungola before retracing our steps. If nothing went wrong— and in Nepal something almost always did—we'd be gone for at least two more weeks. "I already told you, Sanduk. I can't stay that long," Tabin said. "I have to be back in Boston for a speech." I added that with the condition of my ankle I didn't think I could make it all the way to Olangchungola either, but I was determined to reach Sinwa so I could watch Ruit and Tabin treat the people of the region where Ruit was born.

Ruit's face reddened. He scraped his chair back, stood, and began shouting. "David! Khem and I have worked on this plan for months so you could see everything! And Geoff, you know, you can be very, very difficult to work with! Lot of people wouldn't bother and they'd be done with you!" I'd heard about these flare-ups from Tabin but had never seen one firsthand. I coughed and looked away. Tabin blinked rapidly, the only sign that he'd heard what Ruit had said, and sipped mildly at his milk tea. The rest of the meal passed in silence.

Later, in our room, reading by the light of our headlamps during the inevitable load shedding, Tabin said, "Sorry about that. He gets that way sometimes."

"How do you deal with it? It looks like you let it roll right off you."

"Not always. One time we were staying in a guesthouse way out in western Tibet. I went for a hike the morning before surgery that I guess was too long for Ruit's taste. I ran into my room to change into scrubs, and when I tried to leave I found it had been padlocked from the outside and the team was gone until late that evening. I had no toilet in my room and no food. It didn't roll off me then. Ruit tends to make a point in a way you'll remember."

I realized how much I'd come to value Ruit's praise, and how crushing it could feel to be the target of his condemnation. "So you've learned to accept it?" I said. "I feel too upset to sleep, and he hardly said anything to me."

"I guess I have," Tabin said. "Maybe that's why I've lasted so long as Ruit's partner. I try to look for the kernel of truth in his criticism. I do tend to overschedule. But I try not to let others define how I see myself. I want to measure myself against the best. That's why I always play top young tennis players. And that's why I'm willing to put up with the occasional dressing-down from Sanduk. A lot of high-powered medical types wouldn't. I see myself as someone who can get things done. But Ruit's the genius behind everything we do. He's the best. The best surgeon and the best person I've ever met. I try to measure myself against that."

On a small stainless steel table behind Ruit's surgical stool, Ajeev Thapa had set up and calibrated a prototype of the portable phacoemulsification machine Ruit had chosen after extensive testing. It was manufactured by Oertli, a Swiss company that had come closest to meeting his requirements. The device was slightly larger than a brief-case, pale yellow with a sturdy handle on top for easy transport, and rugged enough, Ruit hoped, to accompany him on his travels. The cutting tools Ruit had planned to drop at the hospital in Janakpur, be-fore receiving reports of grumbly Maoists, were nearly identical to the blades in Tabin's lost luggage, so by a lucky accident, both surgeons were well equipped to work.

That afternoon, in a classroom of the Pakhribas school that Til-ganga's staff had converted into an operating theater, Ruit tested his new machine's capabilities on the cataracts of his patients, and Tabin operated manually. Despite Tilganga's advance team having papered the district with pamphlets and advertised on the radio, only 125 pa-tients showed up for surgery. Tabin seemed bored, for the first time in my experience, by his work.

"I haven't seen a mature cataract all day," he said. "These cases are a piece of cake. We've done such a good job over the years that we've cured most of the serious cases in the populated parts of Nepal, and now we're just catching the others before they become too bad."

Tabin's boredom seemed cause for celebration. What was a more tangible sign of success than a shortage of blind people in a country that had once swarmed with them? "It's strange," he said, closing up a patient's wound. "I expected turning around preventable blindness in the Himalaya to take a lifetime. That's why we called ourselves the Himalayan Cataract Project. But we're getting close and it's only been about fifteen years. Now, when I work in Africa, I get the feeling I used to when we were first starting out." Many people would happily hang their life on such an achievement. But it couldn't be bad for the blind of Africa to have an unstoppable force like Tabin turning his attention toward them.

At first, when I'd started traveling with Ruit and Tabin, I'd asked them to point out blind people, so I could be sure to interview them. They'd seemed amused by the naïveté of the question. "Just look for the people who wave their arms and stumble when they have to walk," they'd told me, "or the ones who hunch over as they sit." In many of the places we'd visited, those matching that description had numbered in the hundreds.

I scanned the crowd waiting in the courtyard of the Pakhribas school, most people sitting on the piles of bricks the school had purchased for future expansion. All but four seemed to have enough visual acuity to walk without aid: a teenage boy who sat, slumped, by himself; two older women who'd come from distant villages and were leaning helplessly against their relatives; and a middle-aged man in a clean gray V-neck sweater who was led into surgery, flailing for balance, by local teenage volunteers. The volunteers wore yellow ribbons, like those presented to champion equestrians. And their expressions of pride demonstrated that they enjoyed the duties they'd been entrusted with: feeding the patients and escorting them to surgery.

When I returned to the operating room, Ruit still wasn't talking to me, except when I asked him a direct question. He was speaking loudly and with some heat to Rahan Man Tamang, the patient in the gray V-neck sweater, who'd been placed on his table. I asked him what he was saying. "This gentleman is an alcoholic," Ruit explained. "That's very common among the blind in remote areas who want to escape the drudgery of their lives. But this fellow lives in a prosperous town. He has a trade as a skilled mason and no excuse for not having surgery already, so I'm asking him why it took him so long to come to us for help."

Ruit repeated the question, and Tamang mumbled something in response. Ruit began speaking forcefully, in a tone I recognized from the previous night, and his words clearly found their mark. The man twisted on Ruit's table as if he was already in pain, though the operation had yet to begin. Then he nodded in agreement. I asked Ruit what he said.

"I told this fellow, 'I propose a bargain for you. I'll give you back your eyes. You have to take back your life. You've made a mess of it so far, but I'm going to give you a second chance. When you can see again, do you promise to stop drinking?'"

While Tabin whipped through his unchallenging cases, I walked out, pulled off my mask, and roamed the schoolyard. The teenage boy was still hunched over, with his head between his knees. He wore a dress shirt so faded the original color was hard to discern. With Satenla translating, I learned that he was sixteen and his name was Bhupin. I asked how much he could see.

"If it's bright out, I can see some shadows," he said. "Otherwise, it's always dark."

"Do you go to school?" I asked.

"My parents make me," he said. "But I don't see the point."

Two teenage volunteers tapped Bhupin on the shoulder and led him in to surgery.

Our last morning in Pakhribas, the patients sat quietly on the benches lining the school's courtyard and their families squatted on top of the piles of bricks, waiting for the show to begin. While the nurses laid out their boxes of eyedrops for the patients to take home and prepared for the doctors to begin their examinations, Rahan Man Tamang fell to the ground and began twitching. His wife helped prop him back up and began massaging his legs, trying to ease the tremors from his alcohol withdrawal. Satenla and I spoke to his wife, and she explained that her husband had kept his promise, at least for a day, and had drunk nothing since his surgery.

Bhupin was one of the first patients Ruit unbandaged. Like so many Ruit had operated on, he began to unfold like a plant exposed to the sun as soon as he was able to see. But Bhupin's transformation was the fastest I'd ever witnessed. While Ruit moved on, working his way down the line of patients, Bhupin stood and began walking gingerly, with his arms held before him for balance. Then, as if a switch had been thrown, he let his arms drop to his sides, realizing that he no longer needed to move like someone with an infirmity, and began walking briskly, then sped up still further, skipping back and forth across the courtyard, laughing aloud. His mood affected the other patients, and they laughed along and applauded his every move.

Ruit knelt to unveil Rahan Man Tamang's eyes, and as he looked at Ruit, then let his gaze rest on his wife, who was still rubbing his twitching legs and had wrapped a thick wool scarf around his shivering neck, I noticed for the first time that he was a handsome man. Ruit had prepared another lecture, but he didn't need it. "I promise," Tamang said, first to Ruit, then, lingeringly, to his wife. "I'm so sorry," he told her.

Ruit unwound the gauze from the eyes of his last two patients. Seventy-year-old Devi Maya Khadka was a wisp of a woman who wore her hair pulled back in a pink kerchief; she smiled ecstatically with her remaining teeth when she met Ruit's eyes.

Sixty-six-year-old Devi Rai wore a white cardigan and a finely wrought, flowered gold nose stud that seemed especially fragile on her broad, willful face. "My sister-in-law says she's growing impatient," Rai said after Ruit unwrapped her bandages. "She had to walk me here from my village, and she doesn't want to wait any longer for me to receive my medication and instructions." Rai stood up and stared at her sister-in-law. "Well, get going! I don't need your help anymore. I'll do everything for myself. I'll walk back myself. I'll dance all the way home. Look!" And then she stood up, raised her arms over her head, and began to dance. "I may have the physique of an old lady," she said. "But I've got the heart of a sixteen-year-old now. Come on!" she urged the other Devi. "Our lives aren't over yet. Dance with me!"

She pulled her partner to her feet and began to sing. The two women twirled and spun as the crowd clapped along to Devi Rai's song. "I can't go beyond the river," she sang in a voice far more delicate than her weathered appearance. "I can't cross the water to win your love. My heart will break right here. Sitting alone at home." The two Devis spun to a stop, hugging each other, gasping for breath, as the crowd cheered. Thanks to Ruit, neither one would have to sit helplessly at home any longer. As helplessly as Yang La had withered behind the counter at Sonam's shop down the road, struggling to breathe, waiting for the end prescribed by her banishment from modern medicine.

I looked at Ruit and saw something hard he'd carried since we'd arrived soften and sink without a trace.

We packed up and climbed onto the blue Tilganga bus that would carry us to our trailhead. The people of Pakhribas bowed and handed us bouquets of flowers as we boarded. They decorated the bus with strings of marigolds and tied yellow silk *katas* to its mirrors, knotting them around its grille and lacing them through the windows.

We waved good-bye with our flower-filled hands, and the bus rumbled up the road, deeper into the mountains, deeper into Ruit's past, leaving behind terraced hillsides and cultivated plots, passing patients walking toward distant homes, rolling finally through a wild and empty landscape of clumping bamboo that threw shoots high into the air, shoots that bent and curved in every direction of the compass before exploding into blossoms at their tips, like an enduring display of fireworks.

CHAPTER 27

The Winter Trail

I am of the nature to grow old.
There is no way to escape growing old.
I am of the nature to have ill health.
There is no way to escape ill health.
I am of the nature to die.
There is no way to escape death.
All that is dear to me and everyone I love are of the nature to change.
There is no way to escape being separated from them.
My actions are my only true belongings.
I cannot escape the consequences of my actions.
My actions are the ground upon which I stand.
—The Five Remembrances, the essence of the Buddha's teachings,
as translated by Thich Nhat Hanh

K hem woke me and Tabin well before dawn, easing into our cramped and filthy room in the Yak guesthouse with cups of milky tea. Tabin had thrown his pack onto the more comfortable of the two beds the evening before, and I'd tossed most of the night on a tilting slab covered with a straw mat that threatened to spill me and my slick nylon sleeping bag onto the floor.

Too few minutes later, we stood shivering on Basantapur's main commercial street at first light. A cold mist blew past shuttered shop-houses, and our porters repacked and adjusted the woven baskets they'd brought to carry our loads. Then Ruit marched to the head of the line, holding his walking stick like a band conductor's baton, and waved it, urging us on.

The trail began where the road ended, and climbed gently at first. Tabin had taped my ankle, so I felt reasonably confident as we climbed up a ridge, but the route grew progressively steeper, and we scrambled over slide paths. One section of loose rock was so tricky to cross that I climbed up to a boulder where someone had hammered in an iron cable and, hanging from it, pulled myself across, arm over arm.

Tabin simply jumped down into the gap where the trail had been, bracing himself, in his borrowed shoes, on either side of a sheer drop. Reaching up, he supported Satenla, and then her father, as they tiptoed across a ledge. Tabin's instinctive move was proof of how useful he must have been to Ruit when they were first blazing their path together into the high places of the Himalaya.

After four hours of steady climbing, we reached the crest of a ridge covered in rhododendrons. Pink, red, and the rare giant white rhododendron trees that Ruit remembered from his long walks with his father were in full bloom, and we traveled through tunnels of them for hours, the flowery light filtering through their blossoms, their fallen petals softening the path.

Satenla, her hair pulled back into a ponytail for the trek, was moving more slowly than the rest of us, and her father stayed with her, while the mountain people among Ruit's team took turns helping her over rock slides and boulders that blocked the trail and carrying her light pack. She was winded when she arrived on top of the next ridge, and she sat down heavily, gulping from her nearly empty aluminum water bottle decorated with a Barbie motif. I couldn't imagine her crossing increasingly rough terrain over the next few weeks, but I knew I shouldn't underestimate a Ruit, even one raised in relative comfort.

Past the rhododendrons, the sharp summit ridges of Kangchenjunga carved their way out of a cloud bank, looking more rugged from the west than they had from Kalimpong or Sikkim. "Do you see it, Sat?" Ruit asked. "Do you see our mountain?"

"Yes, Daddy," she said, dutifully aiming her camera.

I kept pace with Tabin and he talked the entire way, telling meandering jokes that lasted as long as the ridges we climbed, and discussing

Ghana, Ethiopia, and Rwanda and his plans to expand his efforts across Africa, and muttering aloud, as if he were walking alone, about the negative effect his extended absences were having on his family.

Twelve hours after we'd set out from Basantapur, it began to rain— gently at first, then whipping up into an onslaught that we leaned against as we climbed. We were still climbing after dark, trying to keep our headlamps focused on the main channel of a rocky path cut through thorny alpine scrub that forked away into side trails and dead ends every few yards. "Do you think we should stop and make sure Sanduk and Satenla aren't lost?" I asked.

"I wouldn't worry about them," Tabin said. "They have half of the Sherpas on Tilganga's staff looking out for them. I'm more concerned about where we are."

I checked my altimeter. We had just climbed above ten thousand feet, and the precipitation, as if it responded to round numbers, changed to hail. It pounded on our hoods in marble-sized pellets, drowning out our attempts at conversation. I thought of a phrase from Peter Matthiessen's *The Snow Leopard*, which he'd written while following another driven madman, the wildlife biologist George Schaller, into this range a few hundred miles to our west. "In the calamitous weather," Matthiessen wrote, "the journey was losing all reality."

We were looking for a town called Gupha, where we planned to spend the night, but my altimeter said we were too high. We'd expected to reach it an hour earlier, and there was no flicker of artificial light or sign of human habitation anywhere we could see, along the entire length of the sharp ledge extending for miles to our north. Then thunder cracked so close overhead that we both ducked, and a bolt of lightning forked toward us with a tearing sound and hit a rocky outcrop a hundred yards ahead of us, precisely where our trail was headed.

"Well, look at the bright side!" Tabin shouted over the storm. "We may be hiking on a slippery trail in the dark, with no sign of shelter in sight, but at least there's an excellent chance we'll both be killed by lightning!"

Just then we rounded a corner and reached a cleft in the ridge where we could see, half a mile ahead and below us, propane lamps the residents of Gupha had hung, flaring like runway lights, guiding us to a landing strip in the storm.

We ducked and walked through a low door into Gupha's teahouse. Ruit, Satenla, and the rest of the team were resting on cushioned benches surrounding a smoking fire box and sipping milky tea. Tabin and I must have climbed above the main trail on a detour that lengthened our trek. The home belonged to a Walung family of Ruit's acquaintance. The matron, a ruddy-faced woman in a striped *pangi*, shoved steaming mugs of milk tea into our hands and stoked the fire. Tabin slid into the last empty seat and I stood against the wall, next to a framed photo of the Dalai Lama. Soon the room was so thick with smoke that I couldn't stop coughing or keep my eyes open, and I slipped out the back door for some fresh air.

The hail had stopped, but the gusts were blowing even harder. We were on a ridge at 9,600 feet, fully exposed to the bitter wind whipping east from the high peaks of the Khumbu. Having left my headlamp inside, I stumbled around in the muddy yard among unfamiliar rounded shapes that looked like crude stupas. They towered over me, two or three times my height, and it was only when I slid on a wet stone and steadied myself against one that I saw they were stacks of firewood. Without them, human life in this place would hardly be possible.

The tin door, banging against its frame, announced my return. Shivering, I picked up my tea and tried to drink without burning my tongue. "David?" Ruit asked from his comfortable seat next to his daughter. "Where's that handsome orange coat of yours?"

I sagged now that he'd said it out loud. "I forgot to pack it," I admitted. My one warm piece of clothing, an insulated belay jacket I'd brought for moments like this, hadn't made the trip to the mountains. I could see the peg where I'd left it hanging in a spare classroom at the Pakhribas school. I'd been chastising myself about losing it all day.

"Are you sure?" Ruit said, his eyes twinkling with amusement as he pulled it out of his pack and tossed it to me. Everyone in the room shared a belly laugh at my expense. I took off my thin wet shell and gratefully zipped the hood of the warm coat over my head. "We couldn't let you freeze to death," Ruit said. "Who would tell our story?"

The next morning, we left again at first light. Scoured all night by rain and hail, the morning sky was washed clean. We hiked up a ridge out of Gupha, and once we'd left the narrow lane between the smoke-blackened homes, Makalu and Lhotse—two of the world's five tallest mountains—jutted into view, directly to our west. They resembled crumbling palaces of vanished Himalayan kingdoms, but they'd been shaped by a hand surer than any human architect and were built to last. Seeing their summits lit by the rising sun made every step we'd taken the day before worthwhile.

Our train of nurses, technicians, surgeons, and porters stretched for nearly a mile, all of them walking at their own pace. Pemba Sherpa, one of Tilganga's most fit orderlies, carried the heaviest load, a metal locker containing one of the operating microscopes as well as two cartons of bottled intravenous fluids. The porters hauled piles of gear that made the light packs Tabin, Ruit, and I wore look weightless. The large woven baskets they carried by plastic straps that creased their foreheads were packed full of crates marked TILGANGA INSTITUTE. Metal surgical stools were lashed to the tops of their unwieldy loads. They sped beyond me as we walked under strands of torn prayer flags at the top of a ten-thousand-foot pass, breathing easily, chattering to keep one another company.

I clambered down slippery rocks on the other side, watching more than forty people descend a saddled ridge while Pemba and the others at the leading edge of the party began hauling their overloaded baskets toward an even higher pass. The immensity of our undertaking struck me. In an age when most doctors are unwilling to even make house calls, the team Ruit had assembled was carrying the contents of an entire hospital over a mountain range to reach his patients.

I was walking with Satenla and her father, telling them how extraordinary the spectacle seemed to me, when Ruit grabbed each of us by the arm, pulled us a few feet above the path, and pressed us hard against a boulder. Around a bend in the trail I heard a faint chiming. "Yak!" warned Ruit, who'd heard them sooner. "You need to give them a wide berth," he said as the animals passed below us, straining at their leads. "They might look like gentle, furry creatures, Sat, but those big kitty cats have sharp horns, isn't it?"

When the yak caravan had passed and we approached our high point for the day, the eleven-thousand-foot Deurali Pass, Ruit stopped short of the summit and rooted around in the thorny undergrowth for a rock with dimensions that pleased him. At the top of the pass he heaved it skillfully straight-armed, like a cricket bowler, and it landed on the very top of a nearby pile of stones stacked into a *chorten*. "Let the mountain rise higher!" he proclaimed, as his father had said to him once, on another long walk many decades earlier. He handed another stone to Satenla so she could cement the tradition.

We walked along a ridge for another hour, then sat on a sunny ledge while Nima Sherpa, a young orderly whom Ruit had asked to pay special attention to Satenla on difficult stretches of terrain, poured us milk tea from a pink thermos decorated with frisky cats pawing at balls of yarn. Satenla was writing rapidly in her diary. Tabin had spotted a cellphone tower on a distant peak and had scrambled up a rocky promontory like a mountain goat, trying to find a signal so he could call his wife. I sniffed my forearm. It smelled like smoked meat after one night in a Walung home, and I understood why respiratory infections were so common in the mountains of Nepal.

With our backs propped against boulders, Ruit and I settled down to wait for Tabin, enjoying the sun.

"I want to say something to you very clearly," Ruit told me. "I know I can be very hard on Geoff. I don't know any other way to be. I have to be straight with everyone I really care about. But, you know, I love him like anything."

I nodded and unfolded my topographical map, tracing the route to our next destination, the village of Dhovan. If I was reading the terrain lines correctly, we had what looked like a steep seven-thousand-foot descent before we'd be there.

Tabin hopped down from boulder to boulder, back to us. "I had Jean for a minute up there," he said. "But I lost her."

"Come, Geoff, we better get going," Ruit said. "It's a long way down to Dhovan."

Tabin and I began walking while Ruit coaxed an exhausted Satenla out of a sitting position and handed her his stick for extra incentive. The trail dropped gradually for the first thousand feet, and Tabin took the opportunity to critique my hiking technique, telling me I was walking too fast, rolling my feet too much from side to side, and wasting energy righting myself after every step. "Try this," he said. "It's called the 'guide's pace.'" I followed his foul-smelling shoes, putting my feet where he planted his. At first I didn't notice much difference, but after a mile or so I realized we were chewing up the terrain pretty efficiently. "Watch the porters," he said. "They walk as fast as they can but fry themselves after twenty minutes and have to drop their loads and recover. If we keep up like this, we'll pass all of them."

The trail turned off the ridge and plunged, far more steeply, down a dry creek bed. Now there was no walking, at any pace. We were hopping or sliding down, from boulder to boulder, and with each impact, my Achilles tendon protested. We traveled like that for five more hours, hopping down slick streambeds and steep, stony trails, stalked by a downdraft of cold air that blew past us like a premonition of disaster.

We had no way of knowing it, since we'd moved so far ahead of the main group, but nearly everyone was struggling. Ajeev Thapa, entrusted to carry the precious Oertli phaco machine in a leather briefcase, had tumbled headlong over a mossy boulder and cradled the device, letting his body take the impact. In the process, he'd badly twisted his knee. Ruit, too, had fallen from a rock, strained his knee, and was moving slowly, leaning heavily on the trekking pole Satenla had given back to him. One of the porters—whom we'd passed, as Tabin had predicted—had also taken a bad fall in a slippery creek bed and had broken his ankle.

Tabin seemed to be the only one immune to the rigors of our descent. Whenever he spotted an exposed ledge, he scrambled up rocks to its highest point, aiming his cellphone fruitlessly in all directions, like a thirsty dowser divining for water, failed time and again by his forked stick. By late afternoon we spotted a suspension bridge a thousand feet below that spanned the Maiwa Khola near the spot where it met the Tamor and led, we hoped, to Dhovan. The last stretch of the trail was lit by fires farmers had set to clear their fields. They burned on the darkening hillside like smoldering pits leading to a subterranean world, and we walked through choking drifts of smoke until we reached the river. Tabin skipped and I hobbled across the suspension bridge to the tent site by the water's edge where we planned to spend the night.

We stripped off our clothes, balanced on boulders in icy pools at the edge of the Maewa Khola, and washed away the smoke and sweat before lying on our backs by the riverbank, waiting for the rest of the group to arrive. They straggled in, limping toward us in small groups, pulled their packs off, and sprawled on the ground. An hour later, Ruit still hadn't arrived.

Ruit's knee was worse than he'd let on, and as he crossed the swaying suspension bridge, he was just allowing himself to picture collapsing at the campsite and calling for a cup of tea when he was met by a party of village elders who'd heard he was coming, waiting for him at the far bank. "They told me a man was in grave danger," Ruit explained to us later. "He'd been gored by a bull and needed my attentions urgently." They led Ruit away from the campsite to the center of Dhovan, where a man in his mid-twenties, wearing a burnt-orange baseball cap with the logo of the University of Texas Longhorns, was lying on a wooden bench, clutching his stomach where the thrust of the horn had punctured him.

"To tell you truthfully, I was terrified," Ruit says. "It had been so many years since I'd practiced general medicine that my mind raced, thinking of what to do."

Ruit couldn't bring himself to look at the wound. He stalled, inspecting the man's tongue and taking his pulse, knowing that if he examined his abdomen and saw feces, that would mean the bull had punctured the man's intestine and, likely, condemned him to die.

Ruit called for a bag of medical supplies and told himself to breathe slowly, think clearly, and be the sort of doctor his siblings had needed when their lives had been threatened in a place more distant than Dhovan. He spoke to the man quietly, calming him, and learned that he'd recently arrived home from working in the Middle East and had married only three days earlier. When the bag arrived, Ruit pulled the man's T-shirt aside. "His intestine was hanging out from his lower abdomen," Ruit says. "But as I probed at it, I could see it was not punctured." Greatly relieved, Ruit cleaned the wound with antiseptic and lifted up the man's abdominal skin, until the viscera slid back inside. He lined up the wound edges and bound them together with heavy strips of Elastoplast, then asked Khem Gurung to fetch a bottle of ciprofloxacin, so he could put his patient on an intravenous drip of antibiotics.

Ruit told us the story later that night as we sat on the ground, eating our dinner of dal and rice in the dark. He showed us pictures he'd taken, and he said that a rescue mission was under way. He had convinced the village elders to organize an "ambulance," a stretcher hauled in shifts by a team of ten men, to carry the gored man up a steep trail in the dark to Taplejung, the district capital, where a jeep could be hired to take him to a hospital. If they got him there before severe infection set in, Ruit said, he should live.

Meanwhile, two of our already exhausted porters had gulped their dinner and begun a four-hour hike uphill to retrieve the load of their colleague with the broken ankle, so the gear could accompany us in the morning. The trail was too treacherous for them to carry him, and they planned to leave the injured man on the mountainside for the night, until another "ambulance" could be organized by the people of Dhovan to fetch him down. Something as simple as a road would have solved both medical emergencies, but the road to Dhovan, shown as a dotted line planned for future completion on my map printed by the Nepalese government, remained a rumor.

It seemed to take all of Ruit's strength to shovel food toward his mouth with his fork. When he'd finished, he pushed his plate aside and stretched out flat on his back. "All day, when we were fighting our way down the mountain, I was worried I'd made a mistake choosing this route, and I was cursing myself for putting my young daughter through such a thing. But because we came this way, I don't think that fellow will die." He looked away from us, up into the darkness, toward the stars shining faintly through the branches of the riverside trees. "I feel," he said, "like I was brought here for this."

Four hours into the third day of our trek, I was wondering whether I could continue. The pain in my ankle had only gotten worse, and our "trail" was a steep climb through thorny scrub on the east bank of the Tamor. We took almost as much time searching for the route as we did hiking on it. That morning, before we'd set out, I'd pulled out my map, pointed to a broad line on the west side of the Tamor, and insisted to Ruit that it must be the main trail. No, he'd said, he'd sent a screening team along the route weeks earlier, and the correct path to follow was on the east bank.

Ruit's father had told me stories about his trade route along the Tamor, traveling with caravans of twenty yaks. But this couldn't be it. Not a single yak could pass this way without slipping to its death on the boulders below. We clung to a muddy route slashed from heavy undergrowth, along a thirty-degree slope that threatened to pitch us into the river if we didn't hang on to the vegetation. Since much of it was barbed or thorny, my fingers were bleeding, and my palms were bruised from thrusting them out, again and again, to break my frequent falls.

We came to a large tributary that entered the Tamor from the east, and we had to wade the shallows and scramble over mossy logs that locals had propped between boulders across the deepest channel. "This can't be the usual route," I said to Ruit.

"You were correct about the main trail being on the other side of the river," he said, pointing to a faint line that traversed cliffs five hundred feet above us on the opposite bank. "It's up there. But I'm told much of it is washed out from the rains. This is the route local people use when the weather makes that one impassable. This is the winter trail."

We crossed so many tributaries that I lost count, and on the far bank of each stream, we had to climb up out of the steep gorges the water had cut. I'd thought our seven-thousand-foot descent the day before would be the low point of the trip, but our third day of trekking was far worse. After wading another tributary, I stood with Tabin, looking up at a steep six-hundred-foot climb that snaked up the face of a granite headwall.

"I don't know if I can do this," I told Tabin. "I'm running on fumes."

"You never know what you're capable of until the bridges are all out behind you," he said. Tabin talked all the way up, while I struggled simply to breathe. "Ruit's really slowing down," he said. "He used to always have to be at the front of the pack, leading the charge. But I'm slowing down, too." Tabin's talk of his diminished powers didn't seem to prevent his powerful legs from churning uphill. They were the source of his physical strength, I realized. "I used to be able to run endless eight-minute miles," he told me. "I mean *endless*. Night and day. Able to keep on at that pace for as long as I wanted. Now I'm up to ten minutes. That's why my days of big mountain climbing are over. My margin for error is gone. But you know what's weird?" he asked, heaving himself over a boulder at the top of the headwall.

I wasn't able to breathe well enough to ask as I clambered up behind him.

"Age hasn't affected my surgery," he said. "Not yet. My hands are still steady. And if anything, I just keep getting better. So my first ascents from here on are going to have to be medical."

We looked down and saw Ruit following Satenla up the trail at the base of the cliff, and continued on. It was hot and windless in the Tamor River Gorge. My water was nearly gone, and I sipped just enough to keep my tongue from sticking to the roof of my mouth. We walked the ledge for perhaps another mile, and then the trail simply ended. We were at the base of an upslanting field of huge, house-sized boulders that looked like they'd been blackened by fire. Tabin scanned the boulder field and found a line he felt we could climb. With ropes and climbing shoes, and without having just spent ten hours fighting our way upriver, it might not have been much of a challenge. But under the conditions, my mind spun at the thought of attempting it.

"Give me your pack," Tabin said, and I handed it over. He shouldered my much heavier bag, full of cameras and books, and wedged his slim bag sideways under its lid, cinching the straps tight. Then, with my eyes locked on his feet, we began to climb. There were crevasses between the boulders, wide and deep enough that a fall into one of them would be, at the very least, a bad idea. People had jammed logs and piled stones into some of the narrower gaps, and after scaling each boulder, we tiptoed across these unsteady bridges, my pulse pounding in my temples. The black rock reflected the heat from the sun, sweat soaked through my mud-spattered clothes, and I resisted the urge to swallow the last of my water. "Hey," Tabin said, standing on top of a massive boulder, holding his wrist with one hand and looking at his mountaineering watch. "Check it out! My resting pulse is only seventy-five beats per minute!"

We finally left the black boulders behind, clambered down a slope of scree, and stood on a wide stone ledge overhanging the Tamor by five hundred feet. There was a small mud-and-thatch hut there, built on top of the rock. I collapsed where I stood, and Tabin sank onto a bench built of stacked stones.

The family who lived in the hut came out to have a look at their unexpected visitors. Those who could see, that is. The elderly matriarch of the family had massive white cataracts and gave off an overpowering aroma of smoke and alcohol. Her daughter and three grandchildren stood in the hut's doorway. All four sets of eyes shifted from side to side in their sockets, like the lenses of cameras trying to focus and failing. "Oh jeez!" Tabin said. "That's just terrible! That shaking of the eyes is 'nystagmus.' I think they have a condition called 'foveal hypoplasia.' The center of the retina doesn't develop fully, and the brain directs the eye to keep searching for receptor cells, trying to send visual information, but the eye can't do it. Can you imagine living in a place like this with a condition like that?"

"Is it curable?"

"Not if that's what they have. It only gets worse."

The thought of a family with a degenerative eye condition living on a rock five hundred feet above a turbulent river seemed almost too much to bear. I took my pack back from Tabin and rooted around in it until I found some candies. The children sucked on their treats happily enough, but they needed so much more. They needed to be airlifted into another life.

One by one, members of our team stumbled in from the boulder field, tore off their packs, and collapsed. Even the Sherpas looked exhausted. Ruit and Satenla arrived last. Satenla looked tired, but her father seemed hardly able to take another step before he slid onto the stone bench next to Tabin. His light blue polo shirt was soaked a shade darker by sweat, and he seemed about to fall asleep sitting up when his eyes fastened on those of the family. Their need affected him like smelling salts, and he struggled to his feet. "What do you think, Geoff?" Ruit said.

"I'd guess hypoplasia of the macula."

"Could be the optic nerve also," Ruit said. "We won't know until we dilate them and have a look with an ophthalmoscope."

Ruit began questioning the mother and grandmother, and his tone got angrier after each of their answers. When he was done interrogating them, he turned to me. "I asked why there are no men around when they're in such a state of need. They said the men went to Malaysia to make some money, but they haven't been sending any home. I told them to follow us to Sinwa, where we can examine them properly. I told the old woman I can fix her eyes very easily. But she said she didn't want to walk so far. She planned to drink herself to death right here. So I got little bit angry with her and told her she can do what she likes with herself. But I warned her not to prevent the children from coming."

And then, as if the electric cord connected to his healer's impulses was suddenly kicked from its socket, his knees buckled and he sat heavily beside me. "Oh, these legs are getting old," he said, gulping from his water bottle. "I'm sorry. That road was really tough. I didn't know. By all standards it was too much. There's a teahouse not far from here where my father used to stop with his caravans. We'll spend the night there. I'm too tired to go on."

It's incredible what water when you're thirsty, a few hours of rest when you're tired, and a plate or two of warm food when you're hungry can do to your spirits when you think they've been shattered. Ruit,

Tabin, Satenla, and I sat cross-legged on the veranda of the teahouse, on a bright Tibetan rug decorated with a phoenix in flight. We sipped spiced tea, picked at fried potatoes, and nibbled hacked bits of chicken fried with chilies. I was unaccountably happy.

"This is a very romantic spot," Ruit said. "Don't you think?"

I did. It was almost impossible not to be caught up in the romance of the evening, on a covered platform suspended over rustling jungle ticking with the impact of raindrops, the glossy fronds of vegetation lit by our oil lamps. And it was harder still not to be swept up in the romance of Ruit's work. I remembered something an Australian management specialist had said to me recently. He'd volunteered to assess the human resources structure of the complicated machine that was the new Tilganga and offer recommendations for how it could be run more efficiently. "The thing about Tilganga, like most organizations built by charismatic leaders, is it's top-heavy, it's all Ruit," he said. "For the newer employees, he's a distant figure and it's just a job. But for those who've been with him for years, who've been through the wars, he's a god. They'd charge through machine-gun fire for him."

It was two hours farther up the river in the dark to Sinwa. And after warming themselves with tea at the guesthouse, the rest of Ruit's team had volunteered to charge through rain, if not streams of machine-gun rounds, to trek on muddy trails in the dark and set up the operating theater so surgery could begin as soon as we joined them in the morning. Ruit pulled the bottle of single-malt scotch I'd handed him at the beginning of the trip out of his bag and held it up for me to see. "Does Your Majesty agree this is an appropriate occasion?"

"I could be convinced."

We had no glasses, so Ruit unscrewed the metal cap and filled it to the brim. He handed it first to me, then refilled it and passed it to Tabin, before helping himself to a capful.

"So, Geoff," he said, after he'd let the scotch linger on his tongue, "are you going to fix things up with your family so they can stand all your absences?"

"I want to," Tabin said. "We have so much fun when we're together, but I've just let it get worse for a long time. There's tension every time I leave for a trip, but I've just been taking the easy way out and stopped discussing it."

"You know, we've had our struggles also," Ruit said. "Nanda has sacrificed. A lot. And my children often couldn't bear it when I was away, especially Satenla here. But I've tried to make them understand leaving doesn't mean loving them less. Just the opposite. So my final word of advice to you on the subject is to trust talk. Trust talk. Trust, trust, trust!"

There was a loud silence after Ruit finished speaking. The rain that had been hammering on the tin roof over our head since we'd arrived had stopped. Satenla took advantage of the silence to say something heartfelt to her father in Nepali. When she finished, Ruit's face was flushed with happiness. "Tell them what you told me, Sat. In English."

"I never really knew what my father did," she said in her soft voice, her eyes cast down demurely. "I mean, I knew he was a doctor who helped people and such like that. But on this trip I've made a new understanding. I told my father I've decided to pursue a career in medicine."

We applauded her decision and toasted Satenla with thimblefuls of scotch, embarrassing her thoroughly enough that she left for her room to write in her diary. In the glow of the oil lanterns and the whiskey, Ruit began talking about the future. He pulled up his pant-leg and tore off the thick knee brace I hadn't known he was wearing. I saw how badly his leg was bruised. "I have to be realistic," he said. "Trekking all the way to Olangchungola is too hard. I'm getting old. But there is one thing I'd like to do while I'm strong enough. I'd like to spend one full year traveling around the world to every eye center we support, and operate at each one, doing about ten thousand surgeries total. After that," he said, "I could really hang my boots happily."

Tabin wasn't having any of Ruit's talk of retirement. "You're not dead yet, Sanduk," he said. "We're just starting to make a difference in Africa and China." Tabin took out his pocket camera and showed Ruit photos from a recent trip to Nigeria. Interspersed with images of women grinning as their peeled-back bandages hung from their cheek-bones, he showed us shocking photos of children with softball-sized tumors protruding from their eyes.

"What can you do about that?" I asked.

"Nothing," Ruit and Tabin said in tandem.

"Get to them sooner," Tabin said.

"I've seen tumors this advanced in China also," Ruit said. "For such a modern country, eye care in rural areas is as bad as anywhere in the world. That's where I really see our growth coming on in Asia." It had taken only a few blurry photos to stop Ruit's talk of retirement and reanimate the impulse I'd seen when he'd noticed the stuttering eyes of the family living on the rock. Ruit began describing the one hundred rural eye clinics he, Tabin, and David Chang had discussed building in China, and the incentives they were talking about with the Chinese government to lure talented doctors to them from their lucrative urban practices.

Tabin changed the subject to the challenge he was most passionate about—Africa—and gave Ruit a progress report on the eye hospitals and training centers in Ghana, Ethiopia, and Rwanda. Tabin sat cross-legged as he talked, hopping slightly and waving his arms with growing enthusiasm about his plans. A wave of exhaustion swept over me then. I excused myself, stumbled to my string bed a few feet away, and crawled into my sleeping bag. Lulled by their excited voices as they plotted the next phase of their global campaign to combat blindness, chattering on with energy no mortals should still possess, I closed my eyes until morning.

Walking along the upper Tamor River, knowing we'd reach our destination in a few hours, was an entirely different experience from our forced march of the last three days. Trails of unstable stone still zigzagged up nearly vertical walls, but I stepped up them deliberately, at a guide's pace, enjoying the view of terraced fields spilling down from the heights and the houses of the families who worked them tacked to hillsides by stilts that seemed too fragile to prevent them from tumbling into the river. Comparing this journey to trekking the crowded trails of the Khumbu, I realized what a privilege it was to travel through the remote Kangchenjunga region. The Tamor grew wilder as we climbed, and I could see it as a young Ruit must have, a live thing, stamping its way down from frozen glaciers to foreign lands, tearing boulders out of its way or bulling over them with its power.

Ruit and Tabin walked ahead, deep in conversation, climbing stair-cased stone trails so high, winding, and treacherous that the doctors resembled figures from Chinese silk paintings, tiny human animals, dwarfed by the magnitude of the natural world. And yet, I thought, the ripples that emanated from them were transforming entire continents. Tilganga now exported the inexpensive lenses produced in its laboratory to eighty countries. They'd constructed twelve regional community eye centers across Nepal and a full-scale surgical center in Hetauda, and they supported five eye hospitals spanning from Tibet to northern India to Indonesia. In Bonsaaso, Ghana; Quiha, Ethiopia; and Kigali, Rwanda, three more treatment and training centers were about to come online.

These two men had told me they were responsible, between them, for training hundreds of surgeons like the Kims, Drs. Olo and Kesang, Hitler Pradhan and B. P. Dhakal, Sona Yonjo, Chris Kurz and Huck-leberry Holz, Matt Oliva, Kunzang Getshen and Dechen Wangmo, Tilahun Kiros Meshesha, John Nkurikiye, and an even greater number of nurses and technicians who were working with them in the countries most cursed by blindness. By my estimate, if you took into account all the other organizations with which they'd shared Ruit's innovations, more than two million sight-restoring surgeries could already be traced to these two men and the motivated individuals they'd set in motion. Pound for pound, footstep for footstep, who was doing a more impressive job of making the world better for those whom poverty had dealt the worst hand?

We walked down through the templed light of a forest of mature golden bamboo, toward Sinwa. The elders of Olangchungola had trekked to meet us at a flat spot on the trail, with a pitcher of tea and a tray of sliced oranges and apples.

Entering Sinwa, through a bamboo gate erected for our arrival, we were greeted by the town's entire population. Once again, we were draped in *katas*, and garlands of orchids were placed around our necks. Ruit let himself be celebrated just long enough to satisfy custom, then rushed over to inspect how well his staff had converted the barren village health clinic into a well-organized operating theater.

The staff had worked most of the night to have it ready and had found innovative solutions to the site's considerable challenges. Sinwa sat on a narrow sliver of rocky land, wedged between the three-thousand-foot walls of the river's canyon, and was unusually windy. The patients' vulnerable eyes had to be protected from insects and flying grit. The clinic had only iron bars for windows, so the staff had nailed heavy woolen blankets directly into each window frame. Ruit pronounced the solution acceptable, and he and Tabin scrubbed in.

I sat on a boulder in front of the clinic, watching storm clouds gather to the west. From my perch I had a long prospect upriver, and I could see patients being carried toward us, down the winding trail from Olangchungola. Many of them were older Walung women, who tended to be broader and heavier than their men, whose work as porters required sinewy strength. I watched the gentle way these slight men lowered their sightless wives and mothers from the baskets on their backs, wrapping them in warm blankets and propping them carefully on benches in the clinic's courtyard, and I wished Ruit could see the gallantry the men of his village exhibited as they delivered their blind down from the heights of his boyhood home to the hands of its most accomplished son.

The storm hit just after surgery began. It started as rain on the clinic's corrugated tin roof, then turned to hail, hammering with such force it seemed capable of bringing the ceiling down. I stepped outside, then jumped back in. Hail the size of baseballs was pummeling the landscape, and a small detachment of uniformed policemen who'd been ordered to watch over the surgical camp put their weapons aside, pulled on ponchos, and hefted sheets of corrugated tin from a stack of building materials to form crude lean-tos for the patients.

In the operating room, Ruit and Tabin worked quickly, side by side as usual, but had to shout to their nurses over the hammering of the hail to request tools. Satenla sat at a child-sized desk, calmly entering patients' vital statistics into a laptop, while Khem Gurung and the rest of Ruit's staff led patients in and out of surgery. The pale yellow phaco machine puttered away on its stand behind Ruit's head, having proved rugged enough to survive Thapa's fall in the dry creek bed. The brilliance of Ruit's system could withstand anything, it seemed. Despite the apocalyptic scene outside, the operating room was running as smoothly as Tilganga's.

Until thunder cracked so close overhead that I thought the ceiling had caved in. Then the lights went out. When my eyes adjusted, I heard Ruit calling to me over the battering of the hail. He was operating on Chung Lama Sherpa, an eighty-five-year-old woman from Olangchungola who reminded me of Ruit's mother, Kasang. She wore the same sort of striped *pangi*, fastened by an identical silver bird-shaped buckle. Ruit had finished pulverizing one of her cataracts with the phaco machine, inserted a lens, and was in the process of widening the wound in her other eye when we lost power. "Phaco is a useful technique. But it doesn't work without electricity," Ruit said. "I'm going to switch to manual surgery so this lovely lady doesn't lose her eye. Can you bring me a torch?"

Tabin, operating manually, soldiered on as if nothing were out of the ordinary, while a nurse held a flashlight over his patient. I felt around in the dark for my pack, found my headlamp, and dialed it up to maximum brightness. "Good luck," I said to Ruit, holding it as steady as I could over Chung Lama Sherpa's open eye.

"This is surgery," Ruit said in a soothing, authoritative voice. "I don't need luck. Only light." In the same time it would take him to complete the SICS he had perfected in a fully equipped urban hospital, Ruit delivered the cloudy cataract out with his cannula and slid the new lens Satenla handed him into his patient's unclouded eye.

A moment later, the hail stopped and the lights flickered on. "That was fun," Tabin said. "Kind of like climbing a 5.12 route without protection. Did yours go well, Sanduk?"

"Of course," he said.

I realized that if I ever needed cataract surgery, wherever these two were—a veterinary hospital, a schoolhouse, or a weathered clinic in northeastern Nepal with blankets beating back the hail—was where I'd want to have it.

In Sinwa, we slept in another teahouse. Tourism was just finding its way to this far corner of Nepal; aside from expeditions attempting Kangchenjunga, few foreigners trekked up this unspoiled river. Our proprietor was prepared for a change in fortune. He'd subdivided the entire second floor of his small home into tiny rooms, with walls built of papier-mâché. After innumerable attempts, Tabin was able to reach his wife and rushed out of our room to the hallway. I would have tried to give him privacy, but there was no point, with walls so thin, so I listened to him apologize for his absences, telling Jean how much he missed her, taking Ruit's lesson of trust to heart.

Tabin crept back through the door and climbed into his sleeping bag. Cutouts in the top of the walls exposed one room to another, so residents of both spaces could share a single fluorescent fixture on the ceiling between them. The switch was on the other side, in Ruit and Satenla's room, but once I heard the volume of Ruit's snoring I wasn't about to ask him to turn out the light. Tabin had pulled a mask over his eyes and was snoring in concert with his colleague, adding a high-pitched harmony to Ruit's bass rumble.

The walls had been glued together with political posters and lined pages of students' homework assignments. Above my head, one student had written, in English, "I am found of helping others. I am found of working hard. I am hopeful of becoming doctor." From a poster by my feet, Prachanda shook his fist at a gathering of rural youths wearing red headbands and expressions of indefatigable optimism. As I drifted off to sleep, serenaded by the two unusual men I'd followed for so long, I wondered if the dreams the poor of Nepal so richly deserved would ever be delivered.

Our last morning in Sinwa, I retaped my ankle and prepared myself for the three-thousand-foot climb to Taplejung; from there, a rented bus would carry us—presuming the way wasn't blocked by a landslide or *bandh*—fourteen hours down a newly bulldozed road, to the flatlands of the Terai. Before they inspected the condition of their patients, Ruit and Tabin crammed into their temporary examination room. The family that lived on the rock had walked down for a consultation, minus the old woman. Ruit hunched over the mother and her three children, peering at their stuttering eyes through his ophthalmoscope. His sigh as he looked at each of them told me all I needed to know. He handed the device to Tabin, and Tabin's groans confirmed the diagnosis. Some conditions were beyond even their power to cure.

Ruit took the mother aside and spoke to her quietly for a long time. Whatever he said made her smile, and her body, which she had held so rigidly upright with anxiety, sagged with relief. "I told her, if she agrees, I'll send her children to the Jamgon Kongtrul's orphanage in Kalimpong. They have experience helping children cope with blindness and continue their studies. They'll be able to train them up and find them a career. As you can see from the lady's tears, she has agreed."

For the last time, I watched Ruit and Tabin hunch in front of their postoperative patients. Despite thunder, rain, hail, and electrical failure, all eighty-one men, women, and children could expect to temper whatever hardships their future held with excellent vision.

As I looked at their charts, I saw that many of the patients and their families had made the three-day journey down from Olangchungola. Ruit removed Chung Lama Sherpa's bandages, unwinding them with the care of an archaeologist until her eyes were revealed. She laughed when she saw Ruit and stuck her tongue out to him respectfully, in the traditional way. "I knew your father," she said. "And your grandfather the *gova*. They were both fat, too."

As she reached out and squeezed his jowls for emphasis, Ruit laughed happily.

I wasn't surprised by what he said next. In fact, I expected it.

"I'm going up to 'Gola," Ruit announced to no one in particular, and his voice trembled as he spoke. "I worried that Sat wouldn't speak to me after I decided. But she agrees. She says we've come too close to turn back now. She's got some iron in her. Not bad for a girl raised in the age of the computer."

We busied ourselves with a flurry of repacking. Ruit would take Khem Gurung, the Sherpa staff, and four porters. The rest of us would begin the long hike up to Taplejung. Judging from the bulging duffel bag of antibiotics, sutures, plasters, and surgical tools I saw Ruit pack, I knew he wasn't just going to climb a mountain of memories. For as long as he could remember, Ruit's mind had raced ten years ahead, toward the obstacles he knew an outsider from these mountains would have to overcome. For once, he was focused entirely on the present, on a single objective at an altitude of ten thousand feet, where he'd be equipped to treat nearly any condition when he reached the village where so many had died from lack of basic medical care.

Tabin had his reeking shoes laced. He strapped his pack over the shoulders of the uniform he would wear, from this point forward, while making his most challenging ascents: blue surgical scrubs. He was eager to go, pacing back and forth in front of the former hospital, now converted back to a clinic. He had to hike three thousand vertical feet up a slippery trail. He had to endure the torturous inertia of fourteen hours on a bus before flying to Kathmandu, where he had scheduled a grudge match with his old nemesis, Krishna Ghale, the tennis pro at the American embassy. The following day he would fly to the other side of the world, give an important speech on a few hours' sleep to an audience of thousands in Boston, push forward his projects in Africa, help reorganize the U.S. military's medical outreach, and attempt to spend more meaningful time with his wife and children. He was going to try, as usual, to do everything at once. He certainly was, as he had once said to me, someone who could get things done. But he was more than that; he was a genius of achievement.

Before he left, Tabin had to do one more thing. "Get over here, Geoff," Ruit said, crushing him against his chest. "And give me a bearly hug."

Then Ruit, with so many gold-colored *katas* from grateful patients draped around his neck that he looked less like a bear and more like a lion with a silk mane, shook hands all around, before fixing his eyes on the trail that spiraled up toward the snow peaks.

Sonam Ruit had walked his seven-year-old son down this same trail once, to give the boy a chance to make something of himself. If Satenla had decided on a future dedicated to carrying on his work, the least Sanduk Ruit could do was take his daughter back up that path, upriver into their shared past, show her where her family came from, teach her what it meant to be Walung, and prepare her for the challenges that lay ahead on her long climb through life.

"Come, Satenla," Ruit said, leaning on his trekking pole and limping north up the trail toward Tibet. "We're going home."

The Future Looks Bright

by Dr. Geoffrey Tabin

One of the great joys of this book, for me, was getting to know David Oliver Relin during the two years he was our travel companion while he researched this story. David had both a wide breadth and great depth in his intellectual interests and knowledge of the world. He wanted his writing to have a positive impact on our world. He was also a darn nice person.

In mid-November of 2012, I spent a wonderful weekend with fine friends camping and rock climbing the immaculate vertical cracks of Indian Creek in the spectacular southern Utah canyon country. There is no cell service in this region of the Utah desert; it was a joy to be totally out of contact. But my high was shattered by the first of seventeen messages my phone received that weekend on the same subject: David Relin had passed away at the age of forty-nine. He was hit by a train in Oregon and killed instantly.

Over the previous four years I had come to consider David a friend. Beyond our shared journeys to Asia and Africa, we had recently spent a considerable amount of time together in Utah and Oregon going over final details and exhaustively fact-checking this book. David was a passionate and compassionate man who cared about people and his world. Before he died, he had just finished and submitted his final draft for *Second Suns*.

In our last conversation David and I discussed book publicity plans and a possible lecture and book-signing tour. He was a serious foodie and knew more about wine than anyone else I know. Our previous travels had centered on David experiencing my world; I was excited to travel with David and experience his. I was also eager to have David as a spokesperson to spread the message that we can overcome needless blindness.

The Himalayan Cataract Project (cureblindness.org) has gained momentum in the five years since David stopped conducting new research for his book. Unlike many other areas of global public health, cataract blindness is a problem that has a definite solution and is a battle we can win: Most people are cured 100 percent by their surgery. We have been working to spread our methods and teach more widely in Asia and Africa, increasing cataract surgery output.

The effects ripple far beyond the individual who gets to see again. I've long studied the psychosocial effects of blindness, but since we began working with the UN Millennium Villages Project in 2007, I've been thinking about the effects of blindness on poverty and how visual impairment impedes economic development, too.

In 2012 we embarked on an economic and social impact study on the effects of sight restoration in Northern Ethiopia. We screened 1,100 blind people, half with vision loss from treatable cataracts and half from other causes. We had a team from Jimma University conduct extensive interviews with all of the blind people and their families to try to assess the economic, psychological, and social costs of blindness in rural Ethiopia.

Dr. Ruit flew over from Nepal with a team of our best nurses and ophthalmic assistants from the Tilganga Institute of Ophthalmology. Working with Dr. Tilahun Kiros and his team from Quiha hospital, we performed 1,133 cataract surgeries in a single week. Our researchers have now been back for one-month and one-year follow-ups with all of the patients and their families, as well as with the blind patients who were not treatable.

The study was part of our broader effort to ascertain how many people are lost to the workforce and how many children don't go to school because they have to take care of a blind parent or relative. We want to quantify both the direct and indirect costs of blindness on the individual, family, and community.

Right now we're still working to finalize the data from our Ethiopia study, but results from a similar study conducted by the Fred Hollows

Foundation are showing a return to the economy of four dollars for every dollar spent on blindness alleviation. Our research also appears to indicate that there is a dramatic increase in mortality when people lose their sight in the developing world; among those whose blindness we couldn't treat in Ethiopia, many died within the first year of the study—many more than among those who had treatable cataracts. Many other studies have also found that blind people have one third the life expectancy of peers of similar age and health in the developing world. Sadly, blind children fare worst, with a majority not living to adulthood.

My hope is that our results will lead to a higher priority given to eye care by governments in the developing world as well as foundations funding global health. In the meantime, Dr. Ruit and I still strive to improve the quality, volume, and impact of our work. Sanduk has continued to oversee an expansion of training and care at Tilganga and watched its influence spread throughout Asia. In addition to Nepal, India, Bhutan, and Tibet, Dr. Ruit has been training doctors and teams from Myanmar (Burma), Indonesia, and North Korea. We also recently signed a new five-year agreement with the Kingdom of Bhutan to further support Dr. Kunzang Getshen's mission to bring eye care in Bhutan to a mature level. And I'm thrilled to report that Bhutan is now starting its own ophthalmology residency training program

At Tilganga we now have subspecialists in all areas of ophthalmology. In particular, doctors Reeta Gurung in cornea, Govinda Paudyal in retina, Suman Thapa in glaucoma, and Rohit Saiju and Ben Limbu in oculoplastics, are now all world leaders in their fields and have established top-quality fellowship programs in Nepal. We have a state-of-the-art refractive surgery center, led by Kishore Pradhan, that is helping support our cost recovery and provide free surgery for the poor. We are working closely with several high-volume cataract centers in southern Nepal and providing training in cataract surgery and subspecialty ophthalmology for Asian and African doctors.

My core team at the Himalayan Cataract Project has grown beyond Job Heintz and Emily Newick to ten full-time and two part-time employees as well as a steady stream of student volunteers and interns.

Similarly, the number of volunteer physicians and nurses working with the program grows every year. Alan Crandall and David Chang have also continued their dedication to alleviating world blindness. Positive results are being seen in all of the countries where we work, and, thanks to international meetings and several fantastic programs in India, our methods and results are spreading rapidly.

We also have a promising cadre of dedicated young American, Canadian, Asian, and African superstars who are capable of carrying the torch when Dr. Ruit and I start to slow down. Huck Holz and Matt Oliva have continued to mature as surgeons and teachers and are increasing the time they spend working in Africa. Matt has become a leader in international eye banking and is now our Himalayan Cataract Project director for Ethiopia.

Rather than slowing down my international travel, I have increased to the point where I now spend more than half of my time working and teaching in the developing world. The chairman of the Moran Eye Center, Dr. Randall Olson, and the University of Utah honored me with the John and Marva Warnock Presidential Endowed Chair in Ophthalmology. So while I teach a course on global medicine at the medical school and also help teach the residents and corneal transplant fellows at the Moran Eye Center and University of Utah, my position also allows me to increase my devotion to global eye care development and reduce my clinical time in Utah. Through the Moran Eye Center we are building a division of international ophthalmology that is the best of its kind in the world. All of our final-year residents are able to spend a month learning how to care for advanced cataracts and other diseases at Tilganga. And the Tilganga residents come to Utah to work on our medical retina and neuro-ophthalmology services during their final year to experience ophthalmology in a high-resource setting. Our faculty is teaching in Ghana, Ethiopia, the South Pacific, Guatemala, and Haiti, and visiting doctors are now coming to the Moran Eye Center for fellowships and short-term observerships. We also work at three free clinics around Salt Lake City and have charity surgery days for the poor and uninsured at the Moran Eye Center. Finally, we are bringing our care and methods to the Navajo Nation. Every two weeks a team from the Moran Eye Center spends a long weekend on the reservation providing care and surgery.

I now have an official international fellow, who spends more than half of the year working in Africa and Asia. This position has become one of the most sought-after jobs among the top young ophthalmology graduates; I have my choice from among the best of the best.

My first international fellow, Mike Feilmeier, is now running his own international fellowship at the University of Nebraska. Mike is bringing our methods of eye care development to Haiti. My next fellow, Matt Bujak, has gone on to set up a division of international ophthalmology at the University of Toronto and is bringing his skills to Uganda. Another former resident, Lloyd Williams, is heading a project in Zambia. Two other recent fellows, Anna Gushchin and Ben Thomas, are working to bring to Africa oculoplastic surgery and retinal skills, respectively. My most recent fellow, John Welling, will join Matt Oliva in practice and direct our programs in Ghana. Perhaps most importantly, we have several young, indigenous superstars who are driving our Asian and African programs forward.

John Nkurikiye has emerged as a true leader of African ophthalmology and is rapidly bringing Rwanda into top-level eye care throughout the country. John married Ciku Mathenge, perhaps the most accomplished ophthalmologist in Kenya. Together they have started an eye institute in Rwanda and are developing training programs for ophthalmic nurses and primary eye health workers, and, in 2017, they will start a full ophthalmology residency program. Meanwhile, in Ethiopia, there are now three ophthalmology training programs, as well as ophthalmic nurse training, and we are in the process of scaling up cataract and trachoma surgery around the country. Dr. Tilahun Kiros continues in a lead role in teaching cataract surgery, while several other fantastic Ethiopian ophthalmologists are cornerstones of the residency training programs. These doctors have inspired a growing number of dedicated young physicians, and we have outstanding doctors finishing residency training in Ethiopia and Ghana who will continue their work. Most of my time is now spent in Africa. In the next ten years we will reach the same level of sustaining eye care that we have achieved in Nepal and in several other countries.

The new Tilganga Institute of Ophthalmology has fully emerged as a world leader for eye care training. In conjunction with the Fred Hollows Foundation and several other partner organizations, we are expanding our training program in Nepal to encompass several very high-volume hospitals spread throughout southern Nepal and a system of primary eye-care centers dotted throughout the hills. In twenty years we have seen an increase in the number of cataract surgeries performed by Nepali doctors increase from 15,000 per year up to more than 300,000 in 2015! (Dr. Ruit has maintained his own remarkable pace; he's now performed more than 120,000 cataract surgeries.) Moreover, the quality of the cataract surgery being performed in Nepal is now uniformly of a very high quality and as good as anywhere in the world. In recognition of that achievement, Dr. Reeta, Dr. Ruit, and I gathered on a sculpted terrace overlooking the ocean in Lisbon, Portugal, to share in the Champalimaud Vision Award, the most prestigious prize in ophthalmology and visual sciences, given for helping Nepal become the first country in the developing world to reverse its rate of blindness.

With all the incredible doctors dedicated to our mission, with all the fellowships, the awards, the support of universities and foundations, and now the mainstream media attention that has started to come our way, I'll admit to feeling, at times, rather optimistic about our progress, to the point that I sometimes believe we're on the road to overcoming needless blindness in my lifetime. But then I'm tragically reminded that eye care cannot be separated from other aspects of development and can be rocked by world events, political unrest, and natural disasters.

In April 2015, a devastating earthquake of magnitude 8.1 shook Nepal, killing 8,000 people and leaving hundreds of thousands homeless. Dr. Ruit and Tilganga's outreach team utilized the experience we gained from outreach cataract missions to lead emergency medical response and reconstruction teams into the worst-afflicted areas in the hills. Unfortunately, the government response has not been as effective. Additionally, political unrest led to an oil embargo and energy shortages that have further crippled the economy of one of the world's poorest countries.

My sideburns are starting to turn gray and Dr. Ruit's knees are getting sore. Sanduk stopped playing badminton, retiring without my ever gaining a victory. But neither of us are slowing in our fight to overcome blindness. Despite political obstacles and a chronic lack of funding, we remain optimistic. We are proud of our cadre of protégés who are furthering our work. Plus, we have reinforcements coming in the next generation. Reeta Gurung's daughter, Alina, is finishing her ophthalmology residency. Ruit's son, Sagar, just finished medical school and will soon start a residency in ophthalmology. His oldest daughter, Serabla, finished business school and works with her dad on the economics of sustaining eye care in Nepal. And his youngest daughter, Satenla, who was only thirteen when she trekked with us in the closing chapters of this book, has just gained acceptance into medical school. Yes, we have obstacles, but the future looks good. David Relin, I'm certain, would be proud of how far we've come.

We still have a long way to go before we rest. Don't ration the passion!

Geoff Tabin
April 2016

Author's Note

Some books you want to write. Others you *have* to write. The book you're holding falls into the second category. When I went to Nepal in the spring of 2008, it was with the notion of writing about a Sherpa mountain climber. But at the insistence of Geoff Tabin, I traveled with his partner Sanduk Ruit to a rural village in Nepal, where I watched the elegant method—and remarkable results—of Ruit's sight-restoring surgeries. There, I had the privilege of watching patients, many of whom had been blind for years, not only regaining their sight but also their chance to live fulfilling lives. I found the experience emotionally overwhelming. So, on that April day in the mid-hills of Nepal, my life changed course and I began this book.

Since then, as I've worked to report and write the story of Drs. Ruit and Tabin, I've come to see their shared effort to eradicate much of the world's preventable blindness as one of the most meaningful ways anyone I know is able to spend their time on earth. I admire these men and their mission, and they've been good company during our shared effort to bring this book to life. That doesn't mean that I haven't found both Ruit and Tabin, at times, frustrating. Tabin can be hyperbolic and hyperactive. Ruit is occasionally moody and aloof. I mention these qualities to make it clear that these men are far from perfect. I believe that makes their accomplishments all the more impressive.

Each of these doctors could have chosen more financially rewarding lives. That's one of the reasons I decided that a portion of my proceeds from this book should go directly to Ruit and Tabin. So is the fact that Ruit and Tabin have not just been the subjects of this book, they have been active participants in the four-year process of creating it. They've each done dozens of interviews, read drafts, and offered corrections and suggestions.

What I respect most about Ruit and Tabin is the decision they both made to stray far from more comfortable careers to focus on one of the world's great, correctable injustices: Of the approximately 160 million blind and severely visually disabled people on the planet, roughly three-quarters of them could easily be cured if they had access to modern medicine. Let me repeat that: Three out of four of them can't see because they're not being offered the same quality medical care people in wealthy countries consider their birthright. That's why the organization Ruit and Tabin founded, the Himalayan Cataract Project (www .cureblindness.org), has concentrated on refining and delivering a simple surgical procedure capable of curing millions of cataract patients for about twenty dollars each. And that's why they've been working for decades to bring the best quality care to some of the world's neediest communities. As I've found, that often means carrying mobile field hospitals on weeklong treks into the hills of Nepal, or traveling wherever their services are needed. Additionally, Ruit, Tabin, and their colleagues at the HCP have made a point of raising surgical standards everywhere they work, and have trained and equipped hundreds of local doctors, nurses, and technicians to perform sight-restoring surgeries without Ruit, Tabin, or other HCP staff present.

Though this is Ruit and Tabin's story, and this book focuses on their efforts, they are far from alone in their quest. There are many other worthy organizations, including the Aravind Eye Care System, the Fred Hollows Foundation, ORBIS International, the Seva Foundation, and Sightlife, working to eradicate preventable blindness worldwide, organizations that have often partnered with the HCP. Likewise, there are a number of scenes in *Second Suns* where I have chosen not to describe other people who were present. Again, my intention was to keep Ruit and Tabin front and center.

In the course of reporting this book, I took eleven separate trips to interview them, research their histories, watch them work, and assist medically in whatever way my limited skills allowed. I've bounced on tooth-rattling twenty-hour Jeep rides across the eastern Himalaya. I've observed Tabin operating with the latest technology in Salt Lake City. I've worked in rural Ethiopian and Rwandan hospitals. And I've trekked with Ruit and Tabin into Nepal's endless ranges, struggling to keep up with these two exasperatingly inexhaustible men.

Like its subjects, the story I tell in *Second Suns* is sure to have flaws. Though I traveled with Ruit and Tabin extensively and saw their work with my own eyes, much of this book must rely on the memories of two fifty-something men who have conducted hundreds of mobile surgical camps. There are days I can't remember what I had for breakfast, yet I've asked Ruit and Tabin to recall and reconstruct scenes from their childhoods, twenty-year-old encounters with particular patients, the complex process of building a charitable organization, and the nuts and bolts of decades of doctoring. Along the way, it's inevitable that I've gotten some of the sequences of events scrambled, and some of the details wrong. I did, however, hire a professional fact-checker, had him interview as many of the people who populate this book as possible, and traveled to Nepal with him to clarify many details of this story. I'm confident that even if I haven't been able to describe more than fifty years of Ruit's and Tabin's lives with absolute precision, I've been able to get the heart of their story correct—that these two men have made an enormous, measurable difference in alleviating suffering. I hope that you've enjoyed reading about them as much as I've enjoyed telling their tale.

DAVID OLIVER RELIN
Portland, Oregon

Reader's Guide

Second Suns is an inspiring story of two intrepid doctors who eschewed traditional career paths in medicine in order to bring life-changing health care to an underserved population. When author David Relin first meets Dr. Sanduk Ruit, Relin wonders if "there was a single person on earth doing more measurable good for others" (25). But the paths Drs. Ruit and Geoff Tabin took were neither straightforward nor easy. This guide takes a closer look at some of the conflicts and themes that have shaped these doctors' journeys.

1. In chapters 2 and 3, Relin heightens the contrast between the worlds of Drs. Ruit and Tabin by juxtaposing a scene in a makeshift, bare-bones operating room in Nepal with one in the sterile, high-tech Moran Eye Center. What other scenes in this story contrast medicine in the West with that in the East? How do these comparisons affect the story?

2. From Ruit's formative years in Darjeeling to Tabin's mountaineering, *Second Suns* is largely a study on what made these two doctors who they are today. Who and what else do you think significantly influenced these doctors' lives?

3. How large a role does religion play in this story?

4. The *tikka*, or third eye, is a recurring symbol in *Second Suns*. Does its connotations change over the course of the narrative? Did you detect other symbols in the book?

5. Drs. Ruit and Tabin perform modern miracles—they make blind people see again. Yet one might argue that this is only one of many results of their work. In what other ways in this story has the doctors' work been a force for positive change? How has it transcended established animosities between countries and peoples?

6. From the charred steaks, frayed shirtsleeves, and white polyester tuxedo to the leech poem delivered to the University of Utah med

students and the wedding-day climbing expedition, *Second Suns* is filled with images and scenes that reveal aspects of Tabin's character. What other scenes and imagery come to mind? Are there moments and images that equally capture Ruit's character?

7. Drs. Ruit and Tabin are the heroes of this story. But are there others? If so, who?

8. What are the greatest sacrifices the two doctors have made on their journey to rid the world of preventable blindness? What do you consider some of their greatest risks? Do you think the doctors ever go too far?

9. Are Drs. Ruit and Tabin a perfect pairing? Is their synergy largely *despite* their differences, or *because* of them? Do the two share any similarities? What are their greatest strengths? What are their flaws?

10. At Golchha Hospital, Tabin learns an important lesson from Ruit: Patience and compassion are more constructive than blunt criticism. What other lessons do they learn from each other?

11. In what ways might Dr. John Nkurikiye's experiences in Burundi and Rwanda have helped prepare him for his work as an ophthalmologist?

12. "Every leading cataract surgeon in the developing world" attends the World Ophthalmology Conference in Hong Kong, Tabin says (279), yet exactly eleven show up for Ruit's presentation. After reading this story, do you feel that the field of ophthalmology should be expected to do more for underserved communities?

13. When Relin travels with Tabin to Quiha hospital, in Ethiopia, he feels more acutely than ever a sense that he is "just a journalist," that "in the face of overwhelming need, storytelling felt like a poor excuse for my presence" (322). Then he rolls up his sleeves and begins to help out in the operating room. Was it fair to call himself "just a journalist"? Does Relin's role in this narrative affect how you sympathize with Ruit and Tabin's mission?

14. *Time* calls this book a "hopeful work." And yet Relin notes that, despite the more than 100,000 patients Drs. Ruit and Tabin have cured of blindness, there are more than "160 million blind and severely visually disabled people on the planet" (410). Do you find *Second Suns* hopeful? Why or why not?

Acknowledgments

Thanks to Sanduk Ruit and Geoff Tabin, for allowing me to follow them and their work across three continents, for enduring my endless questions, and for remaining (mostly) polite and patient over the course of the four years it took to write and report this book. Thanks also to the Ruit and Tabin families, for inviting me into your homes and lives. And a special thanks to Cliff Tabin, a visionary scientist in his own right, for modestly keeping the focus of our conversations on the achievements of his little brother, as well as to Serabla and Satenla Ruit, for their skillful and sensitive interpretation at surgical camps.

In Nepal, I'd like to thank Reeta Gurung, Beena Sharma, Rex Shore, and Rabindra Shrestha, as well as the Tilganga board members for sharing the story of how Tilganga was created. Former Australian ambassador to Nepal Les Douglas was particularly eloquent as he reminisced about helping Tilganga find its footing.

Also in Nepal, Bal Sunder Chansi, Rajluxmi Golchha, Khem Gurung, Ajeev Thapa, Krishna Thapa, and Shanka Twyna all gave me a window into the challenging process of creating world-class eye care in a poor country, as well as helped me to understand the obstacles Tilganga and the HCP faced, and the triumphs they achieved, as they grew into mature institutions. My apologies to anyone else in Nepal I've forgotten to mention here.

At Salt Lake City's John A. Moran Eye Center, CEO Randy Olson and his talented physicians, nurses, and technicians showed me just how well ophthalmology can be practiced when a wealth of resources and cutting-edge technology are combined with a staff that cares deeply about the quality of its work.

Thanks to Job Heintz and Emily Newick at the HCP for helping to explain how they and their small, overworked staff have been able to turn Sanduk Ruit and Geoff Tabin's outsized dreams into grounded